Becoming a Mother

Becoming a Mother

ANN OAKLEY

Martin Robertson

First published in 1979 by Martin Robertson & Company Ltd., 108 Cowley Road, Oxford OX4 1JF.

ISBN 0 85520 206 8

Typeset by Vantage Photosetting Company, Southampton
Printed and bound by Richard Clay Ltd. at The Chaucer Press, Bungay, Suffolk

Contents

for ADAM,
a first child

Preface – and a Personal Note

In 1974 I began an academic research project called, rather grandly, 'Transition to Motherhood: Social and Medical Aspects of First Childbirth'. It was planned as a three-year study of a sample of women having their first babies, and the idea was that it would expose and clarify some of the problems involved in becoming a mother in modern society.

I became interested in this subject I suppose directly through my previous work on housewives' attitudes to housework.[1] I began to see that however much one separated housework off from women's other work, becoming a housewife was synonymous with becoming a mother. Whereas fifty or even twenty years ago women gave up their jobs on marriage, now they do so during their first pregnancies, and it is the moment when she becomes a mother that a woman first confronts the full reality of what it means to be a woman in our society. Motherhood entails a great deal of domestic work – servicing the child, keeping its clothes and its body clean, preparing food. The demarcation lines between this and house- or husband-work blur. It is a crisis in the life of a woman, a point of no return. Evidence accumulated since the 1950s about how the principle of sex equality works in practice shows conclusively that the options available for women outside the home are severely affected by motherhood, and remain so even where 'officially' the commitment is to equal chances for all.[2]

I therefore chose to look at this moment in a woman's history, to catch it and describe it and explore it through the eyes of some of those who experience it. I was interested in every dimension of becoming a mother: changes in life-style – giving up work, staying at home, becoming isolated or making new friends – the impact of, and effect on, marriage, the relationship between mother and child, the medical management of childbirth. I wanted to show that the advent of motherhood is not only an event of importance to the individual woman, but a moment in the history of *all* women.

I am a feminist, an academic sociologist, and a woman with children. I was not a feminist until I had children, and I became a sociologist as an escape from the problems of having children. My first child was born in 1967 when I was twenty-two and had accomplished a university degree, various minor pieces of research for other people and two unpublished novels. I thought it was my vocation as a woman to be a mother. When my son was sixteen months old, my first daughter was born. Both children seemed to me absolutely lovely, and I delighted in them both, but the time that followed was an unhappy haze of nappy-washing and pill-taking, as I found I could not make my dream of domestic contentment come true. I felt depressed and oppressed. I felt constantly tired, I felt isolated, I felt resentful of my husband's freedom, I felt my life was at an end. The pills did not adjust me to my role. In those days – the late 1960s – it was not yet acceptable for women to admit openly to their dissatisfactions. Eventually it dawned on me (and I cannot now remember how) that perhaps I both could and should do something else. I registered to do a doctoral thesis and embarked on my research on housewives. Almost at the same time I encountered two women who were starting a women's liberation group in my area. Joining them I began to understand how my private conflicts were nothing more or less than the legacy that all women in modern industrialised society inherit.

The importance of childbirth itself did not strike me until some years later. In the late 1960s and early 1970s medical intervention in childbirth accelerated and came to the attention of the lay public. Research into various problems in family life increasingly focused on the early relationship of mother and child. On commonsense grounds it seemed to me that the *beginning* of motherhood could be immensely important, and that the way in which a birth is managed could influence a woman's whole experience of becoming a mother. Reading anthropological accounts of birth and comparing them with birth in the industrialised world I was impressed by how *difficult* motherhood had become. Having a baby is a medical exercise. Birth and babies have become mysteries as fewer and fewer people have any contact with either before they embark on parenthood themselves.

Looking back, I could see how all this applied in my own case. What I knew about birth came out of books; I had hardly seen, let alone held, a baby before my son was born. I thought babies made people happy and I failed to realise that you had to make the baby happy first, even if this meant three months of sleepless nights and days with no time to oneself. I imagined childbirth as a time of intense joy and achievement that automatically cancelled out the pain. But when I remember that first birth, I remember myself as a passive patient, bewildered, afraid and alone, controlled rather than controlling, his birth more their achievement than mine. There was no euphoria, the baby in the cot was a threatening stranger, and I felt and looked like the pale ladies in Victorian novels, drained empty of everything. And yet I had a 'normal' delivery. For months afterwards I could not grasp what I had gone through; the only mistakes I could identify were the general problem of unfamiliar people in unfamiliar surroundings and the silly rule that husbands could not see their children being born. I did not understand that I was delivered of my identity at the same time, prevented from being the central figure in the central drama of my life. The baby flourished but it was a long time before I could remove the barrier of his birth from my relationship with him.

I did know that I could not run the risk of another hospital birth – a sentiment that obstetricians, who only count one kind of risk, of course do not share. I caught the last lap of the home confinement tide and produced a girl in 1968. A non-event compared with the first birth, it seemed to me extremely right to have a baby at home (and only in that way could one perhaps be 'at home' having a baby). I did not love this baby immediately either, but I quickly grew into a comfortable relationship with her, and I have never felt the awful sense of division from her that flooded me the first time.

It is a standard sociological and medical joke to have a baby while doing research on childbirth. Early on in the work a doctor whom I was following around with a stopwatch and a notebook said 'I bet you'll have another baby and you won't finish the research'. It was, obviously, a challenge: women can't have professional jobs and babies at the same time – only one or the other. The third birth, nine years after the second, was a hospital birth out of circumstance, not choice. But it was the only one entirely without drugs, the only one in which, equipped with knowledge and determination,[3] I felt I was directing the course of events. I have never been to a natural childbirth or relaxation class in my life (through laziness only) and have come to terms with the fact (or the dreadful discovery) that childbirth hurts. But it does not hurt *too* much, and there is the tremendous comfort of the baby at the end.

This personal testimony is, of course, not intended to be definitive;

there are many ways of having a baby. The point is that academic research projects bear an intimate relationship to the researcher's life, however 'scientific' a sociologist pretends to be. Personal dramas provoke ideas that generate books and research projects. Clearly, all kinds of other excuses can be found for the production of the book or the project; these may get the projects passed by committees, and the books published, but they do not wholly explain why they exist.[4] There were times in the course of the research when I began to confuse my roles – researcher, pregnant woman, mother, feminist, participant observer and so on. I found such confusion disturbing but healthy, for it indicates the artificiality of the boundaries we set ourselves. Human experience is often not as neat and tidy as we strive to make it.

Before I started interviewing pregnant women, I spent six months as an observer in the London hospital from which I selected my sample of women. I wanted to find out what went on in a maternity hospital and, in particular, I wanted to observe encounters between doctors and patients. But the main data used in this book come from interviewing sixty-six women expecting their first babies in 1975–6. Because of the trend away from home confinement, it was not possible to compare home and hospital births or to look at home births exclusively. I chose a sample of women who were all booked for delivery in the same hospital because I did not want to end up comparing the practices of different hospitals: this would have confused the main point of the research, which was to arrive at a picture of those experiences of first-time motherhood that are shared by all women.

The women were aged between 19 and 32 at the time of delivery. I intended to look at first birth when it happens to most women in our society – the average age for having a first child is now 25 years in Britain and 22 years in the United States. All the women were born in Britain, Ireland or North America; I did not include ethnic minorities, since what research is available on reproductive attitudes shows these to vary with different cultural groups. To compare these would have been an entire research project on its own. According to husband's occupation, the conventional sociological index, 64 per cent of the women interviewed were middle class, 36 per cent working class. According to the woman's own occupation, the figures are 91 per cent middle class and 9 per cent working class; two thirds of the 'middle class' mothers had social class III non-manual occupations.

This is a more middle-class population than is representative of the pattern nationally, and reflects the patient population of that particular hospital. Eleven per cent of the women were not married at the first interview; 7 per cent were still not married by the last interview. I saw no reason to exclude unmarried mothers: 9 per cent of births in Britain in 1976 and 14 per cent in the USA in 1975 were to unmarried mothers. When I refer to 'husbands' or 'wives' or 'the marriage' in the following chapters, I know I do some of these women an ideological disservice, but I hope they will forgive me. An appendix, 'List of Characters', gives the pseudonym by which I refer to each woman interviewed, with a brief description of her age, occupation, marital status and housing situation.

Four interviews were carried out with each woman – at average times of twenty-six weeks and six weeks before delivery, and five weeks and twenty weeks afterwards. I also attended six of the births. By the time interview four arrived, the numbers had fallen to fifty-five: four women miscarried, one had the baby prematurely at another hospital, five moved too far away to be interviewed again, and one withdrew from the project because of a disintegrating marriage. All the interviews were tape-recorded and lasted on average 2·36 hours.

When I came to confront the completed interviews I was impressed by the fact that the women said it all much better, and much more clearly and directly, than a sociologist could ever do. I decided to put together a book that consisted as much as possible of the women's own words, to allow them to present their own accounts of pregnancy, birth and the experiences of early motherhood. No single criterion dictated which particular words were chosen to describe the various aspects of becoming a mother; I tried to select those that communicated the experience most economically and most colourfully without being unrepresentative of how the majority felt. I have provided a small amount of text to signpost the reader through these accounts, but my intention has been to reverse the usual text–quotation relationship so that the women's own words make up the text of the book. Chapters 2–12, which reproduce the women's accounts, accordingly reverse normal typesetting practice; it is my comments and not the interview quotations which are italicised. I have included some statistics in a simple form to put groups of quotations into context,[5] but I have relegated the significance tests to an academic version of the research, to be called *Women Confined: Towards a*

Sociology of Childbirth, which is in preparation and will be published in 1979–80. This is for those readers who are happier with a more conventional research report or who want to follow up particular points raised in this book.

Becoming a Mother is therefore a portrait of how it feels to have a first baby in the late 1970s in a large industrial city. It is a book about parenthood through the eyes of *women*; there is a chapter on men and men sometimes added comments to the women's answers, but basically only women were interviewed: as the women described their experiences the role of fathers/husbands was most of the time quite marginal. The key experiences are happening to the women's bodies, their identities, their ways of life; fathers may be more or less involved, more or less supportive, but they are not at the centre of the stage.[6] In this and other senses it is a *polemical* book: a statement of how things are, rather than of how people like to think they might be. It is not a 'how to do it' book – there are enough of those, with their conflicting viewpoints, available already.

Some readers may feel that the portrait of motherhood given here is too bleak, too depressing, an inaccurate rendering of the satisfactions many women derive from having and looking after a baby. I have tried to show the positive side, but of course it is to some extent true that the best news is bad news: happiness doesn't hit the headlines because it is boring. In some ways, too, the picture is deliberately black. What many of the women who were interviewed said was that they were misled into thinking childbirth is a piece of cake and motherhood a bed of roses. They felt they would have been better off with a clearer view of what lay in store for them. I have constructed the book around this conclusion, perhaps amplifying it somewhat, because only in that way are messages made impressive. But the insight itself is authentic – theirs, not mine, even if it does help to interpret the way I felt back in 1968.

My first and last debt is obviously to the women themselves, who listened patiently to questions, who talked openly about their most private experiences, who were warm and welcoming and honest when there was no reason why they should have been. I have of course changed their names and their occupations, so I hope they are only recognisable to themselves. Secondly, I should like to thank the hospital, also anonymous, for tolerating my presence and co-operating with my requests. Many of the staff I 'observed' there were extremely helpful. Thirdly, I must thank the Social Science Research

Council who supported the work financially, Raymond Illsley for encouraging the idea, and my colleagues at Bedford College, particularly George Brown and Margot Jefferys, who provided advice and a sympathetic audience whenever I needed it. Jenny Whyte helped with the interviewing, and did much more work than she was supposed to do, and I thank her as well. Robin, as always, made the whole enterprise possible and supported me through the moments when I despaired that it would ever see the light of day. Adam and Emily endured it patiently and tried to understand why mothers want to interview people and write books. Laura delayed the entire project, taught me how satisfying childbirth can be, and continues to be a great inspiration and solace to all who know her.

CHAPTER 1

Childbirth and the 'Position' of Women

. . . a house without a child is like a garden without a flower, or like a cage without a bird. The love of offspring is one of the strongest instincts implanted in women; there is nothing that will compensate for the want of children. A wife yearns for them; they are as necessary to her happiness as the food she eats and the air she breathes. [A doctor, 1911[1]]

Artificial reproduction is not inherently dehumanizing. At the very least, development of the option should make possible an honest re-examination of the ancient value of motherhood . . . until the decision not to have children or to have them by artificial means is as legitimate as traditional childbearing, women are as good as forced into their female roles. [A feminist, 1972[2]]

THE INSTITUTION OF MOTHERHOOD

Throughout human society childbirth is never just one event in a woman's life. It is always momentous, but in different ways. For culture, the different cultures that human beings have invented as ways of living, defines the meaning of birth, a biological act.

In colonial America, women had twelve or more children; unmarried women in their mid-twenties were economically useless old maids. In Alor, an Indonesian Island, in the 1940s, women's chief role was agricultural work, and men liked babies more than women did. Victorian moralists saw a fully domesticated wife and mother as a sign of a man's social status and a large family as proof of his male power. Yahgan women of Tierra del Fuego go back to work one day or less after having a baby. In England, a woman is paid by the state not to work until her baby is seven weeks old. Jarara women of South America give birth in a domestic passageway or shelter in front of everyone, including small children. In parts of the United States in

9

the 1930s it was against the law for mothers who gave birth in hospital to have their babies with them. Eighty-two per cent of women in a sample of seventy-six cultures gave birth standing up or sitting or squatting, the rest lying down. In Norway in 1974, 90 per cent of pregnant women received prenatal medical care; in Nicaragua 16 per cent did. Among some South American tribes it is regarded as an essential part of womanhood to give birth unaided: death is better than the shame of medical assistance. In contemporary Britain it is illegal to give birth without calling medical help.[3]

Children are important; children are not important. Fertility is admired; barrenness commands respect. Women are put on this earth to have children; women are the breadwinners and babies are a nuisance. Pregnancy means special treatment; pregnancy means work in a field or factory regardless. Birth is a time of medical danger or supernatural mystery; birth is a normal, public act. Motherhood is sacred; women are just people. A woman's achievement is twelve babies or twelve fields cared for, twelve or more years in a factory or office, twelve years of full-time housewifery.

The meaning of childbirth is interlocked with a society's attitudes towards women. Both reflect its economic system. Capitalism, by concentrating production in places other than the home, altered the status of women: mothers working became The Working Mother. The production of capital requires the production of workers: thus women's role becomes not to produce but to reproduce: 'the mother employed out of the home presents a national problem of the first importance'.[4]

One does not have to be a marxist to understand these connections between motherhood and the economy. And it is important to appreciate the history of motherhood as it appears to us in industrialised society today, because our sort of motherhood is unique in history:

The mother gave birth to the child, didn't she? She nurses it, doesn't she? She is, obviously, we conclude, solely responsible for it. Even when she can get help, time off, reprieve, relief for several hours during the day, the responsibility remains hers. During any absence she remains on call. At the theatre, at work, at the party, her ear is always half-cocked for the telephone message to come: the child is ill. If anything happens to the child it is she, not the father, who will be held responsible.

The role of the mother as we define it is almost unique. Motherhood as we institutionalise it is a product of affluence. Few if any societies have ever been able to spare adult, able-bodied women from the work force and specialise them so exclusively for the care of a small brood of children for almost a lifetime.[5]

The institution of motherhood is not identical with bearing and caring for children. . . . Institutionalised motherhood demands of women maternal 'instinct' rather than intelligence, selflessness rather than self-realisation, relation to others rather than the creation of self.[6]

The *institution* of motherhood is the way women become mothers in industrialised society today. And what happens to women when they become mothers reflects what has already happened to them as they became women. Like childbirth, femininity and masculinity follow different cultural patterns: being a woman means something different in fifteenth-century England, nineteenth-century Norway, twentieth-century Brazil. The industrialised world today insists on certain sex differences while having moved towards an idea of sex equality. Equality and difference are compatible, since equality in this ideology does not mean 'sameness'. It means that women should be allowed to do the same jobs for the same pay as men, that girls should be educated as much as (though differently from?) boys, that a woman should become prime minister if that is what she and the country want. Equality applies to the world outside the home. Inside it, difference flourishes (thereby, of course, rendering external equality more of a mere vision).

In the maternity hospital where the women interviewed for this book had their babies two different labels are written out for girl and boy babies: pink and blue. (A reactionary development? Ten years ago all babies had white labels.) On the whole little girls acquire particular ideas about their future roles that differ from those communicated to little boys. Two ideas about women that are still endemic in our minds are perhaps the key ones: the idea that women are not at the centre of their own lives, and the curiously impressive image of women as always waiting for someone or something, in shopping queues, in antenatal clinics, in bed, for men to come home, at the school gates or by the playground swing, for birth or the growing up of children, in hope of love or freedom or re-employment, waiting for the future to liberate or burden them and the past to catch up with them.

The problem is that motherhood is not a passive role. Brought up to regard herself as dependent on other people, a mother discovers that her children are dependent on her. She has responsibilities that far outweigh those she held as a secretary or a machinist or a doctor (for even these responsibilities are limited and doctors do not work every hour of every day every year). She has to make decisions and choices, decide what is best for her child nutritionally, aesthetically, educationally, physically, psychologically, emotionally. Mothers must be strong. In one study of women having a first child, the women who 'adjusted' best were those who were least 'feminine'.[7] Contentment as a mother was more likely among the active and independent women, who more often experienced childbirth as a positive achievement. The greatest difficulties were encountered by 'feminine' women who had more rigid ideas about what mothers ought to be like (perfect and selfless). Trying to live up to this ideal is difficult enough, but being a perfect mother *and* wife *and* housewife all at the same time and without help – this is an ordeal. Again 'ideal' motherhood is perhaps achieved only where people are not typical: a study of mothers in six cultures found that mothers were most 'nurturant' where they had most help with child care (from anyone – older children, men, other women).[8]

First-time motherhood calls for massive changes. Thirty years ago women gave up their jobs on marriage: now the occasion is impending motherhood. The return to work is slow: 20 per cent four years after, 52 per cent ten years after (and it is likely to be a different sort of work chosen for its compatibility with maternal duties). Becoming a mother is more than a change of job: it involves reorganising one's entire personality. For there is a chasm between mothers' needs and children's needs that mothers have to bridge. In a society where children are reared in small, quite isolated families, babies have an absolute need to be mothered (who else will do it?) but mothers, however 'maternal' they are, only have a relative need for their babies. They have a past identity and a future one in which real children do not feature. In the past, when families included grandparents, lots of siblings, cousins, aunts, uncles, etc., these other people filled the gap. Now they no longer do so, the question is of what are women deprived by their maternity?

Surveying the mental health of women, research workers in London have found that one in three women have definite psychiatric symptoms of depression and that the likelihood of becoming depressed is crucially related to motherhood.[9] To Freud and those who follow him, motherhood is an escape route from the handicap of female inferiority: the wish for a child replaces the wish for a penis and is the route to maturation for a woman. Womanhood equals motherhood, baby equals redemption, so that women who choose to spend their adult lives doing something else are neurotic (or masculine). Yet, on the contrary, motherhood seems more often to lead to a sense of lowered ('depressed') self-worth: children take the centre of the stage; the mother is merely a supporting player. Her role is static, theirs dynamic: having no time to herself, her self is quiescent. To talk of 'adjustment' in this context seems wrong. What is the psychological status of those who 'adjust', and what kind of strains are felt by those who fail to? In any case, as the sociologist Alice Rossi has pointed out, we have an apparatus of *ideas* about motherhood, but we know far too little about what 'good' mothering is – from either the child's or the mother's point of view.[10]

Most women now have their first babies in their early twenties, so that well before the age of 30 the biological tie of pregnancy and breastfeeding is over. But the period spent having and caring for young children is the time when men choose careers and advance in them; by their mid-thirties parenthood has firmly wedged the sexes apart. If mothers want careers outside the home they are at a disadvantage. Responsibility for children is the key factor in the non-employment of female graduates, and it lies behind the phenomenon of part-time work (our generation's panacea for the problems of women's role). In Britain, more than a third of all employed women work part-time. Women under capitalism count as a reserve labour force. The double standard continues to apply: men are the breadwinners, women the housewives; the nuclear family supports the nation. When it suits the nation, women are encouraged to work and it is made easier for them to do so. During the Second World War in Britain for example, day nursery provision increased enormously as three and three-quarter million more women joined the labour force.[11] But after the war, reaction set in. In the 1950s maternal employment became once again a thorn in the national conscience, a symbol of women's inhumanity, a sign of failing morality and decaying family life.

'The family', a pejorative term, is part of a conservative ideology. We all (or most of us) think about couples getting married and having children and staying together. Some do. But on the other hand, divorces are now in some countries approaching 50 per cent of marriages; more than half of all households are not of the nuclear family kind; many 'families' are women and children on their own. 'The family' is not always kind to men, women or children. Children are battered psychologically or physically; so are women. Men die earlier than women, of an impressive list of stress diseases.

A baby makes a family. A home is not a home without children. The drive to parenthood is felt, but not understood. Of course the negative side is countered by a positive side; some of the visions materialise: babies *do* smile and smell sweet, children *are* loving and rewarding, the shaft of sunlight does catch the heads of shining hair, the glowing skin, the sturdy limbs and healthy souls. Biological parenthood is unique among all human experiences. To hold the child you grew as part of yourself seems a miracle. And the wonder recurs throughout the years, for it appears that in this most natural activity of reproduction human beings achieve something super-natural, they transcend their simple humanity.

Many children are now the exception and not the rule, but more people become parents some time in their lives.

> Perhaps the most significant aspect of current reproductive be-haviour in industrial societies, and yet one that is so taken for granted that it is rarely mentioned, is the fact that parenthood remains almost universal. Reproduction is statistically normative for the majority of adults within these societies. Widespread parenthood has remained. . . . In England and Wales approximate-ly 80% of adults become parents.[12]

The figure is hard to arrive at, for official statistics so take the fact of parenthood for granted that they provide no basis on which to calculate it.

Altered patterns of reproduction mean that more babies are first babies. In England and Wales in 1976, 42 per cent of all legitimate births in first marriages were first births, and in the United States in 1975 the figure was the same.[13] If more women experience mother-hood, each mother has a narrower experience of childbirth. First childbirth has become more significant, in the first place because it is not the first of many, but the first of two or three (even the only one). Meaning and satisfaction in childbirth are more important. Secondly, the shadow of death no longer hangs over birth the way it did a century ago. Today in England and Wales for every ten thousand live births, one mother and 160 infants die; a hundred years ago the figures were 48 mothers and 1560 infants.[14] Women expect every pregnancy to produce a healthy baby. Embarking on a first pregnancy seems like a safe course, the horizon of that first healthy cry easy to navigate, and the entire journey to desired family size seems well charted and free of the hazards that beset past generations of mothers.

MEDICALISATION

Much of the improvement in maternal and perinatal/infant mortality rates reflects a more healthy population. People eat better and live more hygienically than they used to, and since women have fewer children, high-risk groups of older mothers having their fourth or later child have been reduced in size. Probably about a third of even very recent improvements in maternal and infant mortality are due to these changes.[15] But the tendency is to attribute greater safety in childbirth wholly to better medical care. Doctors themselves have probably encouraged this tendency: obstetricians are peculiar among doctors in having such a clear index by which to measure their success, and they tend to forget that medical care is not the only reason why people survive.

In the past and still in many cultures today women have babies without any medical help. Their attendants are other women, usually those who have had babies themselves. Babies are born in the home, in a family setting, and birth proceeds as the woman's body dictates it should; there is little or no intervention in the natural process. None of this holds in industrialised societies, where childbirth is 'medicalised'. Attendants at childbirth are professional deliverers (for women are no longer their own deliverers in birth, they are delivered 'by' someone); hospital is the proper place for having a baby, which has become an occasion on which the family is split up, not united; trust in nature has been replaced by trust in technology, as tests and machines and instruments become the necessary paraphernalia of birth. This colonisation of birth by medicine is a thread in the fabric of cultural dependence on professional health care. People are not responsible for their own health, their own illness, their own births and deaths: doctors are saviours, miracle-workers, mechanics, culture-heroes. From being necessary to the cure or treatment of a probably quite small number of illnesses, they have been given responsibility for *all* illness, and anything to which, like birth, the label of illness can be attached.

In Britain, childbirth first came under medical management when six 'lying-in' establishments were created in London from 1739 to 1765.[16] Forceps, the ancestors of all birth technology, first began to be used for second stage labour in the seventeenth century. These were fringe developments for a long time, and most women continued to give birth at home helped by other untrained women. In 1902 midwives came under state (and medical) control, and in the following years concern with falling population focused medical attention on the health of mothers.[17] At first, hospital was advocated only for a small number of high-risk mothers; then for all mothers. In 1927 the hospital confinement rate was 15 per cent; in 1974 it was 96 per cent.[18] In 1975, 99 per cent of first babies were born in hospital.[19]

Industrialisation and medicalisation seem to go together, but there are wide variations between countries in the medical management of childbirth. For example, 53 per cent of babies are born at home in Holland, none in Sweden, 1·3 per cent in Japan, 2 per cent in the German Democratic Republic, 3 per cent in Canada and 15 per cent in Denmark. The average length of hospital stay in these countries varies from five to ten days. In New Zealand, physicians are usually present at birth, in the German Federal Republic it is a legal requirement that a midwife attend every delivery, in the United States nurse-midwives were not allowed to deliver babies until 1971. In Norway, midwives are allowed to perform and suture an episiotomy and to carry out forceps deliveries; in England, midwives can perform an episiotomy but not repair it, and forceps deliveries are a doctor's task.[20] International data on intervention in birth (e.g., induction, instrumental delivery, caesarean section) are almost non-existent, but the figures that are available show large differences between countries. Instrumental deliveries, for example, made up 36 per cent of all deliveries in the United States in 1973, 11 per cent in England and Wales, and 4 per cent in Norway. Of these, vacuum extractions rather than forceps accounted for 0·4 per cent in the United States, 7 per cent in England and Wales, but 63 per cent in Norway. Inductions accounted for 17 per cent of births in England and Wales in 1967 and 39 per cent in 1974. In Norway, the two figures were 11 per cent and 14 per cent.[21]

Statistics are bland and boring, but they are clues to women's treatment, insignia of their dependence on, and control by, experts. For the first time in her life since she was a child, a woman having a baby is considered not to know what is in her own best interests. She has to be 'advised' to attend a clinic for antenatal care, to have her baby in hospital, to swallow iron pills, to have an epidural in labour, to breastfeed. Women who do not 'choose' this way of having a baby are 'bad'. They jeopardise the health of their infants either through an outmoded belief in nature or because they are just plain lazy.[22] But this medical management of birth is currently being challenged in a big way. Books are being published, television and radio programmes being made, research projects devised and funded; obstetricians are re-examining their practices and thinking of their patients as more than baby carriages, an assembly line of uteruses and vaginas and competent or 'incompetent' cervixes. (Certain notions about women are suggested by the 'technical' language of gynaecology.) Criticism and self-criticism of current obstetric practice is not yet a tidal wave; but the ripples of each small pebble move out in ever-widening circles. Two questions are the key ones: what is the basis in fact of the methods themselves? (*is* hospital safer than the home? *why* are so many labours induced?); what do current methods of childbirth management do to women (and their babies and family life)? In turn, these stimulate a third inquiry. For, given the extensiveness of childbirth's medicalisation, why has no one complained before?

The following is a list of some common procedures to which many women in industrialised societies are subjected when they have a baby:

Regular antenatal checkups
Iron and vitamin supplements
Vaginal examinations in pregnancy
Ultrasound monitoring of pregnancy
Hospital birth
Enemas or suppositories in first stage labour
Shaving of the pubic hair in labour
Artificial rupture of the membranes
Pharmacological induction of labour (oxytocin, prostaglandins)
Vaginal examinations in labour
Bladder catheterisation in labour
Mechanical monitoring of the foetal heart
Mechanical monitoring of contractions
A glucose or saline drip in labour
Epidural analgesia in labour
Pethidine (meperidine) or other pain-killing/tranquillising
    injections in labour

Birth in a horizontal or semi-horizontal position
Episiotomy
Forceps or vacuum extraction of the baby
Cutting the umbilical cord immediately after birth
Accelerated delivery of the placenta by injection of ergometrine
    and/or oxytocin and pulling on the cord

All of these procedures were introduced into obstetric practice without a systematic evaluation of their effectiveness. *None* of them is without disadvantages or dangers to mother or child or both. *Most* continue to be used routinely and without regard for their iatrogenic (illness-producing) qualities. Practices that undoubtedly benefit a minority of mothers are applied unthinkingly to the majority who do not need them.[23]

> We who care for women at birth must restore some balance between the use of high-risk methods and allowing normal childbirth to proceed. First, we must reaffirm that most women having babies are normal, instead of fostering fear and a mystique of technical superiority over human functions. We see the pattern repeated of high-risk procedures being used more and more until they are routine, even though the procedures themselves cause some high-risk crises. Most births are normal; most babies are normal. . . . Nobody advocates laissez-faire management of high-risk births; but let us keep high-risk treatment for high-risk patients. . . . Doctors almost uniformly find it difficult to acknowledge that most women are fully capable of delivering *themselves* . . .[24]

The goal has always been to improve mortality rates. Both the United States and the United Kingdom are in the bottom half of the perinatal mortality table, doing impressively worse than countries such as Japan, Czechoslovakia, Finland, France, Malta and Israel.

> When a football team finds itself at an embarrassingly low position in the league, there tends to be a flurry of activity – managers are sacked and large sums of money are likely to be spent to buy in expensive talent, and often with little effect. I think that I detect a similar tendency in maternity care both within countries and also between countries at the international level – there is often the unspoken assumption that more expensive facilities and expertise will inevitably improve our league standings. . . . We may have assumed too lightly that more sophisticated management necessarily brings benefits to women, the dangerous argument that more means better – for example, the elimination of domiciliary deliveries, greater access to more antenatal beds, the development of better predictive scores to identify high-risk patients, the use of

more direct measurements of foetal growth and well-being, various policies of elective induction of labour, the acceleration of labour by accurately controlled oxytocics, and continuous monitoring of the foetal heart in labour. This is the face of modern obstetrics. . . . Those of us whose experience and training has embroiled us in the high drama of complicated obstetrics find it difficult to avoid an emphasis on safety, and we tend to retreat into the position that pregnancy can only be considered to be safe in retrospect. However, we have to ask ourselves how effective and costly are our screening and safety devices. What price has to be paid for this safety by the 98% of pregnant patients who have surviving infants? – and, in any case, what do we mean by the use of the word 'patient' as applied to a perfectly healthy pregnant woman?[25]

The obstetrician who made these enlightened comments in 1975 considered that a cost–benefit analysis of maternity care was long overdue. By 'cost–benefit' he did not only include monetary items, but physical trauma and discomfort and emotional and social distress. These measures are not easy to obtain: they are not like deaths or stillbirths or congenital malformations that can be counted. Perhaps for this reason they have been left out of the medical reckoning. Obstetricians deal with death and illness and acute pain, but they do not deal with discomfort, with failures in emotional health and relationships and with 'social' problems. So it is in the field of social science research that we expect measures of the social and emotional costs of current maternity care to be computed.

One effect, disturbed mother–baby relationships, has now been documented, and the 'normal' distance that hospitalised birth puts between mother and baby has been shown to jeopardise the bond between them.[26] The psychological impact of medicalised childbirth is becoming part of the received wisdom of official reports:

Evidence from a large number of sources all emphasises that the birth and newborn period is of major importance for the development of relationships which may have a profound and lasting influence on the future development of the child and the family. . . . Much of our evidence stressed the importance of 'early bonding' between mothers and their children immediately after birth and the need to ensure that the whole birth experience is handled in hospitals with greater sympathy and sensitivity than has been the case in the past.[27]

But what of the mother herself? A pregnant mother, a mother in labour, is two patients: a woman and a baby. Their interests are co-existent but also different. We must not be deceived into thinking that criticism of maternity care centred on the welfare of babies is necessarily 'feminist'; it may be designed to put the baby, and not its mother, at the centre of the stage. It is this area of the effect of medicalised childbirth on mothers as people (rather than as mothers) that is both the most ignored and the least amenable to analysis. How can diffuse anxiety, feelings of unwilling dependence on, and debilitating deference to, medical authority be measured? When anger at medical intrusion and control is by its very nature inchoate and inarticulate, how can anyone else assess it? What is the effect of having one's body 'mastered' by machines and the product of this process handed to one as alienated labour? (The first machine for inducing labour was called 'William' not 'Mary'.) And how do these experiences of first childbirth affect a woman's entire experience of reproduction, her feelings as a mother, her sense of self-worth?

NATURAL CHILDBIRTH?

There is little doubt that technological childbirth is 'unnatural'. But what is 'natural' childbirth? And how is it related to the status of women – as mothers and in general?

The anthropologist Margaret Mead pointed out that in one sense childbirth is never natural; it is always a cultural act, affected by people's beliefs, expectations and customs. One of the meanings of 'natural childbirth' is birth without major intervention. A birth induced with a syntocinon drip or a prostaglandin tablet is not natural: neither is a caesarean or a forceps delivery. But perhaps the central idea in the natural childbirth movement is that women should not have analgesic or anaesthetic drugs when they have babies.

The 'father' of natural childbirth (it had no mother) is usually identified as Grantly Dick-Read, a doctor who in the 1940s decided that the pain of birth is largely due to the effect of fear and tension on the muscles of the uterus. He believed that through understanding, relaxation and breathing exercises women could control these muscles and reduce or eliminate labour pain. Some years later, Ferdinand Lamaze, a French doctor, took up the idea of conditioned reflexes, which had been developed out of Pavlov's work in Russia. Lamaze introduced the psychoprophylactic method of childbirth to the West, a method that entailed distracting the mother from sensations of pain via an elaborate breathing drill. Psychoprophylaxis is taught by the National Childbirth Trust in Britain and has become synonymous in many people's minds with natural childbirth. Popular guides to natural childbirth first began to appear in the late 1950s – between 1958 and 1964, more than a dozen such works were published in England. The use of photographs and pregnant models in antenatal literature generally dates from the early 1960s and is a development that promotes, in a romantic fashion, the 'natural' associations of childbirth: 'The sun is invariably shining and the picture full of summer-time symbols – green leaves, flowers, ducks. . . .'[28] Periodically, other 'new' ideas become associated with the natural childbirth image. In 1974 a Society to Support Home Confinements was founded and for some women natural childbirth and hospital delivery are mutually exclusive possibilities. Ferdinand Leboyer, a French obstetrician, has recently publicised his concept of a 'natural' delivery – from the baby's point of view. He believes that babies should be born into twilight or near darkness, in a peaceful room, and should be placed immediately after birth against the mother's body and massaged by her. The umbilical cord should not be cut until all the remaining placental blood has passed to the baby, and later the baby should be immersed in a bath of warm water, returning it to the comforting wet weightlessness of the uterine environment.[29]

Such advocates of natural childbirth have, however, mostly showed only a narrow concern for the position of women. Their prescriptions are based on a particular diagnosis of the meaning of motherhood. For Dick-Read, childbirth is a woman's biological destiny, her greatest achievement and joy. Leboyer sees the mother's body as a prison, the mother herself as a monster ejecting her helpless baby painfully and forcibly out into the harsh bright world. *She* has no problems with the management of birth, or, rather, the problems she has are the baby's problems only. Lamaze, who stressed the mother's personal need to control birth, advocated control through detachment, taking the mother's mental and emotional awareness away from her body. Much of the heritage of the psychoprophylactic method today has become inextricably interwoven with another stereotype of womanhood: wifehood. Childbirth in this ideology is a *couple*'s experience. Antenatal counselling includes the husband, who is regarded as of equal importance to his wife in the delivery room. Freedom from the pain of labour benefits husbands as well as wives, for it makes women nicer to be with. This is of course a justification not only for psychoprophylaxis but for analgesia, in particular epidural analgesia, which leaves a woman physically numbed but mentally aware. Such freedom from pain, it has been argued, is akin to 'sexual liberation' in placing women more squarely at men's disposal while in no way curing their estrangement from their bodies.[30]

A FEMINIST ALTERNATIVE?

None of these prescriptions for natural childbirth places women as people at the centre of their own experience of childbirth. Patriarchy defines female biology in special ways: women's sexual availability and response to men is important; reproduction within marriage is necessary; breastfeeding is medically desirable but sexually disturbing, for a woman's breasts belong to men not to babies, and exposing a breast to a baby seems like indecent exposure. It is, after all, in the interests of a male-oriented society to play down the achievement of birth and lactation, and the connection with a woman's sexuality that these have.[31]

Thus limited, female biology is not very appealing. It seems something of a burden, or is a sign of inferiority. Perhaps partly for this reason feminists have not been very interested in childbirth. The first murmurs of complaint about the medicalisation of motherhood came therefore not from feminists but from mothers and other sections of the 'lay' public. In Britain, criticism really began to be voiced in a prominent way with the publication of two articles in a Sunday newspaper in late 1974 ('The Childbirth Revolution' and 'The Vital First Hours') and a television programme on the induction of labour that was broadcast several months later.[32] The authors and programme-makers responsible for these prods to the public conscience were responding to a sizeable increase in the technology applied to childbirth that had taken place since the mid-1960s.

Many feminists have been distinctly anti-natalist. The concerns of organised feminism since the 1960s have been with *freeing* women from their child-bearing and child-rearing roles (more abortion and contraception, more state child care) to increased participation in the non-domestic world (equal pay for equal work, equal opportunities and education, legal and financial independence from men). A major theme has been the redefinition of sexuality, its liberation from the constraints of the patriarchal stereotype. Thus feminism has unconsciously echoed the patriarchal view of women; women as sexual objects or subjects condemned by their biology to motherhood. The pain of childbirth has been seen as unnecessary suffering – the heritage of the Judeo-Christian condemnation of women to a punishment from God. The ability of women to grow and breastfeed babies and give birth to them in pain but with satisfaction is only now beginning to be seen by feminists as a valid and valuable aspect of being a woman, a resource to be drawn on rather than a burden to be disposed of.[33]

Woman-controlled childbirth is a fresh vision of an old social arrangement. But there was no golden age in which women gave birth both safely and effortlessly, and it would be a backward step to condemn the whole of modern obstetrics: 'the quality of medical care depends on the extent to which interventions of proven effectiveness are properly applied to those who can benefit from them.'[34] It also depends on allowing women choices, on giving them back the power to decide not only whether they have children but when, where and how they may do it. It means counting the costs and appreciating the benefits, it means seeing childbirth as a momentous time in a woman's life, an act of significance in terms of her own particular life and identity. Birth is an isolated biological episode only to hospital administrators and official statisticians: the women who give birth have a past and a future. So it is in this biographical context that childbirth has its social meaning.

The rest of this book traces the social meaning of first childbirth in the lives and through the eyes of a group of women giving birth in a London hospital in the mid-1970s. Since what is described is a historical transition (from non-motherhood to motherhood), the accounts themselves mostly follow a chronological sequence. Chapters 2 to 4 are about pregnancy from conception to shortly before the birth, looking at its physical, emotional and social aspects: becoming aware of motherhood-to-be, going to the doctor, getting fat, being uncomfortable, giving up work, imagining the baby and its birth. Chapter 5 is about the birth itself: the way it was, the way it was expected to be, the way it is remembered. In chapters 6 and 7 the mothers become familiar with the after-effects of birth and with their babies – in hospital and, later, at home. The next two chapters

('Menus' and 'Domestic Politics') are slightly different in structure from the rest. They follow infant feeding attitudes and practices from birth to five months, and ups and downs in marriage throughout the whole period covered by the research (three months pregnant to five months post-birth). Chapters 10 and 11 focus on ordinary life at five months (the baby's routine, the mother's so-called 'adjustment' to domesticity), and on a summary of what, in retrospect, becoming a mother was like: difficult or easy, the disintegration of a romantic vision, a labour of love. In the final chapter the theme of childbirth's medicalisation is returned to. Are women happy about the kind of medical treatment they get? What do they think of doctors? And how do doctors treat them?

These questions are of more importance in the case of first childbirth than they are in subsequent births. First childbirth has a capacity that other births do not have to brand reproduction with a lasting meaning for the mother, to influence all other reproductive experiences. And it is a turning point, a transition, a life crisis: a first baby turns a woman into a mother, and mothers' lives are incurably affected by their motherhood; in one way or another the child will be a theme for ever.

CHAPTER 2

In the Beginning

It is a good moment when you know for certain that your baby is really on the way. I have known some young mothers who assured me that they knew for certain on the very first day. This may be true for them, and no doctor would ever dispute the highly unscientific accuracy of most feminine intuition. But most young women are a bit more cautious. They have plenty of faith but, not surprisingly, they do like to have a little direct evidence as well.
[A doctor[1]]

Don't get me wrong, it's not that I don't want the baby, but I'd rather we had better circumstances. It's shocked me into the realisation that we don't have a place to put it. It took a while to grow on me; I was pleased, but I wasn't going out of my mind with it – it wasn't till I went to the hospital that it hit me that I was pregnant. I've never thought of myself as a mother . . . I've been doing different jobs trying to make some sort of a career and I've thought of myself more as a working wife than as a mother.
[A pregnant woman]

SIGNS AND SYMPTOMS

SHARON WARRINGTON, audiotypist:
I missed the period in April, so it was just before the one in May that they really started to feel tender, and I know if you sort of rubbed it it felt really sore, but I always used to get that before a period; I never worried, not really, and when I went down to him he just said: oh, gastro-enteritis, how long have you had this? About a week, and I've put up with it as long as I can. He said: what actually happens? I said: it's only in the morning, the sickness. So he said: oh have tea and a dry biscuit or dry toast before you get out of bed. I said, I'm not pushing my husband out, I said, he goes to work all day, I said, as far as I'm concerned it's my place to get up and get him up. Oh alright he said, so I kept plodding along, plodding along . . .

25

I:* He knew you'd missed a period and had sore breasts?

SHARON: Yes.

I: And kept feeling sick?

SHARON: Yes.

I: He knew all that?

SHARON: Yes. Then I let that go and the diarrhoea stopped, and then one morning as soon as I had opened my eyes I knew that I was going to be sick and I ran into the bathroom and I was sick – not being crude, yellow; it scared the living daylights out of me. I rushed into my Mum and I said: Mum! She said: what? I said it's yellow! She said: what's yellow? I said, I've been sick. Where is it? I said it's in the toilet. So she said: well I hope you haven't pulled the chain, I want to have a look – this is my Mum. I said no, I said: go on then. Anyway while she was gone I had to retch up again and there was some more in a bucket. She said: something's wrong with you, she said, that's bile and she said you only ever get that when you're pregnant. So I said no I'm not pregnant. So she said: why not? The doctor says I'm not pregnant, he says I've got gastro-enteritis. She said you don't get bile with gastro-enteritis. I thought oh, you know, and I tried to – you've got to have faith in a doctor 'cos you can't have faith in no one else, so she said: go back and see him. Anyway the next morning it was like someone had cut me, every time you touched it it felt sore, and I thought I'll go and see him, and as I walked in his face was as long as death: he said, oh no, not again. I said: oh, I said, I've got this pain, I said: well, it's not a pain, I said, it's a soreness. Where? I said, in the pit of my back. Hm, kidney infection, he said, water's alright? I said: yes, fine. He said: oh pyelitis. There was no more said – more tablets, more time off from work. . . .

Then I went back again and he said, you know, could you be? And I said – well I don't – I'm not the doctor, you know, I said: that's up to you. He said, well don't get like that. And I said well I've missed March, I've missed April, and I said to me that's unusual, so he said: well alright he said, wait another month. . . .

Some kind of physical symptom, or combination of symptoms, announces pregnancy and is the first warning sign of motherhood. Or at least a woman becomes aware that her body is not behaving as it usually does and wants to know the reason why. But although medical textbooks and books of advice for pregnant

---

* Interviewer. Because A.O. did not do all of the interviewing, the interviewer will be referred to thus throughout the book.

women list pregnancy symptoms, no one knows how normal (not medically or socially special) women first notice pregnancy.

What was the first thing that made you think you might be pregnant? *

JOSEPHINE LLOYD, boutique manager:
Well, first of all, missing my period. And also for a while I thought I had something else wrong with me because I was feeling very sick – not first thing in the morning at all, but during the day at work. What else was it? I really forget now. I know when I went to the doctor's I was explaining to him that I was getting stomach pains and I was really feeling sick during the day, I wasn't feeling like eating, but I'd had a pregnancy test at the chemist's along the road – this was in June – and they told me it was negative. And of course I got worried because I really thought there was something wrong with me. And I thought perhaps it's an after-effect – perhaps it's because I took the pill for a long time, you know coming off it . . . and I just really didn't know what it was. So I went to the doctor. And I told him that I was getting depressed and I told him I had slight backache and I was feeling very sick. I kept going to the toilet thinking I was going to be sick. Never morning sickness, always sort of late afternoon or just after lunch or something. The inability to cope as I normally could and I think, you know, I put it down to a new job because I'd never done accountancy to that extent before, I'd done a little bit before at clerical jobs and at the Building Society but never to that extent and they tried to teach me so much in a short amount of time and I couldn't cope with it and it was getting me down. And the doctor examined me and he said I can't see any sign of you being pregnant.

NANCY CARTER, clerk:
I didn't actually think I *was* pregnant. I went down to the doctor's because I had this terrible itching. He said, oh that's right, he said how long was it since my last period and I said oh ages, but I said I didn't think I was pregnant. And he said, he examined me, and said I think you are, but he couldn't tell definitely then until I had a test.

JOSÉ BRYCE, manicurist:
I'm so regular, it's ridiculous. I know that it's going to be about six o'clock in the evening. It's so funny, because at seven o'clock my husband said: oh, you're pregnant, then?

* *This question, and others like it throughout the book, is taken from the interview schedule.*

KAY EDWARDS, cashier:
I just knew I was pregnant.
I: When did you first know?
KAY: I was on holiday.
I: When was that?
KAY: That was Whitsun, I think. I went to the doctor on the Tuesday, and I just knew when I was holidaying.
I: Can you describe the sort of feeling of knowing?
KAY: I thought there was something different. In fact I knew before I was on holiday, I knew there was something different, but I couldn't pin it down to my period or my bust increasing, I just knew that something different was happening.
I: Had you actually missed a period at that time?
KAY: I think I just missed it as I went on holiday.

MANDY GREEN, hairdresser:
About a week before I was due to have a period, um, my breasts swelled up and it was tender when I touched them. That was a week before.
I: Did you think you were, at that point?
MANDY: I knew I was at that point. I'd never had that before.
I: What happened after that – after you got sore breasts?
MANDY: They really did swell a lot . . . Then after the tenderness had died away, the nipples started to change. But, um, I knew I was pregnant. I even half felt I was pregnant when I had the three-day period on the 17th March because I thought shucks, is it a day late or something? And then when I stopped after three days I thought, ah well girl, you know now.
I: Why didn't you go to the doctor?
MANDY: Well, I don't know. People kept saying you can't be sure, you know, you've just got to wait, and all sorts of things like that. So I thought, oh sod you. I just thought – well I didn't really want to know too soon anyway. I mean, I knew in myself, but it's a period of nine months, and I thought if I get to know too soon it's going to be an awfully long nine months. So I didn't want to go any earlier.

The only 'real' evidence of pregnancy is the birth of a baby. But many women do like to 'know' they are pregnant: pregnancy confers a special status, and motherhood is a role with tremendous implications for a woman's identity and life-style. Signs of pregnancy may be picked up early on if a woman is aware of the possibility of becoming pregnant and if she interprets her symptoms according-

ly. But the body's response to conception may present a confused message, particularly for those women who were not planning a pregnancy.

ANNE BLOOMFIELD, barmaid:
It was really funny. What happened was, my last period was about the beginning of April and from work a girl got married and we went out for a meal. We went to an Italian restaurant and I had a steak or something and I had sauté potatoes and they were in a rather rich thingymebob, and I thought – you know – this dinner's making me feel a bit ill. It's not like me: I usually eat well. But I felt sick and I couldn't be sick and it went on for about four days like that and I kept taking Andrews and it didn't go away. Then I thought I'm late in coming on – perhaps it's something to do with that: I'd better go to the doctor. I never in no way thought I was pregnant: I thought it was the last thing in the world that would happen to me.

A missed period is a first symptom of pregnancy noticed by less than two-thirds of the sample women. One in twenty had a light period instead; one in ten were first aware of breast soreness, and about the same proportion felt nauseous or vomited.

First pregnancy symptoms	
Missed period	62%
Nausea and/or vomiting	12%
Sore breasts	9%
Light period	5%
'Felt pregnant'	3%
Frequent urination	2%
Other	6%

Some women feel they do not need a doctor to identify pregnancy: they can diagnose themselves. More commonly some kind of medical proclamation is demanded: pregnancy, having become a 'medical' condition, requires specialist diagnosis. Yet going to the doctor to have one's pregnancy confirmed does not always seem an appropriately medical exercise.

ROSE WILLIAMS, insurance agent:
I said to the doctor: look, I feel awful. And he said: when was your last period? And I said oh I don't know, I suppose I'm nearly due. I was in an awful state. And he said well you would be – you're two months pregnant! He just squeezed a breast and out popped milk and I said, oh!

DEIDRE JAMES, jewellery assembler:
I told her my symptoms – that I wasn't feeling up to scratch. She

asked me if I'd missed my periods and I said yes. She said it's possible you could be pregnant. She looked through my records and said I'd been regular since I started so I was probably pregnant: come back in two months' time. . . . I was, not upset, but *dubious* I suppose that she didn't examine me or anything. She just took it for granted. But it still didn't ease my mind . . . I wanted to know *myself*. I wanted to tell my husband. He knew that I might be, but he said to go and find out: we didn't want to build our hopes up. But all I could say was 'probably' when I came back. I thought in my mind that I was but there was still a doubt – I wasn't going to go round telling everyone.

These anecdotes express a tension between a desire to defer to medical authority and a feeling that the body's own signals should be trusted. On the one hand it may seem obvious that pregnancy is the only explanation that fits the symptoms, that the person whose body the baby is in should know about it first. But, on the other hand, people are used to going to doctors to have their symptoms interpreted. Why should pregnancy be a special case? After all, women know they are expected to visit a doctor for antenatal and postnatal care and to go into hospital to have the baby, just as they would for a misbehaving appendix or a broken leg.

MOTIVES AND INTENTIONS

Did you want a baby?

Since the advent of contraceptive techniques that are reasonably effective and safe, it is widely assumed that people only have children because they want them – or that this ought to be the reason why children are conceived. But some babies are still conceived unintentionally, so that 'did you want a baby?' comes before any discussion of people's motives for having children.[2]

JO INGRAM, 26, further education teacher, cohabiting for 7 years: I came off the pill because I got thrush and I was absolutely pissed off with thrush and also I didn't mind particularly if I did get pregnant. I think maybe, underneath, subconsciously, I actually wanted a kid: I don't know, I can't tell about that. Not because I wanted a kid for any sentimental reason. It's the sort of thing you think you might as well try because you've never done it. It's not a very responsible attitude at all. But overtly it was because I had thrush and I wanted to try to get rid of it.

LILY MITCHELL, 29, civil servant, married 4 years:
Well, I came off the pill because my doctor said I should come off it because I'd been on it for four years, and he thought I should have a change. So he'd given me six months, and he said he wouldn't give me any more; he just advised me to come off it. So as I say in that six months when I was using up my supply we talked about it and I said we'd just see . . .
I: How did you feel about that?
LILY: Well, you see it was my decision because my husband was all for it from the beginning, whereas I was the one who was favouring the pill, you know. So probably had the doctor not suggested taking me off it we would just have carried on because I think you tend to . . . you just keep putting it off and putting it off. . . . I don't know: I just haven't been one for – I didn't want to get married when everybody else wanted to get married and I didn't get married until I was twenty-five. It wasn't a day too soon. You know, I'm just one of these people who didn't want to get married when I was nineteen, twenty. I just wasn't interested. It didn't turn me on. There was too much to be done in the world. And when we got married . . . because I think once there's children you never really get time again. . . . I think it's really, you know, you've got to make up your mind do you want children or do you want a nice home? You know, it's a big step because once you're twenty-nine and you get into a routine where you've a big social life . . . you see other people having children and you think it's a big change . . . the change would be hard.

ANGELA KING, 26, cashier, married 2 months:
We'd been going together for five years and we never took any precautions so I think we both hoped it would happen, but it never happened for about three or four years and we both thought there was something wrong with us. I was sure there was something wrong with me and he was sure there was something wrong with him. But we were both really pleased.

SANDY WRIGHT, 28, secretary, married 1 year:
We were neither of us desperate. I felt that I was 28 – coming up to 29 – it was now or never.

CARY WIMBORNE, 27, sales supervisor, married 3 years:
Um, yes. It wasn't planned, but yes.

LOUISE THOMPSON, 30, law student, married 10 years:
No, not really. But my husband did.

NINA BRADY, 28, shop assistant, married 8 months:
I didn't want to get pregnant so quick. I thought if I'd a free year I'd
be happy – if I had one year working. But I had just four months – and
as it happens I'm still happy!

JUNE HATCHARD, 29, teacher, married 3 years:
No. We said we didn't want to have children. I suppose the reasons
were quite selfish really. We couldn't really see any *advantage* in
having one. As I was working with children and Ian was as well, this
was the outlet for it.

JEAN CLARK, 24, conference organiser, married 1 year:
No, I didn't. No: I've got no maternal instincts whatsoever. Never
wanted it; I wouldn't have bought a one-bedroom flat. I've said all
along I don't want a snotty little thing hanging round my ankles.

*People do not have clear motives so far as having children is concerned; few
organise their lives according to some overall plan. The subject of children
provokes ambivalent feelings, so that
'planning' is a euphemism for allowing
one particular feeling or pressure to gain
an upper hand. An additional complication is that conceiving a child is not like
buying a new three-piece suite: demand
and supply may not be easily equated.
Although one in five women conceived
straight away, about the same proportion took from seven to twelve months,
and one in ten took more than a year to
start a baby.*[3]

Time taken to conceive*	
Instantly	18%
1–3 months	25%
4–6 months	25%
7–12 months	22%
More than a year	10%

* Among the women who planned
to get pregnant. Fifteen women
were not planning pregnancy at the
time they conceived (eight of these
were using contraception).

Both times as soon as I stopped using a contraceptive I've got
pregnant straight away. (*Elizabeth Farrell, miscarriage 1974, baby 1975*)
We've been trying for a baby for about a year. The last few months
I was beginning to try and not get hung up about it . . . I suppose I was
getting worried. We planned to have a holiday in Italy a couple of
weeks ago and we thought we'll go to the doctor after the Italian
holiday. But we never got to Italy because I had a sort of threatened
miscarriage so we cancelled the holiday! (*Ellen George*)

Why did you want a baby?

Despite its complexity, the question 'did you want/plan a baby?' may be easier to answer than the parallel question 'why did you want a baby?' This taps a vast minefield of unexplored or half-explored motives and reasons. Some women have never asked themselves this question, or when they do the answer is framed in terms of 'always' having wanted a baby: others describe a long process of critical self-examination.

KATE PRINCE, a journalist married to a solicitor:
Well, much as I thought about it and it's nice to be independent and all that – shall we have children? I knew – we *both* knew – that we really wanted children at some stage. We've asked one another why do we want children: oh I don't know! Isn't it stupid? *Why* do we want children? I mean most kids are brats anyway – why is it that our own are going to be any better or nicer anyway? I must say I do quite like kids when I see them and play with them, and so does Mark, but in the long term they are a bind. They produce a lot of worry for you – think of all the lovely things you could do – the nice times you could have together without them. But we just decided that we were probably like everybody else – that we just wanted kids *because* – that we probably are the victims of tradition and everything else. We don't know about this business of reproductive instincts – I don't know whether I go along with that, believe in it or not, but what we thought in the end was let's just have a baby.

I didn't feel: now is the moment! I didn't feel motherhood coming upon me against my will or anything like that . . . I'm pretty sure it's the society . . . I don't know whether it's a biological thing – whether just like fish and birds and bees you just have children because it's the natural thing to do . . . a few times when I was having these irregular periods I thought I would *hate* it if I couldn't have children. But I'm sure that's because of the pressures . . . because I associate people who haven't got children with those couples who've got lots of stair carpets and are always going on cruises. I always think it's a bit poverty-stricken – that sort of existence. I'm *sure* it can add something; they are so interesting, babies: seeing them grow up. Because it is a novelty. There is the curiosity thing about it, *watching*, also, maybe it's pride. I don't know: it could be anything – pride, vanity, seeing your own image, passing something down . . . Whenever I see a birth I find that I'm quite *moved* for some reason, by the physical side of things. All my education tells me I *shouldn't* feel like that – because it *is* quite a sentimental reaction. Which makes me think it may be some sort of *drive.*

GILLIAN HARTLEY, an illustrator married to a musician:
I've always been intrigued to go through the experience of childbirth because it is something that only *we* can go through; and it seems like some sort of experience that people *should* go through. As to having *children,* I think that's just something you choose or don't choose. As long as you've made a responsible choice. . . .

I couldn't even tell you why we're having a child. I don't think we were *pressured* into having a child – certainly not by parents and certainly not by society. I think I like the idea of having a child by my husband. I would like to have *his* child. I think it'll be a very *nice* child; I hope so.

MAX HARTLEY: You say you don't feel under any social pressure but we both feel – not *personally* under it – but we've always talked in the past about how much society *does* push people towards parenthood.

GILLIAN: We were talking this morning about how much we'd enjoy *conforming* for a change – it is very enjoyable for people who've never done anything right before to do the most right thing in the world.

Sarah Moore was infertile for four years, so she and her husband considered both the advantages and disadvantages of parenthood:
I think the reason we want a baby is because it's cementing our marriage and our love. And we want to produce this thing *from* our love. There are all sorts of other minor reasons why we wanted children: we wanted to bring a child up and rear it *our* way because we've got very strong political views and maybe it was just an experiment. I don't know. But I know that before I came off the pill and it's strange, I've spoken to a lot of people about this – when I came off the pill it was just that we wanted a baby: we'd been married two to three years, we were okay financially so that didn't matter: that was okay. And I gave no more thought to it. When I *couldn't* have children – when there was this blockage somewhere – that I *wasn't* falling for a baby, we then had to analyse exactly *why* we wanted children. And I think this is what stopped me from becoming neurotic – you know, weepy at the sight of every pregnant woman, because I really had to analyse exactly *why* we wanted children. We discussed it so much. . . . It's only in recent years that married couples have even been given the choice. More often than not pregnancies are not planned – or weren't planned. And now if you're on the pill you're very definitely given a choice. And I don't think people actually take

that choice seriously enough – I don't think they go into it deeply enough. But we were forced to discuss it . . . we decided that those reasons we put on the disadvantage side of having children were purely selfish but matter a lot. Freedom: that matters to me more than anything.

Other reasons for having children appeal to images of family life – the 'nuclear' family of parents and children, or the wider extended family of grandparents and grandchildren – to the effect of parenthood on marriage, or to feelings that child-rearing might be an essential part of life:

Well you're not classed as a family until you've had one are you? I thought it might quieten my husband down a bit. (*Sharon Warrington*)

It's what we've been waiting for ever since – I mean even before we was married – this is all we talked of, getting married and having children. (*Veronica Pratt*)

I thought you might ask that. It's very difficult to say. I never sort of thought because of this I want to have one. I suppose in some ways it's a bad thing to say but it's a natural course of events. (*Cary Wimborne*)

Lots of different reasons. To do with my philosophy of life generally. I feel it would be nice to have something to leave behind – that it all seems a bit pointless otherwise. Also David and I have always thought that it would be pleasant to have a child or children eventually. And for my parents' sake and David's parents' sake we wanted to have children. (*Lois Manson*)

I've had a family life myself. I want a family of my own with a sense of *belonging* I suppose. (*Barbara Hood*)

Well, I didn't want an *abortion*. (*Jo Ingram*)

It seemed as good a time as any. (*Rosalind Kimber*)

Dunno really. (*Kirsty Miller*)

IT'S ALRIGHT, DEAR, YOU CAN START KNITTING

MARGARET SAMSON is married to a GP:

James kept saying now don't count your chickens before they're hatched; you've got to wait your forty-two days before you can have a test. So I had to wait till then. I think he made me wait a bit longer than that actually – another three or four days just to make sure. Of course he did the test himself. He took the specimen up to work, and he let somebody else do it first and then he did it afterwards to double check, and then he rang up and told me it was alright. I was teaching at the time – all these new girls. I said to him: I can't wait until you

come home at night, you've got to ring me up and he said: well I won't
be able to speak to you on the phone. So he said: what shall I say to the
girl who answers the phone? So I said just say it's alright or it's okay or
something like that, and I shall know what you mean. So he said
alright, I'll do that. So I was sitting there teaching this lesson, and I
thought I shall never wait till the end of the period to see if there's a
note on my desk. So I didn't: I ran out and there was the note, and I
didn't go back for the rest of the period. I sat and cried. I was happy.

SANDY WRIGHT:
Well I work in a family planning clinic once a week. I took the
specimen there and a doctor did it. I stood there while he did it. The
clinic arrangement is we have to take the patients down to the nurses
and I happened to take someone down, and I saw one of the doctors
doing this test, and I said to one of the nurses: is that mine? So she said
yes. I was conscious of my heart thumping while he was doing it – I'd
seen them done before; and he sort of acted about a bit and had to
have a look at it under the light and everything, but I think I knew
pretty well: it goes granular if it's negative and it was staying milky.

ALISON MOUNTJOY:
We went to stay with my parents-in-law and I went to the family
planning clinic there. I surreptitiously phoned them up from upstairs
to get the result – Luke was downstairs – and I flew downstairs and I
thought this isn't the way for a pregnant lady to behave: I burst into
tears and all the rest of it. They told me in such a nice way. The nurse
said: it's alright, dear, you can start knitting.

*In 1975 53,800 illegitimate babies were born in England and Wales; nearly a
third of all women who married were pregnant on their wedding day. The
stereotyped reaction to pregnancy ('a good moment') is therefore bound to be
fictional in a proportion of cases seen by any GP or family planning clinic.
Sometimes a negative reaction can be predicted because a woman is not married or
her contraceptive technique has failed, but not always: June Hatchard had a coil
in when she conceived:*

The doctor didn't think I was pregnant, but he said oh don't worry
if you are: we can arrange an abortion. I was quite surprised. So I
said: I don't want to have an abortion anyway. Then when I went
back [to the antenatal clinic] he examined me again and again asked
if I wanted an abortion. I said I didn't want one: I told you already
once. I got a bit sick of it actually. . . . I think I was surprised as well,
because I thought you had to prove a more positive case to get one.

Eventually her GP removed the coil and she had a straightforward pregnancy and delivery.

Attitudes to pregnancy are not static: they develop and change. So June Hatchard's initial intention to remain childless became positive acceptance when pregnancy happened. But at the beginning of pregnancy mixed feelings are quite common. More than a third of the women felt like this.

Reactions to pregnancy	
Pleased	52%
Mixed feelings	38%
Upset	11%

When you found out definitely that you were pregnant, how did you feel about it?

NINA BRADY:
The first thing I did was cried. I was happy, but I was disappointed if you know what I mean. I was happy, because when I wasn't getting pregnant I thought maybe there's something the matter with me; I thought you get pregnant right away when you have sex with your husband. Then, when I did get pregnant, I knew there was nothing wrong, and then I was disappointed to think I would have to give up my work, dear, because I had a very good job, I earned very good money. It was a smart dress shop, very high class, up in the West End.
I: Did you have any particular fears or worries?
NINA: I'm frightened if anything will happen. You know a lot of people in Ireland, they used to die having children. . . . They told me that in the hospital yesterday; they said if you come here every month nothing can happen to you. That's why you come to the antenatal clinic here. They told me that. I felt better.
I: Anything else?
NINA: Yes, there is, there's one question I'm very worried about. And I didn't like to ask it.
I: What was it?
NINA: That was since I got pregnant I can't have intercourse at all. I just can't. I don't know why. It hurts. I just can't have it. I told the doctor, I told my own doctor, not in the hospital yesterday; I didn't tell them. He said that the womb was enlarged and that's why he said you might find it difficult, he said. Is it natural, I wonder? I've got a little baby book here and it says in that book that you should have no problems. It says you should have intercourse with your husband up until seven or eight months. . . . It doesn't mean there's something

wrong with me? Since I got pregnant I just can't stand it, I just don't like it. And that's why he's so good – he doesn't want it very often either. He's very good like that.

GILLIAN HARTLEY:
Sort of bits of both; terrified and very pleased. I would have been disappointed I think had it been negative. As to feeling absolutely jubilant and on top of the world: no. We have a fairly happy marriage and we've a good set up, schedule; we're used to freedom, doing things when we want to. There are going to be tremendous changes. We've never been parents before. I mean, it's terrifying. I cried that evening, before I rang my parents.

MAX: Yes, but you had three or four hours of euphoria after getting the result before your fears that you'd had before reasserted them-selves. You didn't seem to me at that time to have mixed feelings any more than I did, but I'm sure that after three or four hours I felt the same. I felt: what the hell are we going to be like as parents and how are we going to get through the nine months?

GILLIAN: It was tears of 'my God, what have I got myself into: childbirth is a very frightening thing', as well. All the fears – what if the baby's deformed. All these things.

I: Anything in particular?

GILLIAN: We thought about ourselves as parents, and how it would affect our relationship to each other. You really get frightened about things like that – if the baby is a strain on the marriage. The marriage is more important than the baby.

NANCY CARTER:
I: Feeling sick as you did, nevertheless what did you feel when you were told that the result was positive?

NANCY: Thrilled, really pleased.

I: What sorts of thoughts immediately went through your mind?

NANCY: [long pause] I was surprised to get pregnant so quickly, as we hoped to get the house done out before we had a baby.

I: Anything else that you thought of?

NANCY: Um – that week I was feeling so sick I remember sitting on the stairs and saying oh I wish I wasn't pregnant, I don't want it, because I felt so terrible – but I didn't really mean it, it was just because I felt so rotten.

JANETTE WATSON:
I was really shaking when I phoned the doctor, because I didn't know

whether he'd say I was or I wasn't. I was really happy. I closed the door and I just walked around with a smile on me face – I couldn't stop; I thought I'd better calm down because I couldn't walk out of there grinning.

I: Did you think about anything in particular?

JANETTE: I did think about getting fat and all those things, and packing up work – I'd like to pack up for a while. *He* thinks that's what my excuse is – that's the reason I wanted to get pregnant, so I could stay at home!

I: Did you have any fears or worries?

JANETTE: Well, I did feel frightened. I don't really know – I can't explain it. I had a frightened feeling inside. Strange, it was: I'm okay now. My Mum told me not to worry – she's had seven!

MAUREEN PATERSON:

I don't know really. Because I didn't *feel* any different. I was trying not to build my hopes up – both of us were really. We were just trying to ignore the fact really I suppose. But we were really pleased.

I: Did you have any particular thoughts?

MAUREEN: Looking after the baby I think, really. I think at the beginning I felt a bit apprehensive, I mean when you don't know if you are or if you aren't then when you phone you think oh crumbs, it's really true. But now I am really looking forward to it.

I: Are you worried at all?

MAUREEN: Not worried; you think, oh crumbs, I wonder if I'll be able to cope? Things like that. Because your whole life must alter really mustn't it? It's a different way of life.

Sarah Moore, who had a history of four years' infertility and lengthy (but unsuccessful) infertility treatment, conceived unexpectedly seven months after deciding to terminate the treatment and reconcile herself to being unable to have a child:

I was shocked. And I mustn't say disappointed. I was very shocked. And I had a slight anti-feeling about it – a slight resentment because having worked really hard at work and now I'd got to the point where I was doing what I wanted to do and had just a little bit more authority than I did have. . . . I'd got to that stage and I was enjoying the job so much more, and then I found out that I was pregnant and the first couple of weeks I was almost horrified, because I knew I'd have to give all this up. But then, after a few weeks, I was fine. And the thought of losing my freedom does worry me. . . . It was just an automatic thing: if I was pregnant I was going to give up work. I don't think I've actually reasoned it out; I mean, I think it's most important that a mother should be at home for the first three years. Not necessarily five, but definitely the first three. So that's a sacrifice I have to make – I *have* to give up work. And it *is* a sacrifice.

A married woman pregnant with her first child should be 'absolutely thrilled'. But many have far more complex reactions.

CARY WIMBORNE:
I: When you found out from the test that you were pregnant, how did you feel?
CARY: I was pleased. Well, I was pleased and apprehensive.
I: Yes?
CARY: I don't know whether you're supposed to be sort of bouncing with joy but you know I can never cut myself off from looking at realities all the time. So many people have said to me: are you pleased? And I act indifferently. Then they start saying, why aren't you pleased? And I feel really I should give in to what's expected of me and say yes, I am pleased: I'm thrilled to bits. They expect you to become pregnant, you know, you've been married for three years, and it is the thing that you *should* do, and now you should be pleased.

MANDY GREEN:
I: How did you feel about it?
MANDY: I wasn't overjoyed, you know, because I didn't have to wait, I didn't have to try for it; I didn't have the feeling each month when I came on and thinking to myself, oh dear, I haven't caught yet, I wonder how long it's going to be. I didn't have any of those feelings. It was there before I'd even realised it. . . . So it was just a sort of nonentity really. I was expecting to feel something and I didn't feel a thing. Nothing. The tea lady said, oh you must be absolutely thrilled about it. You know, she said, tell me, are you pregnant, dear? and I said yes . . . Oh aren't you absolutely thrilled, she said. And I said well, I've spent most of my life trying *not* to get pregnant so to me it's nothing much that I am!

So strong is this cultural imperative to be overjoyed at the news of pregnancy that a woman who reacts differently may puzzle the professionals and be labelled abnormal. Lily Mitchell, who had just 'drifted' into pregnancy and was apprehensive about the changes it would bring (pp. 30–1) was told by her doctor that she had a 'morbid fear of childbirth'. Fear of the birth itself, a common worry, certainly figures in her comments:

Well, I think when something big happens in your life you ought to know how you feel. You know if you like something, you know if you don't like something, even if it's the colour of a dress. And I think my God, he tells you you're pregnant and you don't know how you feel about it! It's quite a shock actually not to know where you stand. The majority of people are, as I say, really pleased. I just felt . . . four years and your life's changing, you know. You can't go out any more, your whole life-style's changing. And to me, I just couldn't adjust to it.

I: And you say the doctor found your attitude confusing?

LILY: Well, he just couldn't understand my reactions. But obviously he was afraid medically in case I had problems at home or something. Maybe you're having rows with your husband or something, he said this, you know. He said, I don't really know you or your husband; he said, I don't know what sort of relationship you have. And therefore I don't really know what this news means to you. As I say, I just told him childbirth just doesn't turn me on at all – the actual childbirth thing absolutely put me off for years, you know. I just hated the idea. But having seen how my doctor reacted, I wouldn't say to any of my friends that I had mixed feelings.

Cultural images of pregnancy portray such reactions as abnormal. Yet many women, who become ordinary loving and caring mothers, have them. Worries about abnormalities in the baby, miscarriage, the pain of childbirth, what it will be like giving up work and staying at home – these are in fact common preoccupations of pregnant women.

Fears and worries during pregnancy	
A deformed baby	39%
Giving up work/ change in life-style	35%
Birth	32%
Miscarriage/stillbirth	29%
Money or housing	20%
Looking after a baby	14%
Getting fat	12%
Other	20%

BECOMING A PATIENT

Most women visit their GP during early pregnancy to have the pregnancy confirmed and to arrange maternity care. Because most births now take place in hospital (96 per cent in 1974 in England and Wales), the function of the GP is increasingly that of referring pregnant women on to a specialist for hospital maternity care. Some still do antenatal care in their own surgeries, but few are prepared to deliver babies at home. Some have little or no interest in any aspect of maternity care:

He didn't do any tests or anything. He said well you probably are – here's a letter. He didn't examine me; he doesn't do antenatal care. I had a little bottle with me but he didn't want it. I said, aren't you going to do a pregnancy test? He said to go to the antenatal clinic at the hospital, and of course I didn't want to go up there unless I knew for certain. (*Sasha Morris*)

The image of the GP as a 'family doctor' to whom all problems of whatever kind can be taken, who has the time and the inclination to discuss how a woman feels in and about her pregnancy – this may be an ideal in doctors' and patients' heads, but what happens in the surgery is usually rather different. Only 38 per cent in this sample of pregnant women were examined by their doctors when they consulted them about pregnancy – and these only partially: only 16 per cent received any advice (usually cursory) about the conduct of pregnancy in general. No GP suggested the possibility of a home birth (see p. 277 for the women's own attitudes to this), and 58 per cent of the women were simply told that they would have their baby in such-and-such a hospital; 61 per cent were given no choice as to who (GP, hospital, local authority clinic) would do their antenatal care (and 'choice' here means information, since first-time mothers-to-be usually do not know what the options are).

Becoming a hospital patient is therefore an important part of a pregnant woman's career. Attending the hospital as a maternity patient provides a public legitimation of a private fact; it confirms the pregnancy as a new social role.

VERA ABBATT, canteen worker:
I couldn't get used to the idea of pregnancy at first at all. It wasn't till I went to the hospital and they actually told me I was twelve-and-a-half weeks pregnant that it suddenly hit me that I was pregnant. . . . I went there and at the end the sister said you're twelve-and-a-half weeks pregnant, and I thought I must be or she wouldn't have said it like that. So I came out and I was ever so pleased really – when it suddenly dawned on me. I came home and I think my husband was more relieved than anything else; I think he was a bit worried that I might be disappointed . . . at the back of my mind was the possibility that it might be a phantom pregnancy.

Booking into the hospital involves being processed, categorised, labelled. Gillian Hartley, an illustrator, describes her first visit:
I got up a nervous wreck as usual. Max came with me, which was

nice. The tube was cancelled and the bus wouldn't come so we got a taxi. We got there and we sat there with all these mums and their urine specimens. They started us off – gave the urine samples in, took the blood test. Then they took the medical history and that was nice because I had a student midwife and it was the first time she'd done it and they had another nurse with her. That was really fun; she was really nervous and I said don't be nervous, it's the first time for both of us. I was very impressed with the other midwife – she was a young girl, about 24–25; she seemed very matter-of-fact and very sort of woman-oriented. They said have you ever had cystitis and I said of course and the student midwife said shall I put it on the form and she said no, no. It was very assembly line. I had to get undressed and then I was weighed and went into a cubicle where they did the blood pressure and they were all very communicative. The staff were marvellous – you could ask them any questions. The thing I was a bit put off by was the doctor. He was a young doctor; he seemed about my age – he couldn't have been practising more than a year or two anyway. There were three doctors there and I thought one of the other ones was certainly a bit nicer – I heard him through the curtains; I heard him joking with the ladies. The one I had, you felt he was a bit embarrassed about it. I wanted to know what he was doing with his little chart, you know? At this point we're certainly not planning another child, so this is it as far as I can see. I want to have nice experiences of my doctor! I guess maybe it was embarrassment. For God's sake, if a fellow decides to specialise in obstetrics and gynaecology. . . .

It was very assembly line. They stick whatever it is they stick in you and get the smear and he had a good feel around. He should have been saying well, right now I'm going to check and see that the baby's in the right position, and you've got no erosions, or nothing's wrong inside you. And he said, it all seems alright. But he should have had a better manner especially for a woman who's gone there for the first time. It didn't upset me; I was a bit put off, because I wanted to have a good experience. But it could upset people horribly. . . . If you get a doctor like that, that fact can really colour your entire pregnancy. I did feel annoyed.

The assembly line feeling – I didn't particularly mind that. I think I realised that it has to be like that because of the numbers and they are working very hard. Oh I know another thing that really pissed me off – when the doctor had finished writing everything down on your card they put it in an envelope and *staple* it before you take it to the staff nurse. That really infuriated me. . . . I understand that the hospital is geared to people who have problems – that if you're alright they don't have time for you, which I think is a shame, the system. I came out feeling that I wanted to talk more about my pregnancy – to somebody. They did ask if you have any questions, but they're not really the kind of questions that you feel you want to take up anybody's time with.

In this scenario of tests and interviews and examinations, the spotlight falls very much on the encounter with the doctor. Procedurally, the patients are 'prepared' for the doctor, and, particularly in a first visit, the agenda is geared to the physical examination. Within the script of the doctor–patient encounter is the internal examination, for many women expecting their first baby, their first experience of this. Nina Brady, a 28-year-old Catholic shop assistant, was one of the 29 per cent who found herself in this 'position':

To tell you the truth it was so embarrassing that I wouldn't want to go there again, but I have to go. It was embarrassing, and that's it. But they say when you're having a baby you have no shame, and that's it. By the time you've finished having the baby I reckon you have no shame left. You have shame at the beginning, because otherwise you wouldn't feel the way you do, would you?

I went in and I handed in my form at 8.30 and the first thing was a urine specimen, which I took with me. . . . The next thing was the blood test where I nearly fainted – it made me very weak; that upset me, I wasn't interested in anything after that. . . . The next thing was I was taken downstairs by a pupil midwife and I was asked practically every question you have asked; she asked me about sickness in his family and sickness in my family; about his parents and my parents, and that took a long time. And the next thing was upstairs and get changed – completely undressed – to let the doctor see you. And he asks you questions and examines you and he gives you this eternal [*sic*] examination and that was *horrible*.

I: Why was it horrible?

NINA: I was very embarrassed.

I: Did the doctor know you were embarrassed?

NINA: He did know, because I cried. I was *awfully* embarrassed.

I: Was there a nurse there?

NINA: There was. She had to come. She wasn't there, but she had to come, because I wouldn't do what I was told. He said to put your ankles together, bring your knees up and let them flop; I done the first two, but I wouldn't let my knees go flop. Then he called the nurse in to part my legs – to be truthful, that's why. I cried more or less shamefully, do you know what I mean? Like he said there's two or three thousand more women having babies here like you. . . . He was very nice. He was a young doctor and he was awfully nice. He was very handsome and this is what upset me – if he was horrible-looking, I wouldn't care, I wouldn't be so embarrassed. He was so handsome and so young. I didn't like him to be looking at me.

I: Did the examination hurt?

NINA: It did hurt. I held his hand and he said it won't take a minute, he said. It just took about two minutes. Then he said: was that so bad? I said, it was very bad. After that I had to go and see some other sister or midwife and she gave me the iron tablets. She said everything was okay, she told me that I was in good health and that the baby was coming along fine, and she asked me about any tablets the doctor was giving me, and she gave me those tablets. Oh I forgot, I saw another sister in between which gave me a lot of literature; I asked her about insurance, about how to get a grant and things like that. Then I saw the head sister after that. She said now have you got any questions to ask? Each one would ask me that anyway. Any moans? Any groans? Have you been treated nicely and all that. I said yes to everything. I was treated nicely. I liked the staff, they were awfully nice. And one of them came round to me after it was all over and said do you feel better now? That was the lady that questioned me downstairs after I had the blood test when I was really crying. And she asked me if I felt better now and she gave me a little bottle for the urine – to bring it in next time. She was awfully nice. She said next time you won't be here half as long and she said you won't have as much to do. . . . I was there for three or four hours.

I didn't think there was a need for all this – when you're having a baby to have such an examination? The midwife told me having a baby is a very difficult thing, she said. But she said with the hospital staff they've got, it's nothing. I told her about one lady that had three kids who told me she never went to an antenatal clinic. This girl, I met her at a job, she said it was all a load of rubbish. I had three healthy children, she said, and I went through my nine months without . . . and I told this to the nurse yesterday. I said why should I come here? And get upset over that? And she explained to me that that lady was a very lucky person. Maybe you'll be unlucky, she said.

CHAPTER 3

Remember, Pregnancy is a State of Health

My doctor said just remember that pregnancy is a state of health, not a disease, which I thought was rather nice. That was the one thing that stuck in my mind. I keep thinking about that and it's so true. If you're feeling rotten, you just think you are alright – it's nothing to worry about. Very commonsense.

It's this concern with medicine that seems to override everything else – the natural process, I mean. I mean it is something women have always been brought up to; everybody knows that, okay, it's painful, having labour and everything, but it's very rewarding: it's the one pain we've been brought up to expect and not to be scared of. Before going to the hospital, pregnancy was a normal, nice condition. I'm not so sure it isn't an illness now.

While growing a baby is certainly not an illness like mumps or gastro-enteritis, it is paradoxically a medical condition – a condition to be monitored by doctors. Between seven and eighteen visits to the GP, local authority or hospital clinic were made during pregnancy by the sample women for antenatal care: the average was

thirteen. Going to the doctor suggests illness, and two other features of illness are associated with pregnancy in modern industrialised society: a pregnant woman, like other 'patients', is allowed to give up her normal work, and is encouraged to hand over responsibility for the management of her condition to others (the medical profession).[1] Moreover, pregnancy produces unpleasant symptoms, each of which, in other circumstances, can be a sign of illness:

Drug use in pregnancy	
Iron pills	100%
Indigestion medicines	43%
Anti-nausea pills	38%
Laxatives	21%
Painkillers	16%
Vitamin pills	14%
Sleeping pills	13%
Antibiotics	11%
Pile ointment/suppositories	7%
Tranquillisers/ anti-depressants	4%
Other	36%

vomiting, changes in bowel habit (constipation or diarrhoea), frequent urination, excessive tiredness, abdominal pain, backache and so on. Even in pregnancy some *of these require medication, a habit not normally associated with health. The most common 'drugs' used in pregnancy are iron and/or vitamin supplements, but many women are prescribed or prescribe for themselves others as well, so that the scale of medicine-taking during the process of becoming a mother usually far outweighs anything experienced beforehand. All the sample women took iron pills, more than a third took drugs to combat nausea, two out of five used indigestion mixtures, one in five laxatives, one in ten sleeping pills.*

IN SICKNESS OR IN HEALTH

How do pregnant women in fact think of pregnancy? Is it an illness or is it a normal condition?

KATE PRINCE:
A normal condition. Do some people think of it as an illness?

ANGELA KING:
Not as an illness. But it's not really normal either, is it?

LOUISE THOMPSON:
I think you should behave as you normally would. Women work out in the fields till they give birth. That's what I keep saying to myself. They give you all these things to do, and it seems so ridiculous when most women – probably 95 per cent of women – who have children don't bother.

JO INGRAM:
I don't think it's a *normal* condition – it's not something I'm going to go through for twenty years! Yes, it's normal, in that it's a thing a lot of people go through. It's certainly not an illness. But it's not my *normal* condition – my normal condition I hope is to be unpregnant!

LOIS MANSON:
I think I do think of it as something abnormal. I can't take it completely in my stride. I'm aware every minute of the day that there's something different about me.

NINA BRADY:
Well, my sister treats it as normal. She says it's not an illness. She says it's a natural thing. She was hanging up wallpaper, or doing something decorating her beautiful home I think it was, a night or two before her babies were born. She's very much like my mother – she's

very healthy and she just has her kids, no trouble, you know. I'm different altogether. I think you should rest and look after yourself. Maybe I'm wrong, I don't know. She thinks I take too much care of myself. I don't have to be told to sit down, dear!

JOSÉ BRYCE:
I did feel ill. I was saying to Nick, it *is* an illness – it's like a bloody disease – it's terrible. I don't believe all these stories that you're going to feel·great for nine months. I thought I must be mad: what did I want this for? I felt so bad and everyone – I suppose everyone is sort of pleased when you've waited quite a time to have a baby – aren't you thrilled? what a joyous occasion! – and all I felt was really absolutely lousy. I don't think you can make anyone understand. They say it's only pregnancy – it's such a normal thing, you're not ill – which you're not really, I suppose – but I felt so wretched, I didn't want to do anything: food made me feel ill: every smell made me feel nauseous. I kept saying never again – there'll only be one – I don't know how people can have *two* babies!

Illness symptoms, as José Bryce's remarks illustrate, are particularly likely in the first three to four months of pregnancy. But over the whole span of pregnancy, tiredness, nausea, sleep disturbance, constipation, indigestion and the irritation of frequent urination are the experience of the majority of women. Reminding oneself of the normality and naturalness of pregnancy under these circumstances can be difficult. Other people – friends, relations, work-mates, husbands – can reinforce the idea of pregnancy as a special condition.

Some pregnancy symptoms	
Tiredness	93%
Vomiting/nausea	86%
Frequent urination	82%
Sleep disturbance	70%
Indigestion	63%
Constipation	52%

VERA ABBATT, canteen worker:
My husband's getting ridiculous. The people at work definitely are. At times I feel thankful for it, like when I'm ever so tired I think thank God they're being so gentle. Other times I think oh God I wish they'd treat me as though I'm human and not a bit of china in a china shop. I think you have mixed feelings really.

KATE PRINCE, journalist:
I suppose the men at work are more considerate. They do offer to carry things if they see you humping along the corridor with a tape recorder. It's a funny thing to say, but I think they're less interested in

you, or maybe it's you that becomes less interested in them. Now she's a bloody hen! They make jokes: they're interested, but . . . it's slightly different now. Do you know what I mean? The second they knew, this was: I didn't *look* any different. I got the feeling that before – there was no question of flirting, or anything stupid like that, but they'd talk to you a lot more, chat to you, generally be terribly charming and all the rest of it. And then the very day I said I was pregnant the men who, let's say had less of an interest in you before are still the same, will talk to you as much, for example the married men or the older men, perfectly natural; but the other ones, you begin to think how stupid that they can change just like that. They just must think, oh well, she's a write-off now. Which I find a bit annoying. Not that I want to flirt or anything. Slightly more reverent too. Some of them. That gets on my nerves, too.

ROSALIND KIMBER, social worker:
People even stop me in the street. It absolutely staggers me. Quite a few times I've walked down to the shops just about ten minutes away, people have stopped me in the street and asked me when my baby's due and things, and I've been so surprised because you just get used to English people not saying things. I haven't been so surprised at the shopkeepers, because they all chat, and I expect them to. But when total strangers have stopped me . . . and friends, or even vague friends, react in a funny way, in that people keep coming up and asking me if they can feel to see if the baby is moving. And people keep grabbing me and things – it's very odd. . . . Men, not women so much, but men seem to be totally fascinated. And people I really don't know well keep coming up and saying do you mind if I feel to see if your baby is moving or something like that?
I: How do you feel about that?
ROSALIND: Well, I suppose I'm a fairly reserved person as far as touching people goes, so I found it a bit odd at first. But now I don't mind. But I've noticed that people treat me as though I'm fragile . . . they don't quite understand how I feel in that, you know, when friends come they start off saying no, you mustn't move, put your feet up, sit down, as if I'm liable to break or something and then when I seem like my normal self, they forget about it. And then at the stage when I actually am feeling tired and worn out they've totally forgotten and they don't really realise what it is like. They tend to take a rather extreme view.

I: How does your husband treat you?

ROSALIND: Oh yes, well, he's a tremendous worrier and he always thinks I'm fragile anyway. And he keeps saying you ought to be resting, you ought to be doing this, you ought to be doing that. But he's so excited about it all, he's thrilled to bits.

I: Do you feel you *want* to be treated differently?

ROSALIND: No, except that I want more *loving*, kind of thing. I feel a great need for him to be there and for reassurance – not that I want to be treated as if I'm ill, but I just feel, you know, I just want him to be there all the time. To show that he cares and things . . . but I think that's probably quite natural. At least according to everybody else.

Jo Ingram, one of the two self-confessed feminists in the sample, was particularly sensitive to the connections between pregnancy and womanhood referred to by Kate Prince. Through her involvement in the women's movement, she had learnt that maternal feelings are part of the character attributed to women in our culture.

I: Have you noticed anybody treating you differently since you became pregnant?

JO INGRAM [25 weeks pregnant]: Yes, absolutely. Everybody – virtually everybody. Even feminists who haven't got kids tend to expect me to get softer; I mean they've always known me as someone who's been indifferent to children, but they *seem* to be a bit shocked when I carry on making the same harsh and indifferent comments. They expect me to somehow suddenly get soft about children. And they seem to expect me to talk more about it; they're always very surprised that I carry on exactly as normal. As far as men are concerned they see me as a pregnant mother – not me: it's a different role. I find that very disturbing actually. Because it threatens my image of me.

[35 weeks pregnant] I think my friends have become less interested because it goes on for such a long time that the novelty wears off. I don't know whether this should go on the tape. But I said something to somebody about the possibility of killing the kid – trying to suffocate it or something if it was born deformed. Did you see that programme? [A BBC television play about a woman who killed her mongol baby shortly after birth] It was bloody good. That's how I've always felt. I've always thought Steve would do it, but then after seeing that film I realised it would have to be me if anybody because I'd have a better chance of getting away with it. So I mentioned that to somebody and she was absolutely horrified: she was in the women's movement and you'd think she'd know better. She said – she thought about it for a bit – she said, I'm sorry, I'm trying to put you into some sort of maternal role. Maternal instincts and everything. That's what shocked her – the fact that I seemed so completely hard about it. I'm not.

THE BATTLE OF THE BULGE

During the middle months of pregnancy the private fact becomes more public as it becomes more visible. At the same time a woman's idea of pregnancy changes. Instead of having to tell herself that pregnancy is the reason for a particular symptom, she knows she has a baby inside her. The baby's movements can be felt and seen.

What did it feel like when the baby first started to move about inside you?

PAULINE DIGGORY:
I thought it was indigestion. It felt like food resting – nothing to do with wind because it doesn't hurt, but it just suddenly *falls*. And of course it kept on – it wasn't painful at all: it was very nice in a sense. It kept getting more and more and I kept thinking it was to do with the digestive system. And then I said maybe it's moving and people began to agree with me, and so I began to think it was. And once I began to think it was it was silly to think it was anything else.

ALISON MOUNTJOY:
A fish swimming – or a very large tadpole. But the funny thing was I could *see* it as well. I remember saying to Luke one night that would be it and I hadn't felt it move then but in hindsight that's what it was.

LOUISE THOMPSON:
I can't explain it. Like going on a roller coaster.

DAWN O'HARA:
I'll never forget it: it was great because I was waiting for it to happen. People said to me: oh you should have felt something moving – and I asked that lady with the blondey hair at the hospital and she said the baby's moving but it's not strong enough for you to feel it. And then one afternoon I was doing some shopping and I thought it was my handbag that was giving me a belt, you see. And then I was sitting down that night and my husband was sitting beside me and I felt this

thump. And I gave him a dig – I said don't hit me like that! I was getting a great kick!

MARY ROSEN:
I was very pleased. I was really thrilled. I remember lying in bed one afternoon having a sleep and I felt something move in my stomach and I rushed out – I came in here to my husband and I said I'm sure I felt it move! He said *rubbish*, you can't *possibly* have done. That was about eighteen weeks, and it *was*, now that I look back. It was almost like indigestion, but slightly different. I didn't feel it for about ten days after that, of course!

Despite descriptions offered by friends, doctors or books of advice for pregnant women, it is sometimes hard to identify what is, after all, an entirely novel sensation.

MAUREEN PATERSON:
It started just like fluttering and then I felt it again and then I said to me Mum and then she said oh that's probably what it was. And then after that I felt it moving about quite a lot. One morning Henry woke up and he said the baby's awake, and I thought crumbs, what is he talking about? He must be dreaming. But he must have felt the baby move. It was weird, really!

VERA ABBATT:
It frightened me to death. I was watching television I think – I was lying down there and all of a sudden I felt this little butterfly, and then it came again. I couldn't think what the hell it was. I was frightened to say anything to my mother-in-law [Vera and her husband are staying with his widowed mother] in case she laughed at me – in case it was something trivial. And it went for weeks and weeks before I told anybody. Eventually I felt it really thump one day and I thought oh my God, it's either coming or it's kicking, one of the two. I'll have to ask somebody. I mentioned it to her and she said that's what it was – the baby moving. But it shook me up at first. . . . I really didn't know whether it was the baby moving or something wrong with me. I didn't know what to expect.

The early gentle flicks against the abdominal wall become gigantic kicks and somersaults and tangible changes of position. Knees and elbows, feet and hands appear and disappear: a fascinating panorama. How a woman feels about having a baby inside her depends of course partly on experiences that have little directly to do with the pregnancy: attitudes to being a woman, ideas about herself as a person, feelings about her body, current life circumstances – the work that has to be done, the social and economic circumstances in which she lives. But, given the belief that prevails in our culture about the necessity of child-bearing to feminine fulfilment, 'do you enjoy being pregnant?' seems a reasonable question to ask.

NINA BRADY, shop assistant:
It feels horrible – not a bit nice. I'm going to say that very loud and clear. Because I heard so much about people being pregnant and feeling alright: *it's not a bit nice.* It's very feminine and all that – it makes you feel good when people get up on the bus to let you sit down, but I was never for that – I'd rather stand up than sit down. I'd rather be at my work anyday than be pregnant – I'm all for women's lib: I like to go out to work and have my own money and be independent – I always have done. No, I don't think it's a very nice experience. If you want children you have to go through it – through the nine months – but it's not a nice experience. I wouldn't mind having two or three babies if I didn't have to go through pregnancy.

JANE TARRANT, librarian:
I don't hate it, or anything. I thought I would really love it. But I think in fact it irks me, the restrictions. And the thought of being pregnant again – I don't really relish it, especially not with a little child running around as well. I think that will be quite awful. But perhaps the second pregnancy isn't so bad. Everybody tells me that I have no problems, and I think, if you feel a bit tired and elephantish and you have no problems, what the heck is it like if you're not well?

ROSALIND KIMBER, social worker:
I was thinking that to myself the other day: I do enjoy it, don't I? Most of the time, no, but every now and again I suddenly think well, yes I do. But most of the time no, not really, because I don't enjoy . . . being irritable, being weepy, being clumsy is the wrong word, just cumbersome. I'm normally an active person, and I don't like not being able to do things. And because I'm off food a bit I can't plan proper meals. I just don't feel like eating . . . so no, I don't enjoy that side of it. Though obviously there's a strange sense of fulfilment in that I don't feel as bored as I thought I would do and obviously physically nature is doing something to me to make me feel much more contented. Some days I feel terribly contented and placid, which is a novel sensation, which is really quite pleasant. I like that: and also obviously when I

think of the baby, but I can't really say that I like that until I know that the baby is alright. Because one always has this worry that it's not going to be alright or that it's going to die . . . so I don't let myself think too much about the baby. . . . But I think once I know the baby's alright and then I look back I will look back on it as having been quite an enjoyable time.

PREGNANT PAUSE

Enjoyable or not, at the time or in retrospect, what does being pregnant feel like? Women pick out the nice things – the feeling of being an empire of one's own, the sight of little limbs under one's skin, the imaginary world of the baby to come, and the price that has to be paid – the clumsiness, the physical and sexual incapacity, greasy hair, endless inquiries.

What does it feel like, being eight months pregnant?

ELIZABETH FARRELL, publisher's assistant:
Buoyant. Well sort of fulfilled – awful word. I really do feel that. As me. And amazingly self-sufficient. It's almost as though I don't need anybody. Getting larger and larger doesn't seem to worry me at all. It could do. Things like when I get undressed Robert looks at me and shakes his head. He roared with laughter at this bra which flaps open. I mean if I was in the frame of mind where I was going to get depressed I can understand those things would make me get depressed. But *nothing* could make me depressed at the moment.

HILARY JACKSON, catering manager:
Clumsy. I think, God, if they could only find another way of doing it. It's very *degrading*. That's about the only thing. I think you're so ugly, so clumsy. I mean getting in and out of the bath is an embarrassment in itself.
I: How does your husband feel?
HILARY: He just laughs at me the whole time. He just thinks it's one huge joke. Unfortunately we have a polaroid camera which takes instant pictures: if I could lose the film on the way to the shop, I would.

LOUISE THOMPSON, law student:
I told Oliver I felt like a dried up potato chip. I just can't wait to have this baby.

GILLIAN HARTLEY, illustrator:
I think the nicest thing is being aware of its presence. You see bits of feet or elbows: that's marvellous; life inside you. Yes, it's fun. I'm less bulky than I thought I would be – I'm much more mobile. I can still touch the floor. It's been much more attractive than I thought it would be – I find the shape pleasing. I'm not upset about my shape and Max likes it very much. It's really been very frustrating in a sense because I think sexually it turns him on: he likes it, and of course my libido keeps going absolutely down. I think that's the worst part because you just feel that sex is quite a trial because you can't get comfortable. So you can't relax, so it's not as good as it should be. . . . And I feel guilty about it because after all _his_ hormones haven't changed!

ANNE BLOOMFIELD, barmaid:
Horrible. I don't like it. I don't like being pregnant. I just don't like it. Because I'm vain, I suppose. I have a lot of trouble with my figure anyway. Everybody says, not, how are you? – well, they say, how are you? but they mean: how's the baby? Everybody is really nice, but I just don't like being pregnant. I'm just one of those girls – I just want to blinking have it over and done with because it's uncomfortable. You can't wear nice clothes, you have to wear tent clothes, and you can't fling yourself about; if you go to a party or something you tend to stand still or sit down or something because you can't dance. I just don't like it. I'm not maternal at all. What about the other women you've been talking to: are they the same as me?

SANDY WRIGHT, secretary:
I honestly don't feel much different. I don't know whether it's because I'm not enormous. I know I'm bigger obviously but I think I expected to be like this [gestures] and hobbling around: I'm quite relieved I'm not. The only reason I get aware of it is because people are asking me all the time. You meet someone in the street: how are you? How much longer have you got? As if it's some _sentence_.

RACHEL SHARPE, copywriter:
Well, I'm glad that it's not like bread – that it needs a second rising! I certainly wouldn't like to go through it again. It just feels very

uncomfortable and awkward.

VERA ABBATT, canteen worker:
Heavy and tiresome. I don't really feel any different. I think: I'm going to be a mother shortly. I suppose that makes me feel different in a way. I think seriously about things I used to laugh at before – like me and a house: trying to get a house.

PAULINE DIGGORY, market researcher:
I have to hold onto the mantelpiece when I get up: I feel like an old woman. . . . And I can't do things – I can't *run*: I bounce up and down. The thing I've got over that I was feeling about two weeks ago was the idea that people don't look upon you as a pregnant woman: they just look upon you as a clumsy oaf. You just look clumsy and turn people off. It didn't *worry* me but I thought what a shame. I don't really think that idea exists – those lovely looks, that rubbish. The baby takes all my hair, all the goodness out of my face has gone, I think. My hair's greasy all the time. I have to wash it every two days – before I used to do it once a week.

ALISON MOUNTJOY, fashion designer:
Oh Christ! Large! Very difficult to put your mind to anything else. Like we went out last night and I was happy talking about anything pertaining to the bulge or babies in general, but my mind just wanders when the conversation goes onto anything else. It's most peculiar. And you feel: my God, it's so boring, I'm boring everybody else: I must shut up! It's terribly difficult not to think about babies and things pertaining to babies when you're trying to have a conversation about something else and you get a kick. I mean if anybody kicks you it makes you lose your concentration, doesn't it? The fact that the kicking's going on inside doesn't really make that much difference.

The last weeks of pregnancy are a time for looking forward and for looking back. Thinking about the future is counting one's chickens before they are hatched; it is always, until one holds a live, normal, healthy baby in one's arms, wishful thinking. Contemplating motherhood is contemplating the unknown – the nappies can be bought and the bootees knitted, but one's reactions to the baby and to the new occupation of mother are not wholly predictable; the baby's personality is also a matter for conjecture. Yet imagining the future entails remembering the past, since the restrictions and responsibilities to come invite comparison with the free and carefree life behind one. These last weeks without a baby are also a time for summing up the pregnancy, a process that involves the images women had of pregnancy beforehand, culled from women's magazines, girlhood reading, old wives' tales, or the narratives of friends. More than a third of the sample women found pregnancy worse than they had expected; about half said it was better.

Feelings about pregnancy	
Better than expected	46%
Worse than expected	36%
Same/don't know	18%

Has the pregnancy been anything like you expected?

JUNE HATCHARD:
It's been easier I think.
I: Why did you think it would be worse?
JUNE: I think because you hear – like people keep saying: have you been sick? Have you had this and have you had that? And you think, crumbs, I haven't had anything. And I think sometimes it's all in the mind as well. It's because of what people say and the books say. I think it's like any illness, if you start thinking, if you read a medical book you get all the symptoms.

CATHERINE ANDREWS:
Yes, I think so. I haven't had as many problems as I expected – I've felt better than I thought I might. People kept saying oh I couldn't sleep, I've had terrible this and terrible that. I've had nothing really, apart from cramps and backache. . . . I thought there'd be more *minor* discomforts attached to it than I found.

ELIZABETH FARRELL:
Yes. Well it's been perfect really. Because I haven't been interfered with at all – you know, it hasn't *inhibited* me at all.

VERA ABBATT:
Yes and no really. Most things it's been like I expected it to be. I mean I expected the sickness: I expected the pains in my back: I expected it to drag, which it has done.

NINA BRADY:
No. What did I expect it to be like? I didn't expect to be so awkward. I'm very awkward. Fat and that. Very fat. I'm over twelve stone. You bump into everything. And he's afraid to turn at night for fear he'll hit me with an elbow or something. I didn't expect to be so tired. I thought I'd be able to work till about six weeks before but I couldn't.

JANE TARRANT:
I had no preconceptions except of being rather Madonna-like with a big bump in front and sailing around. No I hadn't thought about it that much. I suppose some of these things like the heartburn: that has been worse. I do find that pretty awful sometimes. If for a whole day you don't keep anything down – that's not very pleasant.

ALISON MOUNTJOY:
Not really, no. It's been I suppose totally different. It's been better in some ways and worse in others. It's something that I don't think you actually know about until you *are* pregnant. I mean it's something you *think* you know about before you're pregnant but when you actually *are* it's a completely different world.

CHAPTER 4

Journey into the Unknown

PATIENT: *Is it too early to ask you if I'll have an easy birth or a difficult one?*
DOCTOR: *You'll have an easy one – everyone has an easy one these days, we make sure they do.*[1]

I don't think you can visualise it or imagine it because . . . it's never happened before, and you can hear about it and read about it, but I don't think you can actually know *what it's like until it happens.* [Pregnant woman]

Having a first baby is a journey into the unknown in more senses than one. Apart from the birth, which is the central drama in the transition to motherhood, three changes have to be accomplished more or less simultaneously: giving up paid work; taking up a totally new occupation – that of mother; becoming a housewife. For a minority of women the break in paid-work career will be short, and the necessary adjustment to domesticity only temporary. But most women stay at home for several years. Some may not 'work' again for a long time.

Unlike other changes of occupation, this transformation of secretary or shop assistant into mother and housewife entails more than small changes in routine: different hours, different work place, different work-mates, more or less money. The language of capitalism – work (paid) versus housework (unpaid) – masks the actual labour of housework and child care. Cultural images of womanhood have the same effect, inflating the grimy floor and the soiled nappy to the status of personal obligations: an extension of feminine hygiene. But while domesticity may be a theme running through women's lives from birth to death, suddenly having no other occupation to call one's own may seriously injure a woman's self-concept, ideas she has cherished for a long while about herself as a person. The housewife–mother's working conditions may pose extra threats to contentment: isolation, monotony, fragmentation, twenty-four-hour-a-day responsibility, lack of money and, for some, poor housing as well. Such occupational hazards of being female may of course have no impact on some women; but in the mind, in anticipation, they hover as grey possibilities on the horizon. To 'work' or not to 'work' is much more than an argument about one versus two incomes; it involves ideas about the needs of babies and ideas about the legitimacy of one's own needs as a person.

THIS AWFUL DILEMMA

LOIS MANSON, 29, university, postgraduate training, research work for seven years:

12 weeks pregnant:

I: Do you plan to work after the baby's born?

LOIS: Well, this is the dilemma. I run a large department and in many ways I don't want to give up work and I'd like to go back full time. But I've got terrific problems as to what I would do with the child if I went back full time. I don't fancy the idea of a childminder and my parents don't live near enough to constantly look after it. It's a big problem. So I've come to an agreement to go back part time. But it's all a bit unsatisfactory – I don't really want to give up the job. . . . Before I became pregnant I didn't think that I'd want to go back to work. I didn't really think about it; I'd assumed that when I became pregnant I would leave and I'd be off for a couple of years – nice – and then I'd go back.

I: So what changed your mind?

LOIS: The actual realisation that I *was* pregnant, I suppose. The awful thought of having to give up the work – the fact that it's been very pleasant . . . and I just don't really want to leave. This awful dilemma. There are so many problems. It really is awful. I've been worrying about this ever since I thought there was a possibility that I might be pregnant; it's been uppermost in my mind.

34 weeks pregnant:

I: How did you feel about giving up work?

LOIS: Oh I didn't want to give up – I was very frustrated about it. And although it was in many ways pleasant to look forward to having all those months of free time, I really was quite frustrated about the whole thing. I wasn't very happy at all.

I: Was there anything in particular you missed?

LOIS: Just about everything, I suppose. I miss very much having something to stretch me in a way – to do at home – particularly at night when David comes home and works and I find I haven't got work to do, although I've been doing quite a lot of reading recently. And generally seeing people; and I always like working under pressure – I don't like the idea of having lots of time to do something in. I'd much rather have to rush around to do something, and there's suddenly no need to rush around; no pressure whatsoever. And I found that most disconcerting. And it's taken me a long while to get used to it. I mean now I can *relatively* happily lie in bed in the morning but it's taken me quite a few weeks not to feel unutterably guilty about doing so. I'm basically a lazy person and I need something to drag me out; I could I suppose get into an awful rut and be very lethargic. I really need to have things to do to keep me going.

I: How would you feel if you'd been giving up work for ten years?

LOIS: Well, the possibility wouldn't have existed. And if it *had* existed, after two to three days at home I'm sure I would have done something about it. I just can't *imagine* what women do if they're at home all day long – I mean if they've got children to look after I suppose it makes a difference. But I just *don't* understand – I'd be *terribly* frustrated. I mean I've been completely confirmed in everything I thought. You could sit at home and eat your way through a box of chocolates and turn the telly on: you could really become an absolute cabbage. I hadn't honestly thought of it as realistically before.

And I haven't thought about what it's going to be like having a baby to look after. Suddenly yesterday – Dave keeps on at me about having driving lessons for this test that's coming up – and I've been vaguely thinking I've got another ten or twelve weeks till I go back to work, and then yesterday it suddenly occurred to me for the first time that I can't possibly think in terms of ten to twelve weeks, because I'm going to have a baby for the last seven weeks of that. And I'm not going to be able to just ring up and say I want a driving lesson from ten till eleven. And really I was quite – I think I panicked for the first time in my pregnancy. It did really occur to me that I was going to have a responsibility towards something and that it was going to impinge upon my life. I think perhaps I hadn't really thought about that. And suddenly I thought well it's not just going to be a question of getting a nice baby-sitter for a whole evening – that's straightforward; there's no problem there. But it's going to be things like an odd hour or so that you would want. It's very natural now to do what I want, I'm completely my own master; and then I thought Christ, I won't be

able to do that: I'd better get on the phone straight away to book up
my driving lessons. And then I started thinking: what are all the other
things that I should be fitting in these next six weeks? Because it's the
last time in my life I'm going to have six weeks free. And I really do get
panicky about it, because I actually thought of it as a child in its own
right with demands that were going to make demands on my life. (*See
p. 245 for Lois's thoughts on work after the birth.*)

SOPHY FISHER, 29, a television producer for seven years:
The classic story is that I met somebody – Matthew introduced me to
a director he was working with and he didn't take me in, he said how
do you do and made a little small talk, and obviously didn't take much
interest. Then Matthew had to go away and we were rather
unfortunately left together. And he obviously with an enormous effort
sort of turned to me and said you're a physiotherapist aren't you? And
I said no, no I work in television. And he said who are you – what's
your professional name? And I said Sophy Bates, and he knew of me –
it's a very small world – and his whole attitude changed, his whole
face changed. And suddenly I was a person and somebody it might be
interesting to talk to. That was awful and I don't like him for it but it
was an absolute indication of how I was not of any interest if I was
Matthew's wife. . . . It was very alarming. . . . I've always said that I
want to go on working when I have children: it's very important to
me.

*Decisions about combining paid work with motherhood are liable to be complex
ones. Kate Prince, a journalist on the full-time staff of a business magazine for
seven years, is bothered by the thought of financial dependence on her husband:*
I like to feel I'm contributing – we're both contributing fifty–fifty
and when I give up work it'll be the loss of a pretty large salary, and
we'll only have his money to rely on, and we won't be able to live to the
standard to which we're accustomed. If I feel at all – and I'm liable to
feel very neurotic about this – that there's anything I don't like about
it, I shall struggle to go out to work. I can't bear feeling financially
dependent.
I: Are you planning to work after the baby's born?
KATE: Well, not straight away. Well I can't; the blooming difficulty is
that I don't want a childminder, I want obviously some time with the
baby on my own just to get to know the baby and enjoy the whole
thing of it, but I can't see myself – I'm 27 and I've worked up till now.
. . . I've always liked to go out to work. I like chatting away and I

always find whatever job I'm doing is quite interesting, no matter for how short or long periods – so I need that stimulation. I want the money, and so I know that however much I enjoy the baby, it's going to come to an end, and I'm going to start getting bored I think. Unless I find that the old domesticity really thrills me, which I doubt, because even those university holidays when I had that university job, after about four weeks, there was only a certain amount you could do around the house. Okay, I could get into patchwork and preserving and all that, but I know all the time I'd be thinking God, I could be doing something a bit more worthwhile than this. And so I'd like to go back to work *when I choose*. But there are no facilities at all that are satisfactory. Either you have some childminder, and most don't seem to be awfully good: there are no facilities for young babies – okay toddlers, and that, but I don't see how I can get out of it. Unless I say, that's it, have another baby more or less straight away – get it all over with, have just a year or eighteen months difference between them and just face up to the fact that I'm going to have to spend five years at home.

It's alright if you've got your Mum down the road, I suppose. I think it's a very difficult problem. I wish something could be done about it . . . I don't know what I'm going to do. It's diabolical, it's terrible that you should have this thing forced upon you where you've got to take this huge cut in income and all the things that go with it – and be housebound if you don't want to be. You probably resent the child and God knows what else. I try to be realistic about it. I also don't want to be in this position that my Mum was in – she was determined to go out to work and she put up with all this business of carting three kids on the bus, and she had somebody that she knew, an old girl, down the road . . . she wore herself out running around with the three of us trying to get to work and all that. There must be an easier way than forcing yourself to go to work. I mean what do these mothers do that have *got* to work?

It should be something that you shouldn't have to fret about. Have you got children? How do *you* cope? . . . I was saying to Mark, he works in a nice calm office, just a few people there, it's a small firm and they've got a big room, and I was sort of thinking when the baby's got beyond the breastfeeding stage and just needs a bottle, could he not . . . ? He says I don't mind. I'm *determined* to get over it somehow. . . . I was saying to Mark, if it gets to the stage where I feel I want the money, I'm not going to just be *imprisoned* . . .

But who will *look after the baby? This conflict, at the heart of women's situation today, may be given a passing thought before pregnancy, but the moment when a woman is about to become a mother is the moment when the conflict becomes real and personal: it's not just women out there who can't find good child care, it's me. The dilemma is not faced by professional women only; Nina Brady has been a shop assistant for ten years:*

20 weeks pregnant:
I: Are you going to work after the baby's born?
NINA: No he [husband] wouldn't stand for that. He thinks when you have a baby your place is with them, and my sister reckons the same thing.*
I: What do *you* feel?
NINA: Well, I don't know. I love going to work, because if I go to work I can earn good money, and I was in one job for five years and the reason I left was that they closed down. I like to meet friends at work, it's very boring at home, that's why I think when I have the baby it'll be very boring here. . . . I cannot picture myself being a mother, dear, I just can't. That's what I'm scared of. I can't picture myself looking after a baby. I can picture myself going out to work, but I can't picture myself looking after a baby.

I've never missed a day's work in my life since I started work. I've talked to him about it, I've talked to my sister about it; I said to my sister I'm going to work, I'm going to put it in a babyminder. I told him as well. I get into tantrums – fits of temper. Some things annoy me, and I say well I'm pregnant and as soon as I have it, it's going to be put into a babyminder and I'll go to work because I love work. He doesn't agree with that; my sister, she doesn't agree with it. She says, well, then, why did you get pregnant? Well, I'd like the experience of being pregnant and having a baby and then putting it onto somebody else and going out to work – that's the way I feel.
I: So what do you think you'll do?
NINA: I'll look after it, I'll stay at home and look after it. I know I wouldn't be allowed to do what I want to and rather than argue and fight – because we don't argue and fight . . .
35 weeks pregnant:
I gave up the first job because of my legs. And the second job because

---

* *Nina has a large family of brothers and sisters (ten in all). Three of her sisters are married with thirteen children between them and the one who lives in London is a particularly important influence on Nina's attitude to motherhood.*

of the heat. There was a week there in August that was very hot. I collapsed: I had to give it up. I was weak. When I gave up I was pleased because I used to perspire an awful lot and I used to feel faint. I get very tired when I wash out a few cups – I get killed out. . . . . I spend most of the time in bed.

I: How do you feel about not working now?

NINA: I feel bad when he has to give me my housekeeping money on Friday. And if I need any money I've got to ask him for it. I've never done that. I had my own money, plenty of it, and lots of clothes and that was it: I had everything. And now I've got to bow down, you know what I mean? I paid £22 for that ring, it's not all that posh, it's just a birthday ring for him, and I had to change what do you call those vouchers for the baby? [maternity allowance] I couldn't very well ask him for money for his birthday could I? He'll give me plenty of money, he's good like that, but I don't like being dependent.

I: What about afterwards?

NINA: Well, I would like to go back to work but in my family none of the girls work. They just don't work. They're not allowed to go out to work. They've got good husbands; they don't *have* to go to work. My sister's got plenty of work to do with four children. I think with one child I'd like to go out to work. I've always been very fond of work – I've always liked work. I'll go out at night anyway – waitress work, up the West End somewhere. He would mind it. He doesn't want me to. I keep threatening. I would like to do it.

Believing, or making oneself believe, that giving up work in exchange for full-time motherhood is the only right thing to do requires an appeal to the psychology of babyhood. Mothers must not go out to work because it is wrong to leave one's child to be reared by someone else – the child will suffer some kind of psychological damage.[2] Or the mother will: for both the necessity of motherhood to women and the necessity of mothers to babies are themes of our cultural attitude to family life.

JANE TARRANT, librarian:

I would say I'll stay at home for three to four years. And then something part time. I wouldn't like to leave the baby with anybody unless it was someone very special.

I: Why?

JANE: I don't know – perhaps I'll change my mind. I feel that it's my responsibility, that's all. I think that leaving a baby at a nursery group when they're old enough to leave their mother – I think that's fine. I think it's good for a mother to have a rest from her baby for a bit. I don't believe in always being with a baby, but I think if you're a mother you ought to look after your baby for the first bit, otherwise perhaps you shouldn't have bothered to have one.

I: Do you think that babies need their mothers?

JANE: Well, I've read quite a lot on this, Bowlby and people. It doesn't really matter they say, as long as it's a mother figure, but I think that young babies are best with the same person all the time – they get to know a person, don't they?

JANETTE WATSON, machinist:

They need their mothers to get to know them. Some mothers, they go to work a couple of months after it's born, don't they? I shouldn't think they can get to know the baby and the baby get to know them if they're never there at all. That's what I want: I want to be with it.

NANCY CARTER, clerk:

Well I think the whole point of having a child – I mean I can't understand these women, they all say I'm dying to have a baby, and then they get pregnant and they have their baby and then they park it with their mother and then they go back off out working again. I mean I can't see the point; you're missing out on it, the most important thing is that the child when it's between one and five, I think it needs you there. And not only then, but when it's older. From my own experience when I was a child I wouldn't go out to work, unless it was really necessary financially.

Giving up outside work and staying at home are one side of the coin; the other side is constant housework.

SARAH MOORE, civil servant:

15 weeks pregnant:

I don't think we realise just how much we do in one day. I'm up at seven o'clock in the morning and, you know, you do so much between when you get up at seven and when you get home at six that being at home all day and just washing the nappies and cooking the meal and hoovering through and maybe doing the windows or whatever seems so much less than what you're *normally* doing. *Almost as though I'm wasting time.*

34 weeks pregnant:

I: Have you adjusted to being at home now?

SARAH: No, I don't think so. I hate housework. I can clean the house from top to bottom in two days, and then I think that's lovely now, I won't have to do it for another six weeks, because that's what I did when I was at work. But then I realise that dust does collect *occasionally* and people do spend *hours and hours* over it . . . I mean I did wash my curtains downstairs which haven't been done for four years and the water looked like a cross between coffee and cocoa. . . .

TANYA KEMP, medical receptionist:
I: Is this the first time that you've been at home all the time since you were married?
TANYA: Yes.
I: Do you like it?
TANYA: No, definitely not.
I: Why is that?
TANYA: Well I don't see anybody. You feel so useless, whereas at work you have always got people depending on you all the time. Decisions to make. But now I'm hoovering, dusting, doing all the housework – which doesn't take very long. I feel lost.

REHEARSING MOTHERHOOD

The baby is the reason why this dilemma of 'work' versus domesticity must be faced. Images of the baby are compounded of past experience and future hopes; a sort of amalgam of what was and what might be, with a spice of ideas about how families ought *to be thrown in for good measure.*

Most women have little contact with babies before they have their own. Three-quarters have held a newborn baby for a few moments, less than a quarter have ever babysat, even fewer feel they 'know a lot' about babies.

Previous contact with babies	
Held a newborn baby	79%
Seen a baby breastfeeding	71%
Changed a nappy and/or bottlefed	23%
'Know a lot' about babies	18%

How much do you think you know about looking after babies?

JANETTE WATSON:
I don't know a lot really.

JO INGRAM:
Absolutely nothing.

JULIET MORLEY:
I get cold feet occasionally, but plenty of less competent people seem to manage it.

NINA BRADY:
I don't know much, dear, about looking after a baby. I'm scared that I won't be able to look after it properly. But my sister tells me that it comes naturally to you.

BARBARA HOOD:
Enough, I think. I can change nappies and things like that. But learning the language of the child – that's the problem. I wouldn't know what was wrong if it was crying because you don't know do you, you can't tell?

SASHA MORRIS:
Absolutely nothing. It's all very well to read about it, but to put it into practice! I worry about the practical things because it *is* a frightening thing – I've never looked after a baby before. And it's in my hands isn't it, to look after it?

ANGELA KING:
I'm very confident. . . . I looked after my sister when she was a baby – I was ten or eleven when she was born. I looked after her a lot. My Mum went back to work. I enjoyed it: I did it because I wanted to. I don't worry about looking after it – I don't know whether that's good or bad. I mean obviously I'll feel a bit frightened when I first have it about handling it, but I feel confident that it will come to me to *be* confident with the baby.

MAUREEN PATERSON:
I went to this class at the hospital and one woman asked, she said I was wondering – I don't know what size clothes for the baby to get; the sister said, well we do most things at this hospital, but we can't really knock out uniform-sized babies!

I mean your own commonsense will tell you surely just to get the smallest – and even that probably will be too big really. . . . But I suppose if you've not had any dealings with babies – I suppose some people haven't . . . I mean my sister's had three, and I've got friends with babies. . . . My sister had her second one at home and I stayed there and I was there when it was born. You see when they were little I used to go down and stay with her in the school holidays and I used to take them out and feed them and things like that. I mean I can't say that I remember *everything*, but I think it does get you used to handling them.

Have you ever seen anyone breastfeeding a baby?

VERONICA PRATT:
No, I haven't. John has.
JOHN: My auntie – I was fourteen – I was just round there. I was surprised: she just done it in front of me.
VERONICA: He just walked in the door and she did it.
JOHN: She had no embarrassment or nothing. She just [pause] had it out and that was it. I come home and told my mother and she said don't let it worry you: it's just one of those things.

CLARE DAWSON:
Yes, my friend. She did it so naturally. I was talking to her about feeding and I turned round and the next moment she was just doing it. My husband was there and her husband and she did it so naturally that we all just accepted it.

CHRISTINA LYNCH:
Only in a magazine.

GRACE BOWER:
Yes. One of my friends actually. I was a bit embarrassed at the beginning but she didn't mind, so I thought I won't. My husband said I hope she doesn't do it in front of me.

Have you ever held a newborn baby?

My niece, she was about four days old. I was frightened, she was so tiny, like a little *doll*, really sweet, I was frightened I'd break her. (*Janette Watson*)

I held my sister's. A bit like a *doll* really. Nice sort of feeling. (*Maureen Paterson*)

Mothers have no professional training for their role despite the enormous responsibilities they carry. Adoptive mothers may be carefully scrutinised for their mothering abilities, and nannies and children's nurses are professionally trained, yet women who simply give birth to babies may not know one end of a baby from the other. But since society relies on women to maintain the birth-rate, it does

provide some informal education: doll play, a feminine activity par excellence, is
most women's only apprenticeship for child-rearing.

I had a doll, well she was nearly as tall as me, Sally, and I always
used to dress her in pink in a little bonnet and jacket and boots and
everything, and I used to dress her and undress her every night before
I went to bed. (*Polly Field*)

I had a doll which Mum gave to me when Anna was born and
everything Mum did I did to the doll. Even the christening; when
Anna was christened so was my doll Susan. It was super really; I can
remember it now. There's a picture of me standing there with her –
my baby's in a shawl and Mum's baby's in a shawl. . . . (*Clare Dawson*)

Women must always have a maternal instinct because when you're
a kid you play with dolls, put them to bed, and all this sort of thing. I
think your maternal instinct starts the first time you see a doll. (*Vera
Abbatt*)

*Growing up involves replacing doll play with baby care. The transition from
pregnancy to motherhood itself entails further sophistication in images of
Mother-and-Baby. The baby-inside, nurtured by the unconscious labour of one's
body, becomes instead baby-outside, independent person requiring voluntary love
and care. At the same time, a woman who is pregnant becomes A Mother in a
society where being a mother has special associations. To what extent do women,
when pregnant, see themselves as mothers? Is the baby inside felt to be potentially
a person with a separate existence, and what is it that women look forward to
about having a baby to look after?*

Do you think of yourself as a mother?

No I don't, no. I haven't really thought in terms of – I'm going to be
a mother. (*Kate Prince*)

I could never picture myself as it before but I'm thinking of it now
all the time. (*Dawn O'Hara*)

I suppose half and half, yes. I can imagine myself as such. It doesn't
feel strange really. (*Janet Streeter*)

No, it does seem a bit funny – when people say – like when I went to
the hospital – it had a little thing about urine bottles: '*mothers* please
take one of these bottles'. (*Deborah Smyth*)

*Do you think about the baby as a separate person, or do you think about it as part
of you?*

KATE PRINCE:
Well, it depends what I'm doing. If I'm sewing something for it, it's a tiny baby. But really it's very difficult because it's still something in your imagination, isn't it? It's something you conjure up.

ALISON MOUNTJOY:
Yes I do now. It's quite a shock when you suddenly realise it's not just a kicking little thing inside you – it's going to be a kicking little thing outside you quite soon. That's quite terrifying.

JANET STREETER:
Isn't that difficult? I think: I can't really envisage it as a baby. Do you know what I mean? I'm really looking forward to it now and I look at other people's babies but I still can't really envisage mine. It's still 'it'; it's a thing, rather than a person.

POLLY FIELD:
I've got a couple of sort of – they're like continental quilt-type sleeping bag things, and they've got sort of hoods which you pull the string in and it comes round, have you seen those? My Mum bought one and I bought the other. And when I was getting the case ready, I sort of got one of these and I was looking at myself in the mirror trying to imagine a baby in it. I put the teddy bear inside it; if anybody could see me, they'd think I was quite loopy, I'm sure.

Is there anything you're particularly looking forward to about having a baby to look after?

Cuddling it. (*Deirdre James*)
I'm looking forward to seeing what it looks like. (*Nina Brady*)
Seeing Barry's face I think. (*Anne Bloomfield*)
He said to me when it's born I'll be dressing it up in all different clothes – he says that's what I'll be doing. (*Janette Watson*)
I picture myself going home to Kevin's Nan and his mother and showing the baby to my mother and everything, you know! (*Dawn O'Hara*)

And what about the first moment of motherhood – that sentimental transaction between deliverer and delivered, as the newborn child is first placed in its mother's aching arms?

How do you think you will feel when you first hold the baby?

Fine. Great. (*Deborah Smyth*)

Who can tell? I think I shall probably be *thrilled*. (*Kate Prince*)

I don't know. I suppose it does depend on how tired you are. I don't say that I'll feel this incredible ecstasy that one hears so much about: maybe I will – it would be nice if I did. But I do expect to feel maternal. (*Alison Mountjoy*)

I don't know but I bet it'll be lovely. All gooey-gooey. (*Pauline Diggory*)

Oh I shall be terribly emotional about it, I'm sure. I shall fit straight into that category of typical reactions. (*Lois Manson*)

I just don't have a clue. I think I will probably expect to feel moderately bewildered. I don't think that at that point I will feel an awful lot. (*Janet Streeter*)

Proud, I should imagine. Tell it off for causing all this trouble! (*Nina Brady*)

I think I'll just be relieved it's all over and done with. . . . That's probably the first thing I'll think of, myself. Getting my figure back. (*Anne Bloomfield*)

I'll be over the moon I expect. (*Janette Watson*)

Oh, I can't *wait*. I get really excited when I think of that. I could nearly cry sometimes when I think of that, you know. (*Dawn O'Hara*)

These anticipated emotions must be measured against reality: see pp. 115–17 for how the women actually felt.

BIRTH IMAGES

In order to achieve a correct attitude to labour it is necessary to educate the woman herself and also those nearest and dearest to her. The converse is likewise true; the interfering female imbecile who insists on recounting, and who seems to take a great delight in retelling, numerous and invariably false or horrifying stories of her own and her friends' experiences in childbirth can do immense damage in a few seconds.[3]

Extract from an antenatal class on labour:

Now, I'll start off with just trying to explain a little bit to you about the actual labour. . . . Now this is a view of the pelvis, and what I want to show you is what happens during labour; down here you can see it's very narrow, and during labour this baby in fact manages to squash itself through that very narrow bit and out through the vagina. . . . Now this slide actually shows a contraction. Now when we look at a contraction, it's rather like a tube of toothpaste. If.you can imagine a tube of toothpaste and you're squeezing the top down; eventually if you didn't take the top off, the cap off, well where would all the toothpaste go?

Now here you can see hopefully one of the things that happens in labour: here you've got the cervix, and it's like a tube, it's quite a. thin little structure, and here you can see it's opening all the time. It's rather like putting on a polonecked jumper, if you can imagine that the poloneck part of the jumper is being pulled over the baby's head all the time. So the uterus is forcing the baby down all the time onto the cervix, and after that it will push the baby through – the baby is being squashed right out by powerful contractions. . . . They start off coming about every twenty minutes usually, but they vary from patient to patient. . . . The great thing about contractions in labour is that you can actually set your clock by them . . . they'll come regularly, they'll come with increasing . . . [long pause] . . . force. . . .[4]

Professional values discredit the colourful imagery of so-called old wives' tales and mistrust the messages of personal anecdotes about labour; the hospital's concern is to 'educate' pregnant women towards medical definitions of childbirth. The hospital attended by the sample women offered a series of four antenatal talks, designed to cover pregnancy, labour and feeding and to familiarise patients with the hospital layout (see p. 278). Women's reactions to antenatal classes are of course partly a function of how much they already knew, and the image of childbirth they had beforehand.

PAT JENKINS, 24, shop assistant:
I went to see a film they showed us at the clinic. I like looking at things like that – it never bothers me, but I nearly passed out. I had to go out. . . . It just put me right off. It really frightened me. The midwife came out after me, and I just burst out crying, and I told her I was really frightened, you know. So she said if you feel that, does your husband want to be with you, and I said yes, and she said, well if you feel that bad you should have the epidural, because I wasn't going to have it, but I think now I probably will. . . . It was seeing the baby coming out, you know, and then – well probably when I'm having it I won't see all that – but she just got the afterbirth, she was really pushing, and then the midwife just got the cord and was pulling it out and then everything seemed to come in on me and I just had to walk out . . . you

know, I could actually feel it, as if you were actually in the bed yourself. I had this feeling in my stomach, you know.

Dawn O'Hara, a packer in a factory, is 21. She came over from Limerick the year before her baby was born, and lives in one room with her husband, who works as a plasterer. She attended local authority classes.

I didn't even know there were such classes. Until I went up and they were really interesting. But when you're doing the actual exercises, you say to yourself well how can they help me when the time comes? But they do, don't they? She's very nice – they're both very nice. There's the midwife, and there's this lady we do the exercises with. And then we have a cup of tea. And we go in and she just asks us have we got any problems? And each week she tells us something different. Last week it was the birth of the baby.

They showed us – it was just slides – they showed us how long it would take and what would happen when you went into hospital. They wash you and what they do to you and how long you'd be waiting. I had a completely different idea – you know what I mean – I just thought I'd go into hospital, I'd probably have pains for a few hours, but I didn't think they – I just thought it would all be over when I got into the delivery room. I didn't understand the stages and everything. I just discovered last week that there were so many different stages. The whole lot anyway is about eighteen hours? The birth of the baby could be about three hours couldn't it? She told us that . . . I didn't even *know* these things. . . . If people don't go to these classes, how do they know what to do? So I know a bit more now.

I: Do you feel you know how to tell when you're in labour?

DAWN: Well I know what to expect, you know. First you might have a show, or else your waters might break, or else you start getting pains in your back. And if you start getting pains in your back there's no need to rush to the hospital; if you get a show there's no need to rush to the hospital, but if your waters break, go straight to the hospital. Because I was thinking about this all the time – what would happen if I was at work or downtown, or at the butcher's, and all of a sudden all this water comes over everything? What would I do? I asked her, does it really happen? And she said, it can! Blimey, I'd die!

But somebody told me that it's terrible to have your waters broken. You know what I really hate about it? I hate the thought of going in – now that I know more – I hate the thought of going in and having a bath and their having to shave you! I didn't know. I didn't know all this was going to happen. I'm stupid, I didn't think. I just thought of going to hospital and having the baby; I didn't think of going in, having a bath, and then having them shave you, and then every few minutes there's somebody going to come over to see how far the baby's down. I really and truly all along thought that I'd get these pains, right, and I'd probably have these terrible pains for about eighteen hours, and then all of a sudden the baby's head would be born. That's the way I had it in my mind the whole time. But it's not! You have pains through the first stage of labour and then the baby's head is on its way, and then the baby's head has to come out. I really didn't know. And then they tell you that the doctor's going to be coming over and they don't want to look at your head, just your bottom. What will I do? I didn't know; I didn't know these things at all!

I'm afraid that I won't just have a normal delivery. Being cut: well most people are cut aren't they? That's normal isn't it? I was asking the midwife about having to be cut – because that's the thing I can't bear the thought of, being cut. She showed us this slide of how far they would cut and when they would cut and sometimes they give an injection, sometimes they don't. Then when I saw the stitches afterwards I'm saying oh God because I think you can feel it, but I know I won't even think of that then, will I? She told us that. I was thinking, could I ask them – well I probably will be cut – to put in stitches that dissolve? The midwife said sometimes they do and sometimes they don't. Did you ever get stitched? You don't mind me asking you that now do you? Because I'd like to know. Is it terrible? . . .

I: Do you think these classes have made you worry?

DAWN: No, because I have no one here really, right? I mean if I was at home I could be asking my mother this. And I would be asking my sister and everyone. Whereas the people here – she's had no children. she didn't have any children, and they're all elderly. And Kevin, he was as innocent as me we'll say, so I had no one to learn it from.

But learning is not the only function of such classes.

JO INGRAM, a further education teacher:
The labour class was absolutely disgusting. I think a doctor should give that talk actually. No, I don't think a doctor should give it; I just think the midwives should be trained to be truthful. All you get is

these ridiculous slides . . . the two pictures they hold onto the longest are daddy holding the kid and mummy holding the kid. Completely useless. I just think that they're a lot of liars. I didn't learn anything at all.

A nurse gave this slide show and she talked and she bristled at my questions and that really pissed me off – the first couple of questions she patronised and then she could see that I wasn't going to sit down, I was being awkward, and she didn't like me. In a way I feel sorry for her because you're put into this ridiculous position. She's only trying to do her job. I raised quite extensive problems about things like epidurals and other things. I asked if the episiotomy was routine and she said it is virtually routine – that they do it 'if it's necessary'. That's the central phrase they use, isn't it? It really annoyed me because she said you needn't worry about it, you won't feel it and it'll be alright afterwards. It's completely contrary to what I heard that it's fucking uncomfortable afterwards. . . . In the feeding talk you're told you'll be very uncomfortable and you're told all the things you can do to relieve the episiotomy before you start breastfeeding!

On epidurals, she started off practically by saying I dare say you've all heard about epidurals, about being paralysed and everything, but I can assure you that it doesn't happen. You can't trust a fucking thing they say, because you know it's just not true. I knew from the beginning that being paralysed was a possibility. I think it's silly that they don't give you the information. Somebody else raised induction. They explained that they didn't unless it's necessary! [laughs] I just thought I'm not going to worry about that, because I'm not going to go in until I'm in labour anyway. This hormone thing – not inducing but speeding up – I was more worried about that. She told me I'd have a stand-up fight with the doctor over the hormones because I don't want them. She said this thing about a glucose drip. I said is it necessary to have a glucose drip? Can't I have barley sugar or glucose tablets? She said no, because we don't want you to be sucking anything because it'll give you more acid on your stomach or something. So I said okay, so you're going to put the hormone stuff in with the glucose? If you think I should be speeded up. She said that's right. I said can I refuse it? She said well yes you can refuse [laughs] but I think you'll have a stand-up fight with the doctor. I said I'm not going to be in any fit state to argue – who's going to argue for me? She said you shouldn't worry about it; it probably won't be necessary. I said that's not the point.

How to have the baby is a secondary consideration; the first is having the baby. When women think about childbirth they are thinking about what childbirth means to them. In their minds it is an idea of fulfilment as a woman, a prop to a failing marriage, a substitute for promotion at work, an experience not to be missed. Birth is also a distillation of what other births have been.

FELICITY CHAMBERS:
I was fourteen when my mother was pregnant and I saw everything that was happening to her, so I sort of knew what would happen to me. I was with her right up until she had the baby; I was with her even when she was in labour . . . she told me a lot of the things that happen because we were very close, and it sort of helped when she was so good in labour and that. It took all the fears off me because she just sat there, well she was lying in the end, she was so calm, and she hardly even moved or made a sound or anything . . . just talking, and then she told me, you'll have to leave now . . . and she said oh you'd better call the sister. So I went out and sister went in and she came out about ten to fifteen minutes later and said I had a brother; I didn't even realise she was so close.

But this is a rare experience. Most women have a less intimate knowledge of birth: they have seen a birth, or selected parts of it, on television, or discussed it in a general way with a friend or relative.

Knowledge of birth before pregnancy	
Seen birth on film	70%
Discussed birth with someone	55%

SHARON WARRINGTON:
I went up to see my friend – the baby was born at half past four in the afternoon and we went up just after half five and I never – her face always sticks in my mind, the state of her, you know. She – oh I thought she was dead, you know, she was grey and no one had combed her hair and where she had sweated it was all knotted. . . .

TANYA KEMP:
I was talking yesterday to my sister-in-law. She said it was just natural, nothing to worry about. Because she has three children and she said when she was having her first one people were telling her all sorts of things, and she said don't listen to them.

DEBORAH SMYTH:
My sister said something about it the other day. She said it was horrible – she kept going on about it. She said I won't have another

one until I've really forgotten what it's like. She said they had to cut you and sew you up. . . . She said they said to her when she was having the baby oh we'll cut you now. She said she saw them coming over with the knife . . .

But mothers are the major resource of birth stories, both good and bad.

NINA BRADY:
My mother had eleven; she nearly had me in a drill of potatoes. She was digging the potatoes – that's very manual work, you know; in Ireland a woman has to do that – used to, not now. And she was digging potatoes and she felt all wet down one of her legs – that was the water breaking. She had her little case packed, my mother always had her little case packed, which a lot of women in Ireland didn't, they were very backward. She used to take her little case and run down the lane about half a mile and thumb a lift from anything that was going along the road to take her to hospital; it was 22 miles away.

JANETTE WATSON:
I spoke to her about it the other day. She told me not to worry. She told me not to listen to anybody that's only had one baby because she had seven and she lost two – one set of twins after she had us. I came out bottom first, I was the second twin, I was the heaviest. My brother was 2½lbs and I was 5lbs and I was underneath him. They didn't know I was in there. He came out and my Mum didn't have any more pain you see so it was difficult for me to be born, so the doctor had to press down on her stomach. The midwife – she knew there was another one in there. There was two midwives and two doctors – there was about twelve people all lining up in the passage – the blood unit, the flying squad, everybody. They were just worried in case anything happened because we was premature; we went to the hospital because my brother just fitted in the palm of my Mum's hand – he was that tiny.
　　She's been through a lot and she just told me not to listen to anybody if they say they'd rather not have a baby. A lot of people have said that – they try and put you off. They say they were in pain. Some people say they were in shocking pain, but they just forgot it and they can't remember what it was like. . . . My Mum said she was in pain a lot but after you've had a baby and you know you've got your baby and you haven't got to go through the pain again she said you just forget it.

Gillian Hartley's mother lives abroad:
She always said before – she gave us a little propaganda: she was always fairly positive about it. I think she really did have easy births. . . . The only pregnancy I remember is that of my second sister. She got nauseous feeding the dog but other than that she really looked great. I've seen pictures of her when she was pregnant with me and my sisters and she really looked marvellous. She must have enjoyed her pregnancies tremendously.

I: What did she say when you told her you were pregnant?

GILLIAN: She was great – absolutely fantastic. She said how good her pregnancies had all been. And she wrote to me, she said I had you, it was four hours and it was a joy. The second one was even shorter and the third one she didn't get to the hospital in time. She had an easy time; she said you'll probably be the same. It gave me a lot of reassurance.

It is easier to listen to mothers than not to listen.

KATE PRINCE:
I'm not going to listen to my mother or my mother-in-law because they do go on. In the nicest possible way. They just describe how awful it was for them. . . . Everyone immediately launches into their own experiences of the various pregnancies they've been through. The first thing my mother-in-law told me was that she was in labour for thirty-six hours with her first one and that they left her in this room with the door locked and every time she called out nobody came, and she rang the bell for the nurse and the bell didn't work so she was just left there lying on the floor and she just wanted to die . . .

My mother said oh it was terrible; I had such a rotten time, of course it was because I've got a contracted pelvis: that was the trouble. I didn't listen. They rather *enjoy* telling you about it. I said to Mum, I said the amazing thing is when you ring me up or anyone rings me up the first thing they say is how are you? They want to hear how you are, and you open your mouth to answer and they say of course when I was pregnant . . . and they completely forget and you just sit there with the phone and they go on and on. God knows what we'll be like when we're 40 or 50. I'm determined that if I have a daughter, when she's pregnant, I'll just shut up about it.

Out of these anecdotes an image of birth crystallises: pleasant or unpleasant, dignified or degrading, intensely painful or merely slightly uncomfortable. The

way in which sexuality was learned about and acted out, a woman's awareness of
body sensations, her encounters with doctors and hospitals and medical technology
– these also contribute to her anticipation of childbirth. Running through the
scenario in her mind's eye the film may be frozen at several points: the shaving of
pubic hair, the episiotomy, the legs in stirrups, the stitches, a deformed baby. All
the sample women had some anxiety about birth, though the degree of this anxiety
and its focus varied.

SHARON WARRINGTON:

I went through a stage, not so long ago, about babies being born dead
and babies being born without arms and legs and that and I spoke to
my Mum about it and she said it was natural and that everyone thinks
about it, and then when I see the baby on the ultrasound and I saw his
arms and legs and it has got them all, that is all I think about, not the
actual birth.

MANDY GREEN:

If I can carry it through the way *I* want to carry it through I think I
would look forward to it. But if I'm told what I'm to do and told no,
you can't do this . . . I'm afraid I might panic because I would feel I
can't control the situation.

CLARE DAWSON:

I think one of the things that worries me is how much it's going to
hurt, and how you react to the way it hurts. I think that worries me a
bit – that you might make a fool of yourself. I think I'm a bit worried
about how I'll react to it. I think that *really* worries me actually.

NINA BRADY:

I: Do you have any particular worries or anxieties about the birth?
NINA: The delivery. A lot of people gets cut and has stitches don't
they? I'm awful scared of that. I know its bad: they tell you it's
nothing but you won't tell me it's nothing because anybody that has
to be cut is *bound* to be sore. I like to know the truth but they won't tell
you the truth. I was brought up on a farm back home and I was
thinking a woman is very much like a cow; she has her baby the same
as a cow has her little calf. And you should see the care we used to take
with the poor cow when she was about to have it and her water burst
and all this. She used to be so ill; and that big calf coming out of that
small little place. It was cruel . . . I can't understand how the baby can
come out at all. But she explained to us today that it opens up, it's
flexible, the uterus? It opens up, it's like that [demonstrates]. But I

still can't understand how it's big enough for a seven pound baby. Another thing I didn't know, and I was amazed. And that is that a baby doesn't come out of where you pass your water. Is that right?

JULIET MORLEY:
I suppose there are a couple of things which still worry me a bit. The first one is having a shave and the enema which I find extremely distasteful. And the other thing is this business about being cut and stitched which I don't particularly fancy. In fact I dreamt about it one night. In the dream I was sort of sitting on this chair giving birth [laughs] and the baby sort of got stuck in the perineum so to speak and the doctor came along and cut it and it came out so quickly that I had to catch it but it didn't hurt at all. Is that wishful thinking?

VERA ABBATT:
The pain . . . I think the idea of going into the unknown. I don't know what I've let myself in for – or I don't know what my husband's let me in for – whichever way you like to put it.

ANNE BLOOMFIELD:
I'm getting a bit scared of when my waters break. I'm not scared of having it – I'm scared of whether I know when it's happening. But I'm sure I will because of the pains and that. I'm scared the waters will break when I'm walking down the High Street or something like that. Well you hear these things. A friend of mine, hers broke in a taxi and she said – well I mean it's like when you pull a cork out isn't it?

LOIS MANSON:
Not fears about the actual *childbirth* but fears about what people *do* in hospitals. . . . And I'm worried that my pelvis isn't going to be large enough and I'm worried that the cord's going to strangle it. I *am* worried, no doubt about it, that I'm going to give birth to a baby that's dead or abnormal or something. That *is* something that worries me . . . I suppose inasmuch as the pregnancy's lasted that much longer now I feel that it would be – I mean it's the whole thing, it's not just the idea of a dead baby which is horrific. It's the idea of the nine months that you've been through and what have you and I suppose the further through one's pregnancy one gets the more attached one becomes . . . I'm sure it's a *normal* fear.

KATE PRINCE:
Everybody who's had a baby says afterwards I'm not going through

that again. . . . I wish I'd known about so-and-so and all that. But when you go in you say, well, you take over, to them don't you? Everything is vulnerable about you – physically and everything. . . . I'm trying to establish what sort of *feeling* it is, not out of morbid curiosity or anything but so I'm *prepared*. Everybody's pain threshold must be different, but is it like – people said – my sister blithely said it's no worse than, it's like a bad toothache or something like that, and other people have said it's like a physical sort of *effort* pain. . . . I can understand that kind of pain, it's not a lingering sort of pain like a cut, say, I mean once you've made the actual effort, it's over and done with.

But what about this swearing business? Why in the old days did people scream? You'd never scream with a bad period pain or a big shit, would you?

Imagining the pain of childbirth is an impossible feat. Penetrating the easy assurances of antenatal educators and doctors, women may suspect that childbirth hurts, but the closest analogy that is offered is that of bad period pains. These images are best approached retrospectively – by asking after the experience of birth about the gap between expectations and reality. The same is true of the information shown in the tables, which should be compared with that given in chapter 5 (p. 86, p. 105).

Ideas about birth	
Birth will be:	
Pleasant	29%
Unpleasant	30%
Inbetween/neither	41%

Pain relief planned	
None	20%
Entonox and/or pethidine	21%
Epidural	29%
Don't know but *not* epidural	20%
Other don't know	11%

LADIES-IN-WAITING

I feel disoriented most of the time in that I don't really feel that I'm living any kind of a life at the moment. Because I can't visualise the future at all, I've given up my job and I'm not sort of committed to anything else. I mean you can't be committed to a baby that's not here yet, so I feel I'm living in a kind of limbo from day to day. (*Rosalind Kimber*)

*In the 'kind of limbo' that marks the last weeks of pregnancy, one sign of the
approaching drama is below the surface and cannot be reached or measured
through questions and answers. The unconscious mind produces scenes of horror
and disaster only some of which seem to be about the impending birth.*

ELIZABETH FARRELL:
This particular one was about my father. I love my father very much
but I was horrible to him, and in this he was going blind very slowly
and he hadn't said anything about it to anybody. And he came home
from work one night and put the car in the garage. It was Christmas,
and there was a Christmas tree and we were having a party. And he lit
a match and on this Christmas tree there was a butterfly; he lit a
match and he put it right up to the butterfly, obviously to see what it
was, because he couldn't see it. And I saw him doing this and I
shrieked at him. It was at a party with several people there, and I
think Mummy had half realised what was happening – that he was
losing his sight. But I had no inkling at all. And after that I think he
went out for a walk and shot himself. . . .

KATE PRINCE:
I keep dreaming, by the way. The last two or three nights. Two nights
in a row. The first dream – I know I'd been to relaxation classes for the
first time on Friday, and the district nurse had this doll thing made of
chamois leather, with a doll's head – plasticy stuff. And it was
supposed to be the actual size of a foetus. And she had a sort of plastic
pelvis, and she said now this is how it happens: when the head
engages it goes down – she was thrilled with this doll, which she'd just
taken delivery of [laughs]. And she said it goes just like that, and it
turns its shoulders and all that. And I dreamt I had my baby, a proper
baby, a girl, a daughter, but it was delivered just like that – while I
was, I don't know, I was in a pub or something and there was a whole
load of people there and it was a funny little thing, and it grew very
very quickly, and it was sort of smiling and all dressed up in no time –
within five minutes.

There was that – that was the Friday night – and the following
night, the Saturday night, I had another dream. I've got two sisters
and we were all pregnant at the same time – my elder sister was
pregnant, and my other sister had just had her baby but it was three to
four weeks premature and it was delivered in a supermarket. You
know these polystyrene trays you get meat in, with sort of cling film
over the top? It was in one of those and it was a tiny little thing and it

was face down and it was only that long [gestures] with a tiny little bottom and everything and there it was: the hospital or someone had wrapped it in this cling film. My baby was due on a certain day and it just went on and on and it never got born, you know. My Mum said oh for God's sake what's happening? And I said well it was due, everybody's had theirs except I haven't had mine. And she said oh dear, that's very bad. And I never actually had the baby. . . .

CHAPTER 5

The Agony and the Ecstasy

I thought it was so bad, I thought if it was a question of having the baby or stopping the pain I would stop the pain. . . . No wonder women died in the Middle Ages. . . .

It was just amazing. It was like a miracle. It could be a religious experience. Now I know it's superior to be a woman.

How can the experience of childbirth be described? Does it defeat words? Or is it twisted by being trapped within words so that an event powerfully experienced is reduced to a technical account, a recitation of medical manoeuvres? Some people find it easier than others to put their feelings into words. Questions provoke answers, but the answers may be only clues, signposts. Statistics sketch another kind of partial picture; to know how many women had what kind of pain relief during labour is not to know how much pain was relieved; to be told how many babies were tugged or persuaded into the world with forceps, is not really to know much more than that.

Certain themes run through the accounts of birth gathered in this research; the problem of recognition – is *this labour,* is *this a contraction; the clash of* expectations *and* reality – *now I know how it feels, I know how I expected it to feel; the question of* control – *am I doing this myself, or are other people doing it to me? How to recognise symptoms of impending birth and how to square these with the images collected from mothers, antenatal classes, television programmes, Victorian novels and so forth – these are the classic dilemmas of women having a first baby. But the issue of who controls birth is part of childbirth today in a more general sense. In entering hospital to give birth a woman becomes part of that great and growing debate about who is having the baby: the mother, the medical profession, the hospital, the family, the state.[1] In the role of patient a mother is vulnerable, but she is vulnerable twice over, for she has not only her own interests to defend but her baby's. Hospitals are made up of rules and set procedures; certain things must be done in certain ways at certain times and in certain places. One does not have a baby in the admissions hall, an epidural in the lavatory, a baby without prior removal of pubic hair. This proper way to give birth may seem improper, but as a patient it is not the reasoning behind the rule that matters, only the existence of the rule itself. How to defeat the depersonalisation that results – the feeling of being a cipher, of being one amongst many machines mechanically programmed to produce a baby, like a cup of coffee or a pop song – this becomes a massive, and often unreachable goal.*

These statistical statements about the sample women set the birth accounts that follow in their technological context:

79 per cent of the women had epidurals* (with or without other analgesics)
20 per cent had other analgesics only
Only one woman had no analgesia at all

52 per cent of the women had forceps or ventouse deliveries*
98 per cent of women had episiotomies*

41 per cent of women had induction or acceleration of labour with syntocinon*
59 per cent of women had their membranes artificially ruptured
69 per cent of women said they did not feel in control of themselves or what was going on during the labour.

BIRTH PASSAGES

ALISON MOUNTJOY, 27, fashion designer. Labour accelerated, 16½ hours, epidural, forceps delivery:
I'd better tell you the whole story. Do you want to know the whole story? Right. The doctor had said at the hospital that if nothing happened I might as well come in after the weekend to be induced. Which was alright, because I thought by then I'll be two weeks late and I can't keep hanging onto it forever. But you know when you've finished at the clinic, and you have to see the nurse and get more iron pills? Well, this nurse and a woman doctor who was also sitting at the desk, when they heard that I was going to be induced – having the membranes broken – which I hadn't been nervous about previously, but the way those two went on – they were sort of half joking, saying ugh how uncomfortable it was, and I was getting a bit worried, I said well you are joking aren't you? Well, it's not *too* pleasant, you know!

---

* *These figures are representative of practice in this hospital in managing first birth.*

So you can imagine what I felt then. And of course it got worse as the days went on, as Tuesday approached and nothing happened, and then Tuesday morning I woke up with piles. Just the day I had to go into hospital. That just about *finished* me. I was *terrified* by then of being induced, *terrified* of going into hospital, *terrified* of just about everything, and with this bloody pain up my backside . . . I couldn't even get any toilet paper anywhere near my backside . . . I mean, why did they have to come the day I had to go into hospital?

I went into hospital in the afternoon, and I was *so* terrified: Luke stayed with me, he went home for supper and he came back and they let him stay. I asked the sister what it was going to be like, whether it was going to be as bad as everyone made out, and *she* didn't put my mind at rest at all. Yes well, it *is* a bit uncomfortable. You know when doctors say something's going to be a bit uncomfortable you know it's going to be bloody awful. Anyway, the doctor who was going to do it came to see me about ten o'clock at night and he could see I really was in a state by then, and he said, if you can relax it's nothing. So I said well how the hell can I relax? He said, well look, if you really are this worried, I can give you an injection and you'll just be nice and woozy – you won't *care* what we're doing to you. So I said well why didn't anybody tell me that before? So we arranged for me to have this injection at about six o'clock in the morning, because they wanted to do it [rupture the membranes] at about six thirty.

They came and gave it to me at six o'clock and I drifted off feeling absolutely wonderful . . . and while I was lying there feeling wonderful I started feeling these wonderful twinges starting and I thought no, no, nothing's happening – too good to be true. They couldn't take me up then, because the delivery rooms were so crowded, they'd had a busy night. So there I was starting off by myself: I felt so proud of myself, and I didn't tell anybody for about an hour. I can't *tell* you how pleased I was that I started off myself: I was *so* chuffed. And eventually I thought I'd better tell somebody because I had a show and everything started happening, and they came and timed the contractions and they said yes, you actually *are* in labour. And I was so pleased: that set the day off right!

So when they did take me upstairs, they didn't do anything. Until about twelve when they decided they wanted to monitor the baby which apparently they do *routinely* there. And the bag [membranes] hadn't broken by then so they had to do it – I said why, what for? But of course they didn't listen. By then these pains were coming quite fast and they were pretty painful. You're not allowed to call them pains, are you? They're contractions. It always made me laugh when I read that because I *knew* they bloody well hurt. Everybody kept asking me every ten minutes whether I was going to have an epidural. And I had been in such a state the night before that I was in no mood to be firm about anything. Also the breathing wasn't working – it's a load of old codswallop, that breathing. I mean it works when the pains aren't so bad that you can remember to do it, but once they get to a certain pitch it just doesn't work – well, it didn't with me. So when the tenth person asked me if I wanted an epidural, I said yes. They did it just after the membranes – that wasn't that bad, it's no worse than an ordinary internal.

The worst thing about the whole of the day, the only bad thing, was that at the same time they did the epidural they wanted to put me on a glucose drip. I wouldn't have the other – the drip that speeds it all up. They wanted to do that straight away when they broke the membranes, I don't know why, I suppose because they didn't want me to be in labour for very long, for their own convenience probably. But I said no: I'm doing alright, aren't I, I said: I'm having good strong contractions aren't I, so you're not going to do it, are you? I had one nurse to start with who was on my side. She talked two doctors out of putting me on the drip. She said this patient is *in* labour. She doesn't want to go on a drip and there's no need to, is there? I think because I'd gone into hospital to be induced they hadn't really worked themselves round to the idea that in fact, although I had been, in fact things were a bit different. I thought they would just take me up to the delivery room and let me get on with it. I couldn't understand *why* they wanted to put all these monitors in – and when they started talking about putting me on this drip to speed it up, I said what on earth for? Anyway they wanted to put me on a glucose drip and I felt I couldn't argue with that because they always do with an epidural for some reason. And *that* was painful. It took three goes to get it in because I've got narrow veins, so eventually Luke had to help her and that was the only time he nearly passed out.

If you count from when I started having contractions, which I suppose was seven o'clock in the morning, and I had her at eleven thirty at night – sixteen and a half hours. At four o'clock they did put me on the other drip. They said look, you're doing very well, but it doesn't seem to be progressing much, so do you mind if we do this? So I said no. Well as I had the drip in, I said you're not going to put another needle in are you? No, no, we just attach it to the same tube. Anyway I had so many tubes coming out of me by then – the two down there, the epidural, the drip – so it was the fifth thing altogether. You feel so strung up, you think, well what's one thing more?

It was what I *feared* was going to be the case. I think they have actually gone round the bend there. And I think that was why, knowing that hospital was so keen on sticking tubes into you and injections and all sorts of things, I think that was one of the reasons I had the epidural. Because to be honest, when I asked for the epidural, when I finally decided to have it, it wasn't *totally* the pain, it was also the fear of – they're so used to doing all these things to people who've had epidurals and who are completely numb – what's it going to be like when they start doing things to me forgetting maybe that I can actually *feel* everything? I was aware at the time that I asked for it that I felt I was coping . . . I was just scared. It wasn't just the pain. I didn't mind the contractions really. The pain of somebody doing something to you is worse. I had decided beforehand when I got so scared about being induced, I had more or less come to terms with the fact that I'd probably be asking for an epidural. I know my own emotional capabilities and it wasn't anything to do with the pain by then; I was just scared of what *they* would do to me and how much *they* would hurt. . . . I thought, I've had enough, I just don't want to feel it.

Having said that I definitely didn't want an epidural before going into hospital and then deciding eventually to have one to make life easier – for them as well as me – it was actually super; I mean I don't regret having had it, I mean having decided to have a baby at that hospital the best thing to do was to have done what I did . . . It's terribly unlikely that I'll have a baby there again, because we'll be moving out of London, so presumably I will be somewhere where they will have the attitude of encouraging you and helping you to get over the pain, instead of saying why put up with it, we can give you something for it. [And this in fact was what happened – her second child was born twenty months later without an epidural in a small country hospital.]

And I had a forceps delivery. That was a bit unfortunate because the last time they topped up the epidural was about nine o'clock in the evening, and about two minutes later they were due to do another internal, and they did it and all hell broke loose because they suddenly realised that I was completely dilated whereas before I'd been only about four centimetres, and they rushed off and got a doctor and it was this nice doctor that I'd liked who'd been on duty again by this time which was rather nice, so he also had a look and said, right, okay, start pushing! And the unfortunate thing was that this last top up left me *completely* numb from the waist down, whereas I'd been topped up about four times and each time it'd left me with *something*. But this time I really did have to look at the machine to know when I was having a contraction.

I was *very* disappointed that I couldn't feel to push. I was really *furious*, not with them – I was furious with *myself*, and I suppose it was a good thing that I had been to some classes because I did know *how* to push, but it was a question of getting it right – obviously if you can't feel your bottom, you can't feel it. Sometimes I knew I was doing it right; this little nurse was scratching the sheet to try to get me – there was only one nurse, actually the whole thing was so funny, because I had one nurse on one leg to push, but they were shortstaffed and of course I needed somebody on the other leg, so of course Luke had to come down off my shoulder and hold my leg. And it was so funny because at one point in the middle of a contraction when I was heaving and panting she said to him: oh look, you can see the baby's hair! And he said, well actually I'm not terribly sure what I'm supposed to be looking at! And I just burst out laughing, I just had fits, which I suppose is quite nice because it's not often that you can lie there in labour giggling.

But I suppose the most disappointing thing about the whole procedure was not being able to feel her slither out . . . I would *love* to have felt her slither out or whatever the feeling is that you do have when they come out. I really would have liked to have felt that. I was furious that they topped me up, I was never shouting to be topped up, they topped me up without even asking me: I said what are you doing? I don't need it, I don't want it. They just put it in: I mean you can't really move away. He let me push for an hour which is quite a long time for them because normally it's ten minutes and that's it. But maybe it was because the doctor, because he liked me as well, and I think maybe he was happy to let me go on for as long as he thought was safe. And eventually he said you just can't get the head round the corner. So he said you're going to push it out, but I'm just going to ease it at the same time – good psychology! I mean I don't know whether that's a typical forceps delivery. . . . It was one pull, one push, and out she came; she didn't have a mark on her. I suppose I can't tell until I've had another child and hopefully I won't have an epidural – I suppose you miss that feeling of pushing them out yourself. I could feel the pressure of the forceps and I could feel that he was doing something that did in fact hurt, even through the epidural I could feel that, and I could feel it stop, but I didn't know that she'd come out. And then suddenly everybody was saying oh you've got a little girl and all the rest of it, and I said I can't see it, I can't feel, where? And Luke had to pull me up and she was only half out and she was already crying and I was so relieved to see her: she was so obviously all in one piece and crying and . . . I just felt immense relief. She looked totally *right* when she came out: the right size, the right length. I held her all the time they were stitching me up. They just plonked her on my chest. It was totally amazing. Looking at her and thinking – well I suppose it was terribly difficult to believe that she'd come out of *me*. I sort of half thought that she must have come from under the table somewhere, because having *not* felt but seen the direction she was coming out of, I sort of wanted to go and look under the table to see what was going on under there. It felt very strange. I mean yes: it was *my* baby, and I loved her, but I think I was just so shattered by then that whatever I was feeling I couldn't feel much of. I mean I was totally aware that she was my baby and I loved her and I wanted to hold her but I felt so sick I couldn't react to *anything* by then. I could hardly believe that she'd come out of me.

SHARON WARRINGTON, 21, audiotypist. Labour 18½ hours, epidural: It was six o'clock on the twenty-third and I got backache, not a bad backache, but it was annoying. It went on all night and I woke up at four in the morning. It got worse, but not that bad; I didn't know, I'm not ignorant, but I just didn't know: I got up, and started pottering around, I didn't know what was going on really. My Mum said I don't want to frighten you, but I think you've started labour, and I laughed. She said, right: you wait and see. She said my face was so flushed. I didn't think I was in labour, I expected it to be painful. It was right at the bottom of my spine, as though someone had got their knuckles into it. My Mum got up and sat making tea and coffee and seven o'clock came and I felt tired, so I got back into bed about seven fifteen. I just moved in bed and as I moved I got a terrible thud in the back, and the waters broke. So up I jumped, ran from the bed into the kitchen, gets to the toilet, and finds what's happened. I told Mum what had happened and by this time my tummy had started to tighten and that. So I got washed and dressed and my Mum rang the hospital and said I was on my way. I said to Alan, would you get up, and he looked at me out of one eye and said why, what's wrong? He didn't know what I meant. So I said my waters have broke and the baby could come at any time, and he said you are joking, and I said I am not: he thought I was joking. And within five minutes we were off. He didn't even have a wash.

Got to the hospital and from the reception they took me up to the admission place. I was upset: I cried when I said goodbye to my Mum. I was alright going in the car, but once you are in that delivery room and you see all these things . . . I was thinking oh God, if when the baby is born it has to go on that machine or this has to be done . . . then I got a little bit scared. I got examined and then I went straight into the delivery room because I'd already started to dilate. Then the doctor came in and then the pain started really to come about lunchtime and I wanted that epidural so I had it done, and it didn't work. Alan went out for his lunch and he said what time did they think the baby was going to be born, so they said about four. Anyway up comes four and I am still there, so they gave me an epidural again, and it still didn't work, so I gave up. They examined me quite a few hours after I was admitted and I was still only about three and a half to four centimetres, and then they examined me about five, and it was seven centimetres, and then they examined me again about half nine and it was completely open. . . . When they examine you they write in the file and give a special stamp and I asked her what it was and she said I can't tell you. She said all I can tell you is that you are progressing. She said what is written in the file is strictly confidential.

He had this thing on his head [an electrode to record the baby's heart-rate]. I was worried in case it could harm him, and they don't ask your permission to do it which I think is all wrong. But when it came off – it took long enough to be put on, and it darn well hurt, because the girl who had done it hadn't before, and it took quite half an hour to get it properly in place; anyway, within half an hour of being put on it fell off, because you have got about four tubes going inside and they keep turning you from side to side and each time you turn you pull, you can't help it, and I said I don't want it again, because I said it might damage his head when he is born, and they said it doesn't harm him, they said if you look at this, this records his heart, this records your contractions. So, well, you can't really say no to them and yet they say that they only do it with your approval. But they don't ask.

He was the only baby born at Christmas. The only one, all Christmas Eve day and all Christmas Eve night, and all Christmas day and night. There was only me, and this other woman having a race. About half nine they said that I was ready to push, so the nurses and all that come in. I started pushing about nine forty five and he was born at twenty past ten, it was all over. I was propped up, but you've got your legs on the table and you have a foot on each nurse's shoulder, so you have to rick your neck to look down and you can't do it, because you are trying to breathe at the same time. Alan see it. When the actual birth came, they went and got him from the room and they brought everything in and got all ready and I started to push and push and push and his head sort of got stuck, it just wouldn't come out.

You feel like your whole bottom half is going to split, literally, you can feel this bulge and as they say the urge to push is terrible. They say don't push, don't push, and they tell you when to push. I always thought you could push when you wanted to push, but you don't: you have to wait for their command. They feel your tummy and your face is all crinkled up with agony and they say oh you've got a pain, you can push now, and you push and then you relax.

Anyway the sister who was on duty came in and said how was I doing sort of thing, and I didn't know what they was doing, but they got this big blue sterile pad and I knew she had something in her hand, because she kept her hand down there, but Alan could see, because she was on the same side as him and she said right push, push really hard. And as I pushed I hear snip, snip and Alan went white, and they cut me down and across like a hot cross bun, and then his head was born and another push about a minute later and he was completely out, and Alan was half way up the corridor, gone. It was a darn shame that he had to go, but if he hadn't have gone, he would have been out on the floor. He saw the head, it was about half out, and he said that all he could see was like the back of his head, and then he said they cut you and I said to him, how did you know, and he said, well I see didn't I? And the nurse ran after him and got him and he came straight back in again, and the baby was just lying in between my legs at the bottom of the bed. They wrapped him up and put him in his crib and Alan just went straight over to him. He didn't want to know me!

Now I am glad the epidural didn't work, at the time I wished it had done. I think I appreciate what I done, I am pleased with myself, that

I could do it. I think some people have that just for the sake of having it. Ninety per cent before their pains even start have it, and even a couple of days after I was so pleased to say I had it but it didn't work, that I took the full brunt of it, whereas these people who had had it said that they couldn't feel a thing. Well to me that isn't having a baby. What's the point? I said it was awful. But it's not awful really. What you suffer for an hour or two is all gone. What you suffered for the whole nine months and the last few hours is sheer hell really. But it is all worth it, once they give you the baby, it's absolutely marvellous.

I held him for a couple of minutes and they asked Alan if he wanted to hold him and he said no, and that upset me. Then not long after a nurse from the ward came up and took him down, and that was all I saw of him . . . I would have liked him exactly as he was born, for them to have cut the cord and given him to me. But they've held him first, that's the way I look at it. You are not the first. I think a mother should be the first one to hold it. A couple of days after we was talking about it in the ward and one of the women was saying that she didn't hold hers for about twenty minutes and they were mucking around with it and that, and I said I had him about five minutes after, so she said I don't think it is fair, I think you should have them raw sort of thing, just as they are, and I said yes. He was such a sweet little thing, he was wide awake with his eyes open looking at me, and looking at Alan, and although they can't see, he was staring all the time, he didn't blink once. They commented about that; he still does it now, he still stares.

I had thirty stitches, I had thirteen inside and all the rest were outside. It was about one o'clock before he came along, he was singing to me 'God rest ye merry gentlemen'. It was Christmas Eve. It was funny, as the contractions were getting bad they came in and they turned all the lights off and I thought what on earth are they doing? And they moved me and all these machines and everything into the door and I got this pain and I'll never forget it as long as I live. I was swearing under my breath and there was this whole mob of doctors and nurses singing 'Away in a manger' and I'll never forget that as long as I live. I cried my eyes out. I hadn't cried all the way through, I'd bitten my lip, but that really broke my heart.

LOUISE THOMPSON, 30, law student. Labour 4½ hours:
I tell you, I almost had her at home. That was the funniest thing. I had a show at six thirty in the evening, but the contractions came

every five minutes or so. I phoned the hospital and they said oh don't worry; it's your first child, it'll take twenty hours or something. Eat dinner, stay calm, and come in, you know, tomorrow morning. So I actually was cooking dinner – it was about seven – but they just got, they didn't hurt that much, they were just coming very often. And I said well you know, maybe I should pack my suitcase. But we'll stay calm: right? Oh and also we were moving that Monday so the flat was such a mess. Then at seven thirty I was starting bleeding, like a period, and I said I'd better phone the hospital. And they said, yes, you'd better come in. But if I hadn't started bleeding I surely would have had her at home. Because I got there at eight fifteen and then I had her at ten to eleven. When I came in, after they examined me, I was put into the labour room. I was five to six fingers dilated. But it didn't even hurt at all – not at all – until right before I was in the second stage of labour. I tell you, if I hadn't started bleeding I would have waited till the pains got really bad and it would have been half an hour. They got quite bad at the end of the first stage. I mean I didn't have any drugs or anything. It wasn't terrible.

When they said oh it's a girl, I said oh good, I am so happy! . . . I held her after a while. Actually she fed right away. Oliver said – let her feed, let her feed.

It was just amazing. It was like a miracle. It could be a religious experience. Now I *know* it's superior to be a woman.

PAULINE DIGGORY, 25, market researcher. Labour 12 hours, epidural, forceps delivery:
A few days before I had the baby we had friends round and we were talking about the epidural. And this friend said, you know it's ridiculous, in the Middle Ages it was excruciatingly painful to have a leg off, and it was excruciatingly painful to have a child. He said these days it's only excruciatingly painful to have a child: why should it be so? I said for the joy at the end. He said oh balls. Which is very true.

So I had this epidural and I felt guilty. I felt I should feel cowardly about it. But the amount of women who felt cowardly about it made me annoyed. There was this woman in the bed next to me and she was an intelligent woman and she said if you do the breathing exercises you can cope. I said well, why should I bloody have to cope? She was all for having it naturally. I think that's disgraceful, you know. I've really changed. This idea of these women saying if you learn to breathe you can cope . . . !

I had the epidural after the first hour. I came very fast you see. Wednesday night I started getting period pain type contractions very slow and they built up and they were coming very very fast but very irregularly. And then I had a show and Jeff said I'm not having you like this all night; this was about one o'clock. She said come in, stay the night, and we'll see what the doctor says at nine o'clock. Whether to send you back home again or . . . So Jeff went back home again which was good, because I wouldn't have slept, I would have kept him awake at home because I was just writhing all night, you see. That was the worst part really, all on my own. They asked me if I wanted sleeping pills and I said no I don't want anything – and they put me in this ward with three other women. And at seven o'clock in the morning when the new staff came on they decided to break my waters, the new sister did, and she said it was four centimetres, and they started to wheel me away to the labour room and I started every two minutes which I think was quite quick. Oh it was dreadful! And that awful gas! It made me sick! I tried it, but I knew I wouldn't like it . . . so I had the epidural, and it has to be topped up every hour, so at the end of the hour I was going come on, come on! I thought it was dreadful, I thought it was so bad, I thought if it was a question of having the baby or stopping the pain I would stop the pain. Honest to God! It just takes over your whole nervous system, doesn't it, really. I mean it's not like a *pain* pain, it's not like period type contractions. . . . I just said I think it's a disgrace, no other operation in the world does one have to go through so much pain! And they were going yes, but it's not so bad if you learn how to breathe – learn how to breathe! Can you imagine my Mum – eight, and a pair of twins! I think about that now. I look at women all differently now if I know they've had kids.

They do tend to make very casual conversation over you. Like when my epidural was due, this man came round with his students. That was the worst thing. Some doctor. What do you think of this one? He did talk to you as though you weren't there. And also his students seemed pretty dopey. He said shortly after lunch she should have it, and I said that's good: what time do you have your lunch? He was right – seven minutes past twelve.

You see, it wasn't very long – only four hours. I had a bath at seven and she broke my waters at half past seven. From eight o'clock till twelve I'd say the labour was, really.

They had to forceps her you know because their bloody machine broke down. They've got this ancient machine that's meant to monitor the heart. Well it took them half an hour to work it. And then they lost the heartbeat. And I'm sure, because all the way through my antenatal they'd all said how strong her heartbeat was, and I'm sure it was their machine rather than her. They lost it, she was virtually out, but they had to whip her out quick. They sent Jeff out – why did they send him out? They lost the heart and then they all started looking at each other and pretending it was alright. Well really, quite honestly, I didn't think anything was wrong. They started fiddling with the knobs, but they were always fiddling with the knobs – that machine's terrible. I had no confidence in it.

They said oh it's a little girl – like in the films. They gave her to me: I felt bewildered. She was looking at me – I was looking at her. She looked very bewildered herself really.

I wonder what would have happened if I'd stayed the night at home and hadn't gone in. I wish my waters broke like everyone else's seemed to. That would have been quicker than lying in bed all that night with that pain.

I thought it was very unpleasant. No wonder women died in the Middle Ages. I'd have an epidural again . . . I mean it *is* a disgrace you know! They wouldn't cut off your leg and say sorry we don't have any anaesthetic in this hospital: you'll have to put up with it. I mean they wouldn't, would they? I think women ought to be told that it's painful. I suppose if I recall all those films of women in labour – which I didn't at the time recall until it happened to me – holding onto the bedstead and all this sort of thing – I suppose if I'd recalled that . . . I don't think about it much now, it's fading a bit. But the first two weeks I did, definitely. I remember telling a girl in the shop who hasn't had a baby yet and who asked me. And I told her: I said it's very painful. And she was really shocked. And I thought well I'm sorry you're shocked but I wish somebody had told me if I'd asked them, because I said it really is painful, it's terrible in fact. No wonder women die in it. She went: my God, really? What kills you – the sheer pain?

VERA ABBATT, 28, canteen worker. Labour 16 hours, epidural, forceps delivery:
Well, it was a Sunday, we were just sitting here and I had pains in my stomach.
MOTHER-IN-LAW: She always laid about, didn't do anything, just laid about. But this Sunday morning, she was just the same. She kept laying about, didn't you? Frank said to her, don't you feel well? She

said I'm alright, I'm alright. He said shall I make up a bed for you over there? She did lay on a bed. This was the day time.

VERA: No, it was night time, six o'clock.

MOTHER-IN-LAW: This went on all day, this palaver with her. About seven she goes upstairs and she tells him she's had a show. He called me upstairs and when I saw their bed, straight away I said phone for the ambulance, it had been there all day.

VERA: I lost it during the night, and I didn't realise it. And yet I went up and I went to the toilet and I had a show then and I called Frank and I said – because his cousin was running us up – I said you'd better go and get Dave, I think we have a bit of a problem here. Anyway I was taken to hospital. But when we got up there we didn't have any problem – they took me right into the labour ward. Then they took me into another ward and they gave me two sleeping tablets. Because apparently they thought I was going to go on till next morning. And just as she gave me the tablets she said she was going to test the contractions, and as soon as she put her hand on my tummy she said oh never mind the tablets. By this time I'd taken them. She said get her down to the delivery room. So I was in there about eleven o'clock and he was born at half past four.

I mean I was all that time in labour, all day, and I didn't know anything about it. I felt pains in me stomach but it didn't dawn on me that's what it was. I thought it was wind actually. That's what it felt like to me. I thought I was full of wind. . . . It was about an hour after we got to the hospital it started to get really bad. And then they gave me the epidural for the birth. So I felt nothing during the birth at all. In fact I slept during most of the delivery. It was terrific.

I had a forceps delivery. He was stuck in the neck of the womb, he got stuck coming round the corner. They told me that. And of course as soon as they told me they were going to have to do a forceps delivery I was up in arms again: what's wrong with him? She said there's nothing wrong with him, he's just stuck. It was a bit degrading. But I didn't feel it so it didn't really make much difference. I was alright until they put my feet up in those slings that they use . . . it was a female doctor, which wasn't too bad.

I didn't even know he was out – he was crying his eyes out and I thought – there was another lady in the next room having a baby – and I thought it was hers. I didn't know he was out! She picked him up and said you've got a baby son! Oh God – is he mine? Where did he come from? I didn't really feel anything, I was so tired: I was glad it was over, that was it. I couldn't think of anything else.

JULIET MORLEY, 28, rebate officer. Labour 9½ hours:
I woke up at seven o'clock in the morning not feeling sure about it and
I had him at half past four in the afternoon. I wasn't even sure I was in
labour for the first four hours. I was awake at seven, and I had, you
know, a few twinges of backache, and I was expecting to get something every half an hour; it wasn't a textbook labour at all. If I'd gone
on what they told me I would have had him here, because I didn't
have any of the things they tell you to wait for. In the afternoon I rang
them because I was having sort of much stronger twinges round the
back, then I started having some that came round the front, so I rang
them up about twelve. No show – no waters breaking, and no
regularity: don't come in. I rang them at two – I'd just had a very little
bit of a show – oh don't come yet! I said I'm coming in . . . My
contractions had no regularity at all. I had one at the top of the stairs
and one at the bottom sort of thing, so I suppose they were about
every couple of minutes at the end. But none of this every half an hour
building up to every ten minutes . . . I mean labour was nothing like I
expected.

When I got there the sister came into the admissions room and I
was sort of leaning on the bed having a contraction, standing up, and
she put me down and had a look and said you're nearly fully dilated,
and got me whizzed along on a trolley at top speed. I've never known
anything happen so fast. They said I was too late for an epidural. And
virtually too late for pethidine. But I didn't want them anyway. I had
a bit of gas and air to help me over that stage when they were wanting
me to lie down . . . Standing up and leaning on the wall I was perfectly
alright. As long as I was *sitting* up I was alright. I sat up on the
delivery bed for the last few really strong ones and I was perfectly
alright. But when I had to lie down, that was useless – you couldn't
concentrate. I didn't feel much pain really: with back rubbing it was
quite alright.

About three thirty I just said I wanted to push and the pupil
midwife said right, carry on. It wasn't nearly as strong as I'd been led
to expect from all the books and from what people had told me. And
also the pushing was quite different from what I'd expected. It just felt
like passing an enormous motion – the pushing. I was expecting to
bear down from above. You know the Sheila Kitzinger book? [*The
Experience of Childbirth*, London: Gollancz, 1972.] Well that says it's

similar to the feeling you get during orgasm, that it's a sort of bearing down feeling similar to that. At the relaxation classes they tell you to push down from the top but the midwives tell you to push down into your bottom which is a very silly way of putting it. If they said what they meant you'd know what to do.

I had to have an episiotomy. I saw him waving this syringe around and I said what's that? Because they just do these things without telling you, you know. The pupil midwife I was quite happy with, she said I wouldn't have pethidine and I wouldn't have the epidural and she'd get me some gas and air in case I wanted it. So I wasn't worried about that. But I saw this syringe and I said what's that? And I'm sure they were just going to give me the local and the episiotomy without telling me. And he said what it was for and I said do I have to have it? And he said well, in case we have to cut you. And I said do you think you're going to have to? And he said yes. So I had it then. Because I've never had stitches or cuts or anything: I didn't know what it was going to be like. And then I heard the pupil say something that I didn't catch and then he said something – he said lengthen the episiotomy; it must have been something like the heart's going down which she said quietly, I think. Afterwards she said the baby's heart was going down and they had to get him out *very* quickly. And if they hadn't done that it would have had to have been forceps and I think it was because his head didn't engage and it had the extra distance to travel . . . and I think he must have just got tired because he's a big strong baby. I did feel it was rushed, I'd rather have done it without the episiotomy and I think I could have done if I'd had more time to think about it and relax.

I opened my eyes just in time to see the head come out. That looked just like the pictures in the books actually. When he was sort of lying there somehow he looked exactly like the baby in a book. It was funny. They said it's a boy. I hadn't looked actually; I was sort of looking at the whole baby rather than the sex. I hadn't noticed it was a boy until they said. I kept on about holding him, so I got him. I think they got the placenta out first and then I held him.

I felt – you know – just, I don't know – over the world. I couldn't believe it. It was a feeling of exhilaration, that's the best description I think. The baby himself didn't really enter into it. I wasn't thinking of him as an individual. I think it wasn't till I got him in the ward that I began to realise he wasn't just an extension of myself. I certainly didn't feel at all as I expected to feel. I wasn't prepared for him to be so strongly an individual. . . . Having carried him for nine months as part of yourself you don't expect – I mean it's almost as if he could have been *any* baby.

ELIZABETH FARRELL, 28, publisher's assistant. Labour 3 hours: It was unpleasant. I felt more pain than I've ever felt in my life before. I really know now that I was expecting it to be virtually painless; I think I was. And oh my goodness it wasn't.

Afterwards I thought about it a lot. I mean I remember thinking I wonder if I shall ever want another baby. I wrote it all down: here it is: 'It was like Richard or Edward II – I can't ever remember which it is – they wanted to kill him without it looking like murder, so they stuffed a red hot poker up his rectum and the screams could be heard all over Gloucestershire!'

It woke me up from a deep sleep – such a sudden, strong pain. Robert and I had just had an awful row, that was another thing; that was the only reason he stayed, I'm sure. I went to sleep in tears. We hadn't made it up and so when I woke up I had these great swollen eyes from crying. I woke up at 2 a.m. and she was here by five. I woke up with a stabbing pain as the waters broke and from then on the contractions were more or less continuous. I could hardly get dressed. In fact the way I woke up *shocked* me, I was suffering from shock after it and I didn't really know what to do in spite of all the preparation. So of course I mechanically thought I should have a bath. But I couldn't move. I was standing in a plastic bowl dribbling, so I woke Robert up and he said wake me up when it's all over, and I said no, you'll have to get up and put some newspaper on the floor from here to the bathroom. So he did that and I had a bath which was completely pointless, because I was still dribbling away. Got dressed and put on endless disposable nappies and sanitary towels and two pairs of knickers. And it came all the way through all these disposable nappies I had on to my dress. And Robert took me in and they examined me and I think it was two fingers dilated when they first examined me, and so they wheeled me straight into the delivery room.

My goodness, that was a struggle: when I said I don't want anything [i.e. no analgesia] the midwife, she got, well, not exasperated with me, but I could read what was going through her mind. She thought I was stupid. And I hate to inconvenience people and have them ill-disposed towards me so then I sort of said well maybe I'm being silly; then she was getting it [an injection of pethidine] ready and I said no, I don't think I will. I suppose that must have been a gap between contractions: I definitely decided *not*. And then I mean I didn't get a chance to get into the breathing rhythm at all. It seemed to be meaningless – I didn't have enough time to think myself into it. The contractions weren't, the build up wasn't *gentle* enough, they were just too sudden. I mean I've never had a baby before so I don't know whether they were exceptionally strong and violent contractions.

Time meant nothing. It could have been one hour or twenty-four hours, I don't know. And then there was that awful stage when they were telling me not to push and I couldn't. You can't prevent yourself. One minute they're telling you that your uterus is an involuntary muscle and the next minute they're telling you not to push. I don't know whether you push with your uterus, I don't suppose you do. To me if the uterus is pushing, it's nature working properly. I don't know *how* you can damage your cervix. I wonder whether that's not a fashion as well.

I couldn't help it; I couldn't *believe* how strong they were. And well they'd given me that enema thing and I hadn't been to the lavatory – I hadn't had a chance. And that was another thing I now realise – that was sort of coming out along with everything else, which must have been awful for everyone else. I didn't feel embarrassed at the time – I couldn't think of anything else except the contractions! And I do like to be helpful and co-operative and do what they say and it really distressed me at the time that I couldn't prevent myself from pushing.

And during the transition stage they put me on my side and at the breathing classes for the transition stage I was told to pant and sit up and so that flummoxed me – I couldn't do the rhythm. And they kept telling me to breathe deeply, and we'd been told to pant, in stage D. And so that was awry. And then when they said I could push they rolled me over onto my back and sat me up and I had no desire whatsoever to push then, and anyway we'd been told to push down at the front and they said push down towards your bottom as though you've got a large motion. So there was something wrong there. I felt like going back to the lady at the breathing classes and saying so because her reasoning was that if you pushed as though you'd got a giant turd to get rid of that closed up your vagina. We tried it and felt it and were convinced that it did close up your vagina. I didn't push very successfully I know because I was scared of splitting myself. I suppose that was another thing. And then they gave me a massive cut, it really was a huge cut, I'm certain. It goes all the way to my back passage and there's a little lump by my back passage . . . I do think they gave me much too big a cut, I mean I know she had a big head.

From the researcher's notes:

ELIZABETH: What's the time?
PUPIL MIDWIFE: I don't think you'll be long.
ROBERT TO ELIZABETH: Is it painful?
E: I can't describe it. . . . Can I have some water?
PMW: Can I listen to the baby, please?
E: How much longer till I can push?
PMW: I don't think you'll be very much longer now. Right, over on your back, let's see if I can see the baby's head.
E: No, no [she's in the middle of a contraction]. No, not yet . . . I'm sorry.
PMW: That's alright. You're doing very well.
E: Am I in the transition stage?
PMW: Yes, you are, that's why it's so difficult.
E TO R: I'd like you to stay, but if you don't feel you want to . . .
E TO PMW: Keep shouting at me, it helps me to remember what I'm supposed to be doing.
PMW: Are you hoping for a boy or a girl?
E: I don't mind.
PMW: Don't push.
E: You've no idea how hard it is, it just happens, I can't control it.
PMW: I just want to have a look, lift your leg up.
E: Am I making progress?
PMW: Yes, I think I'll get staff, I can just see a few strands of hair.
  [Elizabeth is propped up ready for pushing.]
PMW: There's going to be a time when I tell you not to push, just to pant, alright?
STAFF MIDWIFE TO R: Are you going to stay?
R: Yes, alright.
SMW: Can you sign this form please?
PMW: Now, push down towards your back passage.
E: At the classes, they said push down towards your stomach.
SMW: No, that's wrong, you want to push down into your back passage, as if you're constipated and you're dying to go to the loo.
E: But at the classes, they said that was wrong.
SMW: No, it's no good pushing into your stomach . . . you've got to

give some longer pushes, short ones are no good. . . . If you give us
some nice long pushes, it'll be out in half the time. . . . That's it, a nice
long push. Down to your bottom.

E: Is that right?

SMW: Yes, yes. Another deep breath . . . that was better.

E: I'm beginning to get the hang of it. Can you touch it yet? Is its head
on the outside?

SMW: Yes, it's got lots of dark hair. . . . No, put your bottom on the
bed, love. That's it, push. . . . We're just doing a little injection now,
alright?

E: Oh I want to push.

SMW: Okay, push, put your bottom on the bed.

E: Are you going to cut me?

PMW: We're going to have to give you a little cut – you shouldn't feel
it too much because we'll do it during a contraction and you've had an
injection. [Episiotomy done.] Now push, push. . . . Keep your pushing up now, nice and long – with the next contraction the head'll be
out.

E: Really?

SMW: Okay, stop pushing now. . . . Just a small push, a little one
again. . . . I'm just feeling for the cord, right there's no cord . . . there
we are: the baby's head is out.

E: What do I do?

SMW: Push down.

PMW: It's a little girl.

E: Gosh.

PMW: [looking at clock] Not bad: from two till five, just three hours
in labour.

E: It's long enough. [Watching PMW and SMW handling baby.]
What are you doing to my little girl? What are you doing to it? [Is
handed baby.]

E: Oh Robert she's *huge*. . . . Do you want to hold her?

R: No, I don't think so.

E: Oh Robert, I'm sorry you haven't got a son . . . [to PMW] You'd
better wash my bosom [undoes delivery gown, puts baby to breast,
baby very mucousy, won't suck].

PMW: Don't be disappointed, Mrs Farrell, if the baby doesn't suck –
she will later.

E TO BABY: Well, feel my skin anyway [holds baby very close, strokes
her cheek].

Birth is a trauma in every sense of the word. Physical lacerations ensue, but the mind and the emotions are wounded as well by the immensity of the physical sensations felt and by their meaning: another human being. 'Shock', a word used by Elizabeth Farrell, appears over and over again.

I was in a state of *shock* . . . time had stopped.

It is a state of *shock*. I was unaware – I mean I'd like to have another one, just to be aware of what's going on.

I woke up in the middle of the night and I couldn't believe that I'd actually delivered him. It was such a *shock*. . . .

He was so big . . . nine pounds six . . . I was absolutely *shocked* out of my mind.

I felt it was lovely holding her and everything but I didn't really feel anything . . . because I was *shocked*.

I felt depressed in hospital. It was partly *shock* really, and being away from home. . . .

Asking women to summarise their feelings about birth reduces these images to a standardised response. But it is useful to see how the individual fits into the general picture:

42 per cent of women said the birth was better than they expected.

47 per cent of women said the birth was worse than they expected.

49 per cent of women said they felt more pain than they expected.

34 per cent of women said they felt less pain than they expected.

Picking out the highlights and the moments of agony adds substance to this outline.

What were the best aspects of the labour and birth from your point of view? And the worst?

There weren't any best bits at all. It was just no fun. It was a right drag from start to finish: a smelly horrible experience in a smelly horrible room. (*Kate Prince*)

A nice feeling was him coming out. I took it that I'd passed the head and now it was the body twisting round. I thought: that's nice. The worst bit was all the time I was shivering and being sick. I was like jelly all the time. And me husband come in: he said what's the matter, try and relax – I couldn't, couldn't keep calm. I put it down really to me being nervous. (*Michelle Craig*)

The best bit, well there weren't any best bits. Well the best bit was my husband being there. I liked that, that was nice. The worst bit was just the pain of it all I suppose. The first hour before I had the epidural. (*Pauline Diggory*)

The best bit was when he was born really. The worst bit was the bit after, just waiting to be stitched up. That was the most boring. (*June Hatchard*)

When she was born and when they cut me. (*Ellen George*)

There were no best bits. That catheter was horrible. I think I could feel it. She said you won't feel it, but I'm sure I could feel something, and then the bloke coming round to stitch me up and *that* is embarrassing. That's more embarrassing than having a baby as well. (*Anne Bloomfield*)

Whereas an episiotomy is rarely experienced as pain at the time (the perineum is anaesthetised both naturally and by the injection of a pain-killing agent) the ritual of stitching can be most unpleasant. Like a big baby, a lot of stitches become a hook to hang the account of birth on: look at the enormity of what I have suffered. (It is pedestrian to have had only some stitches, but no stitches at all warrant a different kind of pride.) But it isn't only the symbolic importance or the pain: the act of stitching brings the doctor into the closest confrontation yet with the mother's perineum. Inches apart, he sews in silence, regretting his lost sleep or pondering on the next day's work, like the lady who knitted through the French Revolution.

I: Stitches, how many did you have?

MANDY GREEN: About half a million. I don't think they counted after the first, but it was a lot. It seemed like an endless time. The doctor passed me over to his second because he had to go somewhere else for an interview, but he said you finish off, I've done this and that and he told the other doctor, a trainee, where he had got up to more or less. And this doctor seemed to be stitching for ages and I asked him, no I think I cried then, I had just about passed out by then, and I couldn't feel my legs because they were still strung up, oh it was terrible, and he said it's alright, I'm on my last inch, and I thought Christ almighty if he's on his last inch, how many inches has he done?

SHARON WARRINGTON:

They helped him put on his sterile gown and then they put them up. And that to me, when they take that bottom piece away and your legs are up in the air, and the doctor sits there, is more embarrassing than anything I can remember. I mean he is about that much away from you, and you could literally die with embarrassment.

I: Did you feel that at the time?

SHARON: Yes, and he knew it.

I: Did he, what did he say?

SHARON: He just kept singing. I started counting and because I could feel them, the nurse was holding my hand and I'd look at her and go oh, and she'd look at him and he'd go like this [gestures], and I'd think oh my God, it seemed to go on for hours.

The details of what happened coalesce into a memory. Part of this memory is weighing images versus reality.

In general, was having the baby anything like you expected it to be?

No. I mean yes. No, it wasn't really. I'd never imagined it like that. You read things about what it's going to be like but words can't convey what birth is like; it's just something completely different from anything you've ever done before. (*Jo Ingram*)

Well, I knew it was going to be pretty painful, but in fact I think it was worse than I thought it was going to be, I don't think that I've experienced anything quite like it. It was quite incredible. (*Clare Dawson*)

It wasn't as easy as I thought. It was tougher on you, you had a rough time. But it wasn't bad or anything. Nothing to put you off . . . it was longer, it was more tiring than I'd expected, and there was more pain than I thought . . . and there were so many things that you don't even think about that they do to you, like examinations and everything. You don't even think of them. You just think you go in, you lie down, you have your labour pains every now and then and out it comes. And that's it. But there's a lot more to it. Breaking the waters and all this, and all the monitors they stick on you and all the drips and everything. You know I didn't even know you had a drip. . . . (*Felicity Chambers*)

No. I don't know – quicker. I don't know, you can't *imagine* having a baby. My friends say to me – a lot of my friends are still single and they all come round to see her and they all think she's beautiful and that. . . . And they come round and they say what's it like, having a baby? And I say you can't explain it. You can't, can you? I just said it's foul. (*Anne Bloomfield*)

Yeah. It wasn't bad. That's what it had in this book – how every woman is afraid of the pain of labour, but I wasn't afraid. This crazy friend, she has a child, two years old. And she had a forceps delivery. It was very painful, and she had about a thirty-hour labour. She said: Yeah, you have a natural childbirth – you have it once, and you'll see, ha ha. (*Louise Thompson*)

It was what I expected really. I mean it was what I'd been waiting for, for nine months. Because when you see this baby, if you were cut all over you wouldn't think about it. (*Dawn O'Hara*)

Well I thought it'd be worse. Having the epidural as well I didn't feel a lot. Well, I didn't feel anything really. So I don't really know what the real thing's like. (*Janette Watson*)

AFTER BIRTH

One aspect of birth that is often omitted from antenatal education is the placenta: the organ that nourishes the baby in the womb and grows to about a sixth of the baby's weight. (Some women go into labour ignorant of its existence.) Many of the world's cultures treat the placenta with special care, even regarding it as the baby's twin,[1] but in our industrialised society the attitude is strictly clinical. Under half the sample mothers saw their placentas.

CHRISTINA LYNCH:
I saw it afterwards in a plastic bag. It was quite revolting. I said what on earth are you going to do with that? She said we're going to put it in the fridge for a little while. I thought what on earth for? She said to test it, test the blood, make sure that it's all there. It did look funny: a mass of red and this knotted cord.

MARY ROSEN:
My husband was absolutely *fascinated* by the afterbirth. He couldn't believe it. He really sat up when he saw that. It was absolutely *enormous*. He tells people – you know they put it in a bowl, a kidney shaped bowl – he tells people the way it flopped out because it was so huge. And he tells people more in detail about that than about the baby!

DEIRDRE JAMES:
It didn't hit me straight away what it was. It was on the side in a plastic bag. I looked at it and thought: ugh. It looked really like liver. Imagine me having that!

Birth is evaluated, can only be evaluated, in the light of images absorbed beforehand. In this sense, expecting the worst is the best guarantee of a positive experience. And of course the opposite is true.

KATE PRINCE:
I'm disillusioned about it being so wonderful to give birth, and I'd be breathing my way through it. It just didn't work for me at all. And I thought I was quite tough, could put up with pain, and so on. That's obviously not true, I learnt quite a lot about myself. I'm a coward – no pain threshold at *all* when it *really* comes to pain. I thought the pain was *excruciating*. Don't you think? What did you think about it? I really thought this is absolutely *awful*. I was trying to think how to describe it, and I think it's like when somebody twists your arm up your back – have you ever had that done to you? Such agony. It's like having that done time and time again. But all over me. There's no way you can get out of it.

I think I had all these illusions because all these friends of mine had such an easy time.... I thought I don't want to hear people like my mother who said it's like nothing on earth. If people had said it's either going to kill you or it's not and you won't know till it happens . . .

Now I just recount it, I say that it was awful and that I'm disillusioned, but *then* – a couple of days afterwards – I felt I'd been *tricked*, actually *tricked*, by the health visitor, by the books I'd read – by the Gordon Bourne book, because he says that the word 'pain' should *not* be applied to labour contractions. And somebody had said well it's not like it is in the films or something. And I thought well it's *exactly* like 'Gone with the Wind' – it's *exactly* like those old movies when they're all writhing about in agony: that's *exactly* what I was doing.

The whole mental thing, the whole physical bit: the lot in fact has been completely different. They all lied to me! I mean all these myths that it's like shelling peas – our family's never had any difficulty, *that* sort of thing has been shattered. Our family *has* had difficulty, even if I'm the only one. These books, they should say: right girls, it can either go well or badly.

All that sort of silly nonsense, rubbish, forget it. Don't write things like that to people because it did a power of *bad* for me. Everybody said you'll forget terribly quickly what it's like, in a week's time you'll say oh it was okay. That's supposed to be the thing about childbirth. But I've been determined *not* to forget, so next time I don't make the same mistakes....

Do women forget the pain of childbirth? That is one of the legends, passed down from mother to daughter. But this is the fate of women in our culture: they are imprisoned, labelled, disposed of within stereotypes, and this is how the labour of women in childbirth is disposed of – the suffering, for suffering it must be, is forgotten:

KATE PRINCE, four months later:
I think that it isn't a question of women forgetting about the pain of having a baby. I think that you forget about the actual sensation of *any* pain. You can't describe pain because I mean if I pinch myself now, I know it bloody hurts. But then I've forgotton about it; that's all there is to it.

How much do you think about the actual labour and delivery now? [five weeks afterwards]

LOUISE THOMPSON:
Not much. Afterwards I discussed it with this friend, the pregnant one. I don't re-live it; maybe if it's a bad experience you do.

JANET STREETER:
I do think about it. I often do. I thought one would forget about it. But I often find myself – in fact I dreamt about it the night before last. Really horrible, worse than it was: I *keep* rerunning it. I sit in the bath; I always think in the bath, and I find myself thinking about it without meaning to. I just find myself going through it again.

JOSÉ BRYCE:
I did have nightmares afterwards about having her, about the forceps. I had quite a few nightmares, horrible dreams about these forceps. I kept thinking, I don't know, it was just horrible, you know: a jumbled nightmare, and always at the end a baby was dead or something was wrong with her. Never anything clear-cut. Just a horrible bit about the forceps. I just thought you'd be pushing away and it would just sort of lever it out and you wouldn't feel it. But it felt like a huge suction – as though everything had come out: as though I was all *empty*. Like everything had come out with it. I certainly think my brain was born at the same time. I said to Nick for days I was like a lunatic.

JANE TARRANT:
Right at the very end when they'd sort of gone away and somebody

was coming to wash me down I remember thinking gosh I don't want to go through this again in a hurry. But now, six weeks later, I look back on it with interest. You forget the unpleasant bits: well, you don't forget them, but I think the thrill of giving birth to a baby and everything doesn't strike you at the time, but now it does.

GILLIAN HARTLEY:
I try to push the birth out of my mind. It's over and it's done with, and I don't think it's the be all and end all of . . . I mean he's growing now and he's smiling and he's doing things – the fact that he was born, I mean he obviously *was*, but I'm not going to hold it against him that he tore me or anything like that: that would be ridiculous. No, the birth wasn't this great emotional experience.

SARAH MOORE:
When I think about it I think about them actually giving the baby to me and then Keith nursing it. . . . But as far as thinking about the pain, no I don't: I've forgotten the pain. I look back on it with – nostalgia is not the word, but I feel quite sentimental about the birth. The scenes that I remember are pleasant scenes.

JANETTE WATSON:
No, I don't think about it at all really. Well, I was smiling all day long so it couldn't have been bad, really. I kept myself cheerful, it'd be silly sitting there crying your eyes out.

SANDY WRIGHT:
No, not now. I thought about it in respect of – I thought about having the epidural rather than the actual labour. I thought, should I have persevered, and so on. I think that was almost slight guilt feelings because I'd promised myself I wasn't going to need it, I wasn't going to have it, and then I did have it.

CLARE DAWSON:
Suddenly to see her there and to see her head coming screaming out, you know it was super . . . In a way I wish I could do it again. If I could sort of watch it again, or do it again, and really take notice of what – remember it detail by detail. It fades away, you don't quite remember all you would want to remember.

As these extracts suggest, there may be many reasons why a woman re-lives the scenes of her baby's birth. Joy can be recreated, the importance of the moment recaptured, the whole drama re-enacted, not just as it happened, but as it should have happened. A bad experience can be recited time and time again in a search for meaning: why *did it happen;* what *went wrong? Regret and guilt are both spurs to thought; a birth marred by dissatisfaction seems to be an enduring blow to a woman's self-esteem.*

But, finally, the most pernicious memory a mother may be left with is that she simply was not there: she missed the experience, and was a mere spectator during one of the most important dramas of her life. This feeling is only present when drugs and technology intervene in the relationship between the mother and her experience of birth. Epidurals act by removing sensation from the waist down; pethidine can blur the mind so that a mental absence counteracts the physical presence. Any kind of medical 'assistance' (induction or acceleration of labour, forceps or ventouse delivery) runs the risk of turning the mother into passive object rather than active subject.

KATE PRINCE, epidural, pethidine, forceps delivery:
When I think about it now, it wasn't me having the baby. I was looking at it all through – in a daze almost. I was so tired and in such pain, just not with it at all. In a perverse kind of way I'm looking forward to the next experience because I think I missed out a lot last time. I'd like to take more part in it next time.

MANDY GREEN, epidural, pethidine, forceps delivery:
I didn't really feel anything very much at all. When I became a bit more conscious it was an experience, but I wish I'd had more of that experience. I was never sufficiently aware of myself, my surroundings or anything right from the beginning because I was stupid with the pethidine, absolutely knocked out.

There was nothing best about the birth – you couldn't sort of pat yourself on the back and say haven't I done well because you haven't really . . . there was no feeling, there was just I think nothing really. Just something I had to go through and I went through and that was it. If I'd been more compos mentis, yes I would have liked to have seen the whole thing and be aware of what was happening . . . I would have kept my eyes peeled. I think it would have been very interesting. *I wish I had been there to see it all.*

CHAPTER 6

Mother and Baby

I couldn't believe it was over, it took so long to really click that he had been born . . . I had to keep reminding myself that I had given birth.

Depression, mood changes or fits of crying occur for no reason. Everything is going well, but suddenly the patient bursts into a sobbing fit, and after the episode feels better. She knows that she is being silly . . .[1]

In a sense, a woman's relationship with her baby begins not only before birth but before conception; it has roots in her own babyhood, in the way she herself was 'mothered'. Also important are the messages sent and received throughout childhood and adolescence that, decoded, read: women need babies, babies need mothers. Myth, fantasy and the economics of reproduction under capitalism are all jumbled up, but the effect is powerful. Most women by the time they achieve motherhood have, from these various sources, some idea about how mothers do (or should) feel about their babies.

FIRST ENCOUNTERS

Bloody, messy, screaming, demanding, the emergence of the baby throws cold water on old ideas. A mother's first opportunity to confront the reality of the baby occurs as he or she comes out of the vagina.

Did you see the baby being born?

CLARE DAWSON: Mary, 6lbs 12ozs
There was a head there one minute and the next minute – one minute it seemed to be just a little bit of her head and the next minute she was there. Before she was fully born, she cried. Yes I remember that: I

remember her head coming out and I could see her just screaming her head off, it was just incredible, she wasn't even born and she was screaming . . . I think that is when I began to cry and I thought I've done it! It is a very emotional moment, that is.

JOSÉ BRYCE: Suzy, 8lbs 6ozs, forceps delivery
I saw her when the head was born and the sister came and sucked stuff out of her mouth . . . and then I saw her when she was actually *out* and I saw this bloody little thing going over there . . . I didn't *care* anyway.

ANNE BLOOMFIELD: Jessica, 7lbs 6ozs
I just saw her pop out, that's all. She just flew out – the minute they cut, she just flew out. She wasn't as revolting as I thought she was going to be; I just thought oh my God, she looks like Barry, because she *really* did – even when she was born. It made me really sick because I did all the work and she doesn't look like me. She grabbed the scissors on the side. She picked them up on the way out and she would not let them go; little cow she was, the moment she was born. She grabbed hold of her cord and she wouldn't let it go. She was screaming like this, and they were laughing their heads off . . . she didn't want to be born, I think.

LILY MITCHELL: William, 7lbs 2ozs, forceps breech delivery
. . . then the sister was right in front of me and she said oh go on, go on, keep on, and all of a sudden there was a cloud of blood going up all over the place, on her face and mask and everything else, and Kenneth went to turn my face away because he knows that I can't stand anything like that, and then after a minute or two I looked and you could see his whole body upside down, and I thought oh they are never going to get his head out, you know, and it felt like an eternity before his head actually came out, but Kenneth was looking and had obviously gathered that he was a boy and once I could see him I was interested because I knew the worst was over and I didn't mind looking, but he did look a mess, it was terrible. But I thought I would burst into tears, but I didn't: I just couldn't believe it, I was just lying there looking at him, and then he started crying. . . .

But although three-quarters of the mothers wanted to see their babies being born, only a fifth did so.
I wasn't sitting up enough. Next time I'm going to watch the whole thing. Make sure. I was disappointed. I was very disappointed. (*Mary Rosen*)

I wanted to see her born but I was so – I had my eyes tightly closed trying to push and then she came out. I just sank back with relief, and forgot to look. I *meant* to, but at the time ... I had a pethidine injection, if I hadn't I might have seen her born. ... I *should* have watched her. (*Nicola Bell*)

I couldn't have seen him born even if I'd wanted to. They had a sheet over the whole lot: is that because of forceps? Did you see yours? Do you know that's something, because I didn't see him coming out, I'm sure if I'd seen him I would have felt he was part of me. But because I *didn't* see him, one minute there was that excruciating pain and then suddenly there was this baby that came from somewhere over there – he didn't seem to have any connections with me at all. Perhaps that's why I had so much less feeling about him, because I didn't feel he was part of me at all. (*Janet Streeter*)

Holding the baby for the first time has for so long been the light at the end of the seemingly endless tunnel of pregnancy: the mental image that has sustained the mother through all sorts of trials and tribulations. It is this moment that symbolises the achievement of motherhood. The birth is over: mother and baby are born. Yet the moment when it arrives is strangely discordant with the image.

Can you describe your feelings when you first held the baby?

NICOLA BELL and ANNETTE:
Well everybody says it's the most wonderful feeling, but I didn't feel, I felt pleased and everything, but not as much as I thought I would have done. In fact I was quite surprised; after they'd washed me and cleaned me up they took me straight to the ward and I couldn't really have cared less about her. I didn't really feel anything for her, not really. I thought it wasn't natural to feel like that, I thought then I didn't have a maternal instinct.

ANNE BLOOMFIELD and JESSICA:
When she was born they went oh you've got a little girl. And I went oh [flat tone], will you go and get Barry for me? I had *no* reaction; I didn't even ask was she normal – didn't ask what she was; well I *saw* what she was; didn't ask anything, just looked at her. It was really weird. I had no reaction, I didn't feel anything. I didn't care about myself, I didn't even care about the baby. They put the baby in my arms and I just looked at her. It was really weird.

MARY ROSEN and DANIEL:

I was very pleased. But I was very tired. And I didn't really – I mean I would have been upset if they'd rushed him off without me holding him I suppose, but on the other hand I felt I'd done all my bit at that stage and okay, I had a healthy baby and that was it: I wanted to go to sleep, really. I wasn't worried about him . . . I can remember thinking that I was a mum and that was quite nice. But I don't think I was – I mean the actual minute he was born was very emotional, but afterwards and apart from feeling happy and pleased with myself that I had a lovely baby and it was a boy and everything else – I mean I didn't feel quite soppy, or anything, I wasn't really interested. In fact I was a bit worried that I wasn't interested. I thought I've got postnatal depression immediately!

After such hard labour, is anyone in a fit state to fall in love? Drugs used to kill pain may act as an extra barrier, numbing the emotions as well as the nerves. Sasha Morris had an epidural, but she uses the phrase 'completely numbed' to describe her emotional reaction:

I was absolutely stunned. I couldn't say that I felt anything for her for a while. The next day I was reluctant to admit it to anyone – I said oh I was delighted, but I wasn't . . . and of course Ben was very moved by the whole thing. He had tears in his eyes which is most unusual for him, because he's a very tough businessman – he wouldn't have tears in his eyes for anybody, he's not the emotional sort, but he was *extremely* moved. Which pleased me: I was delighted by his reaction. But I had none of my own. I felt nothing. I couldn't relate myself to her at all. And I never asked if she was alright. I said *nothing.* Everybody said she's a girl. I thought oh: how tremendous. When I looked at her I thought she was lovely. When I held her I said to Ben, you take her. I didn't want to hold her for a long time. And when they took her away I wasn't saying where are you going with her? And I think the same night they brought her for a feed and I put her beside me and I thought she was lovely, but I didn't want to pick her up and hug her. I just wanted to go to sleep. And I couldn't: I was so tired.

I was very amazed at my own reaction when she was born: I was completely *numbed*: I thought I'd be delighted. I think a lot of people won't admit to their feelings. They say they're absolutely delighted, but I'm sure half of them aren't. It's quite normal, isn't it?

Lois Manson had a caesarean; her baby was in a breech position, and too large to negotiate a small pelvis:

Well I've tried very hard to reconstruct that night many times since, and perhaps it's awful, but I really can't remember much about it. But I don't think I felt this sudden gush of love and warmth that apparently one's supposed to feel. And I put that down to being very drowsy and what have you. But I remember examining her and I remember being horrified looking at her navel and there was this great long piece of umbilical cord still there. I thought Christ, she's got a penis – they've lied to me! And I thought what a rotten joke to play on someone who's just had a caesarean. I wanted a boy so much. And I was absolutely convinced it was a boy. And when they brought her to me and said it was a girl I said no, you've got the wrong one. It couldn't possibly be right. I was very drowsy, but I really thought they'd made a mistake. . . . I'm sure having a caesarean made a difference. This sort of detachment. Not actually seeing her born . . .

Even if maternal love fails to arrive ready-made with the baby, pride, euphoria and amazement are other reactions reported by 30 per cent of women.

Feelings on first holding the baby	
Not interested	70%
Amazed, proud	20%
Euphoric	10%

Oh cripey. It was the best moment of my life. You know if I ever see that advertisement for Sterling Health on television it brings back memories, you know? I could cry! (*Dawn O'Hara*)

I felt that it was a miracle, full of wonder at it. That it had been achieved and there she was: and she was lovely and fine, and she had all the necessary bits. I felt more the *wonder* of it than actual sort of *tenderness* for her at that point. She didn't look particularly *beautiful*. She looked like a very new baby. I was just *awed* by it really. (*Sophy Fisher*)

It is almost as if what has been achieved is too much for the mind to grasp. From having a baby inside to holding a baby outside – that incredible feat for the body to accomplish cannot be absorbed by the imagination either.

I just really couldn't believe it. It was really difficult to believe. It took me weeks to realise that it had all happened. After you live with this great bump you can't imagine what it's going to be like. It's all a bit too much. I thought she was tiny, and she was all purple . . . I really felt she was a stranger. It took me really a long time to get to love her really. It's such a funny thing, that suddenly you've got this person that you've got to get to know. . . . (*Sue Johnson*)

BOYS AND GIRLS

Most women spend months imagining what the baby will be like. They may conjure up mental pictures of the baby's appearance, its personality, its habits, its behaviour in later childhood, adolescence or adulthood. Such pictures cannot be formed without some notion of the baby's sex.

LOUISE THOMPSON, 35 weeks pregnant:
Did I tell you I wanted a girl last time? Well for some reason I am sure I'll have a boy. . . . First of all because we can't think of a name for a boy. And second I am against having it circumcised. In America they circumcise *everyone*. [Louise and her husband were born and grew up in the United States.] You see Oliver, because he's circumcised, he said oh how could you *not* have the child circumcised. But I'm definitely against it. I mean to come out into this world and then to have a major operation – it's a *horrible* thing. But that's why I want a girl, for these two reasons. [And she had a girl.]

Most women have definite ideas about what sex they want the baby to be. It is a common finding of research on parents' sex preferences that boys are more popular than girls: this is especially the case with first babies.[2] Over half of this sample of women did in fact want boys – and the quarter who said they didn't mind included some who admitted afterwards that they did want a boy but hadn't liked to say so (because a wish thus stated might not come true). A comment on the social evaluation of femininity in our culture is that 44 per cent of the women who had girls were disappointed to have daughters (compared with the 93 per cent who had boys and were pleased).

Sex preferences and reactions	
Wanted girl	22%
Wanted boy	54%
Didn't mind	25%
Had girl: pleased	56%
Had boy: pleased	93%
Had girl: disappointed	44%
Had boy: disappointed	7%

JANE TARRANT:
11 weeks pregnant:
Well I suppose to be really honest, people think it's a bit more thrilling to have a boy. They feel it's a bit more clever to produce a boy. I'm sure if I have a boy and somebody next to me has a girl I'll feel oh I did a bit better than you. Of course if I have a girl I wouldn't admit that to anybody.

When Christian was 6 weeks old:
After he was born I had all these cards saying congratulations: you've got a boy, you've got a son and heir. I got a bit annoyed about it in the end. I keep thinking well if he'd been a girl I suppose we wouldn't have been so pleased. I suppose I feel more pleased because everybody else is pleased too. You think you've done your duty.

CATHERINE ANDREWS:
14 weeks pregnant:
I think Justin would make the most super father and for that reason I'm really quite hoping for a boy. It would be such a pity if we didn't have a boy at some stage. He'd be an awfully good father for a boy. Not that he wouldn't be for a girl, but he'd be *wasted* on girls in a way.

Seven months later when Fleur is 4 weeks old:
I think for the first few hours after she was born I was just *faintly* disappointed. I mean she was such a beautiful baby that I didn't mind at all, but I think *underneath* I felt well it is a pity. It only took a day and after that I thought: why did I ever worry about it? There was somebody in my ward who *desperately* wanted a boy and she had a girl. When they said it's a girl she said oh. And for about two days she kept going on about how she wanted a boy. But by the end of a week she was quite reconciled to the fact that she had a girl. My mother says they're easier to deal with, anyway!

JO INGRAM:
25 weeks pregnant:
I don't want the awful problem of bringing up a boy, a sexist child. I really feel I can't take that. I really have problems with that whole thing – knowing that I'm bringing up something that's going to oppress somebody: I can't see how to stop that. And it's probably going to oppress me at some stage – like I'm only its Mum, and I'm a woman.

At the birth:
STAFF MIDWIFE: It's a boy! [Held him up for Jo to see; no expression on Jo's face, she burst into tears, tears streaming down her face. Baby's face wiped, baby wrapped up and handed to her. She refused him.]
SMW: I'll put him down, and you can have him later. [Jo vomited, placenta was delivered. SMW hands her baby again. No expression on her face as she looks at the baby; she pulls the cover down and looks at his face.]

JO: I wish he'd stop crying.
When Sam is 3 weeks old:
I still would have liked a girl. But as I say I'm just getting on with it, really. . . . The only time I was aware of it [the baby's sex] was when I was getting this material for cot sheets. I wanted the pink because it was pretty. But I thought I'd get some blue as a concession. That's the only time. He's just a baby at the moment. He's becoming more of a boy, slowly. I *feel* that he looks more like a boy. I'm sure he doesn't – I'm sure he just looks like a baby. But I'm beginning to recognise him as a boy. I just hope it's not going to make too much difference.

I was waiting to see the doctor and she came out and said oh you've had it then! What was it? I said it's a substitute girl. Oh she said, poor little thing!

BIG AND LITTLE

Along with the baby's sex, the other item of information the mother receives about her baby is its weight. This can be regarded as a mark of her achievement, a status symbol.

CHRISTINA LYNCH, baby 7lbs 15ozs:
I think I was a bit disappointed because they said he was going to be a big baby, and I imagined a nine pounder. But he was very long – twenty-two-and-a-half inches. When I got the tape measure and saw twenty-two-and-a-half inches – I thought oh God. I was a bit disappointed that he wasn't a big whopper . . . I wanted to boast, I'd had a big baby.

RACHEL SHARPE, baby 9lbs 6ozs:
I was *shocked* – not surprised. I never expected to have such a big one. Especially since I'd only gained seventeen pounds so he was more than half that.

JULIET MORLEY, baby 7lbs 12ozs:
They don't weigh them until they get them down to the wards, and they come in with these little labels on their cots, it's hilarious! I thought that was more or less average – seven and a half pounds is average isn't it? My husband took far more pride in the whole weight thing than I did.

LOUISE THOMPSON, baby 6lbs:
I was curious. The midwife said a little one, six pounds, but I think two-and-a-half kilos is less, I'm not really sure. I even asked the doctor and she had a chart but the chart didn't go as low as two-and-a-half kilos – I know I was less than six pounds when I was born and they say you usually give birth to the same weight as you were.

AFTERMATH

I think it takes a tremendous toll. It's like a real *illness* isn't it? You need a period of convalescence. (*Kate Prince*)

If the birth is the climax, after the birth is anti-climax. The physical deflation is matched by emotional deflation. The excitement of producing a baby gives way to an awareness of discomfort, as the after-effects of birth – pain, constipation, loss of bladder control, haemorrhoids, engorged breasts – set in.

SANDY WRIGHT:
You see I didn't *sleep* – I went to the ward in the middle of the night. They wouldn't give me a tablet, it was half past three. I had to stay up in the delivery room for a while because I was running a temperature. So they kept me up there. I didn't sleep at all. I couldn't. I felt too uncomfortable and sort of *deflated*. I felt quite sort of 'up' after the delivery and after the stitching I was chatting away to the pupil midwife. And then I got down to the ward and collapsed.

ANNE BLOOMFIELD:
I didn't go to sleep. And then I started crying about an hour later. I went down, I felt lonely, and they pushed me into this ward and everyone just sort of stared at me and I'd just had her and I was a bit tired. They said you'll have a lovely long sleep but I didn't. I couldn't. I just started crying. I felt really lonely. I thought what an anti-climax. Well it is, isn't it? And then Barry came in and I started crying again because I wanted to get out of hospital and I knew I had ten days of it.

JOSÉ BRYCE:
And then they all disappeared and I felt so ill, because I was still on this thing [a drip]. And then she came and got rid of that – that was horrible; I hate injections, especially when I can see them. And she

said oh you are – something about me bleeding a lot – and it was all going down her arm just from my hand, on the floor, and I thought this is bloody ridiculous: every orifice in my body, there's something coming out of it! And I was thinking my hand's hurting, and I said I can't put up with all this – it's all too much. And I was too uncomfortable, it was so narrow, that bed.

It was really a horrible night. I went to the ward: I think it was about a quarter to twelve when I was in the ward. And it was so *hot*, it must have been about 90 degrees in there. And I was in bed and they kept saying do you want anything – tea or anything – and I didn't want anything: they gave me a sleeping pill, and I should have asked for seven. It was mogadon, and I thought it *wouldn't* be mogadon, I thought they're not daft in here, that was why I asked for one. And all the action was going on in the ward anyway, because all the babies were in that ward and I could hear various babies crying and being trundled about. And I can remember the best feeling of the lot was going to the loo in bed because I hadn't gone. They tried to put me on a bedpan beforehand, and then I couldn't go, and I remember it flowing all over my legs in bed and thinking what a relief, and then I felt so comfortable and wet that I just lay there, I didn't ring the bell. I just thought I'm going to leave it until I feel really bad. Then I think I went to sleep. And I can remember doing it again actually, I must have been absolutely *soaked*, and then eventually it was all getting cold and a bit nasty after an hour or so and I thought I'd better ring the bell now. And then they changed everything. I think it was about four – oh yes it was four, because I said can I have another sleeping pill, and she said well not now, because it's four o'clock and they wake you up at half past five: it's not worth it.

A bleeding nuisance

JOSÉ BRYCE:

Afterwards Nick couldn't *believe* the blood, it wasn't that much in fact, not enough to have a transfusion, because the girl next to me, they said it was just over a pint, but the girl next to me said she'd lost two pints, so she did have a transfusion after a couple of days. So I thought it can't be that much. But it *looks* so much. Nick said it was just like something out of Monty Python. It was everywhere. Down his little wellington boots and all over the floor. If someone had told me, it looked like someone had murdered someone. . . .

DEIDRE JAMES:
I remember laying there and thinking oh it aches . . . I was really aching. That was the worst part. I had really bad pains, like period pains. And I was surprised at all the blood I lost. They said yes you will, for a few weeks. You see it's these things that I hadn't been prepared for at all. I carried on losing for three and a half weeks, and it worried me.

The worst thing was that day after. When they put me in the ward, about half past four, I couldn't sleep; they gave me a couple of sleeping pills, but everything was wearing off; I was really sore, couldn't get out of bed, they wouldn't let you get out of bed. I kept losing all this blood everywhere. Every time I moved or they changed the sheets there was all this blood.

Sore points

SOPHY FISHER:
You get to the stage, as I said to somebody in the next bed, where you discuss your bowels and bladder with any passing stranger. If the window cleaner had come through the ward and said how are you, I'd probably have told him.

JULIET MORLEY:
They had these rubber rings for you to sit on and they didn't tell you about them because they didn't have enough to go round. So until one of the other patients told you, you didn't know about them. I found one got very *primitive* about these things; I wasn't parting with my rubber ring for *anything*. . . .

SASHA MORRIS:
I had cracked nipples; I couldn't get her on and then I couldn't get her off when she was on; I almost had to sit on her head to remove her. I had to go down to the nursery to express them, this was what really got me down, of course I *couldn't* do it by hand. I thought that was the most *awful* thing to have to do and one of the sisters nabbed me one morning and said I suggest you express some for twenty-four hours, and she came and got the most enormous amount – about four or five ounces – just by hand, and I was sitting there thinking this is *dreadful*. Will she *ever* stop? And she wouldn't let up. And she was saying, look I've got all this milk. And I was sitting there: I felt just like a cow.

JANE TARRANT:

I had piles. The trouble was, you were alright when you were sitting down, but to try to get up – I suppose you're pressing on some muscle somewhere – it's *agony*. It was real murder and people aren't very sympathetic. And trying to go to the lavatory – it is worse than having a baby: it takes a lot of courage, I think.

VERA ABBATT:

It was more constipation than anything else that was painful. They couldn't do anything about that with the stitches. I just used to scream and spend hours in the toilet. And of course with the stitches it was agony. I don't know whether it was worse for the doctor or worse for me – I was driving him nuts. I kept saying for God's sake, can't you do anything about this?

JOSÉ BRYCE:

She said that's your red hair again, that's why you're so badly bruised – and that's why it's not healing up as quickly: everything was attributed to having red hair and fair skin. At the end of the stay in hospital it was so painful whenever I sat down. I thought this is ridiculous, and I asked the sister to have a look and she said it's knotted, and they were sticking back like a thorn. And she said I'm going to have to cut them. And she cut one, it was like a piece of fishing wire, a great knot. I swear to you. And she held it up, and she said that's why you were uncomfortable. It was such a relief. It wasn't the stitch itself, but the fact that it was still there, and it didn't come away in the bath, my ninety-fourth bath of the stay. I said to Nick, I could sell my body to Smith's at the moment, because it's like a crisp, it's all dry and salty.

In these days following birth, having a baby most resembles an illness. Being in hospital, a place of illness, accentuates this feeling, but the symptoms are real enough, and are treated with a barrage of drugs, reinforcing the notion impressed during pregnancy that having a baby is a medical phenomenon.

Drugs taken in hospital after the birth	
Painkillers	91%
Sleeping pills	84%
Laxatives	55%
Iron pills	41%
Ointment/suppositories for piles	30%
Antibiotics	16%
Indigestion medicines	5%
Other	34%

They dish it all out like Smarties in there – they come round with the drugs trolley and ask you what you want. It's incredible. They give you painkillers for headaches – anything. (*Juliet Morley*)

The sleeping pills they just leave. I'd never taken sleeping pills in my life before and I thought I wouldn't need them. I said oh I don't need any of *them*. But they said you might as well take them: they're meant to make sure you have a night's sleep. I said I'm sure I shall do that. But they said no, you'd better have them. I had them and I think nearly everybody came in saying I'm not having sleeping pills, but we all had them in the end. (*Clare Dawson*)

For those who do feel ill, hospital routines provide no rest; and for those who have recovered from the birth, hospital is not the place to be. Lack of sleep plus forcible separation from husband and home plus the strain and anxiety of getting to know and care for the baby equals misery. A place of safety becomes a prison.

BABY BLUES

Many antenatal advice books describe a phenomenon called 'third' or 'fourth' day 'blues'.[3] The causes of this are variously named as tension, hormones, tiredness, or problems in accepting the maternal (feminine) role. Symptoms listed include sudden mood change, crying for no apparent reason, irritability, irrational misery. Estimates of the frequency of 'baby blues' vary from 5 per cent to 80 per cent.[4] Most (84 per cent) of the women in this sample suffered from them.

I: Did you feel at all depressed at any time during your stay in hospital?

PAT JENKINS: Oh yes, I think it was on the second day that I cried.

I: How long did you cry for?

PAT: Well I cried one day in the morning, and then after that I cried again – everyone had a different day!

I: How did you feel when you were crying?

PAT: I don't know. You just feel an emptiness. It was really big sobs, you know, crying hard sort of thing, but I didn't know why.

I: Had you expected to feel depressed?

PAT: Well they say you do, so I thought it was probably natural you know. Everyone was doing it, you know.

NANCY CARTER:

I think it was on the fifth day her crying, her screaming, it just went right through me and I just could not cope. I was lucky, a very nice sister on at that time took her away from me for the day. She said I was to have complete rest, and she kept her in the nursery. When I got her back next day I was fine. And then I got depressed again, that's right, it was on the day I was due to come out, and I couldn't wind her, and I got hysterical in the end: it was awful. I really hated her and wished to God I'd never had her. I wasn't getting any sleep at night because they took the babies away for so many nights, but then, even without your own child there, all the other ones kept you awake. I think they said our ward was the worst. I'd get up in the night and it was the same old babies that would play up, and first of all it would be one of you out of bed and then you'd get back and settle your baby and someone else's baby would start and yours would start again. It was really terrible in the end. I thought that was very bad actually, to have the babies with you. I'd find myself going to sleep, and I'd think oh she's due for a feed in two hours and I'd be so pent up and scared that I'd sleep through her feed that I wouldn't sleep. One night Joanna was screaming her head off and I must have been so tired and in such a deep sleep the others thought that I was letting her cry it out, and they realised in the end that I wasn't and when they came to wake me I just screamed and screamed and screamed, so pent up I suppose, with shock. I just screamed and woke everybody else up!

She seemed to be very good during the day. After the visitors had gone, we'd all have a laugh in our ward, and when I look back I think most of us were on the verge of hysteria really. It wasn't proper laughing, we all knew what was coming to us that night. I changed her one night, got out of bed and changed her again, and I knew she was clean and dry but she just wouldn't stop crying, and I realise now that I probably hadn't brought her wind up, you know. I just didn't know what to do with her. It was awful. I took her into the nursery and as soon as I got her there she was quiet and I booed my eyes out. The nurse came in and she said what are you crying for Mrs Carter, she said what are you in here for? Your baby's quiet, and Joanna looked as if she'd gone to sleep again. As soon as I got her outside back to the ward she'd start crying again. It was terrible.

I: Did you expect to get depressed?

NANCY: Yes, but I didn't think it would really hit me that hard.

I: How did you think it would hit you?

NANCY: Well just like an ordinary depression. I didn't really think I'd hate the baby like I did, you know, and wish to God I'd never had her.

HILARY JACKSON:

I just feel generally depressed. General weeps and that. If anyone says anything, that's it; I either have a go or just walk out. It started about two days afterwards – I was quite amazed really because a lot of the women in the ward felt like it and it seemed to be that nobody *knew*. None of the nurses and that *knew*. It was the girls in the ward that knew, and it was amazing that they could go through such an emotional happening and nobody knowing – and how they could cope with it. Because I mean the nights were *death* in there. Absolute death. And these women were really at breaking point and yet nobody knew. It was only us, amongst ourselves, that knew, and we coped between us. Because there's only one staff nurse and one auxiliary, or one of these agency nurses, on at night, and they just haven't got time for you. There's so much for them to do. If you've got a child that's screaming through the night . . . it was the nights that we all hated. I mean the day staff were so fantastic and we all coped very well, but we all just used to dread the nights because when one cried nobody would know if it was theirs so we'd all six of us get up, and of course five of us could go back to bed. And then of course about half an hour after it, another one would cry and we'd all get up again. So this is what it was like. I mean the ten days was far too long to stay there. Absolutely. I mean the girls that were doing this forty-eight-hour thing – we were just envying them. I mean towards the end literally, I mean I wanted to ring my husband and wake everyone up about four or five o'clock in the morning because I was so cheesed off and I literally felt that I would have just rung a minicab and discharged myself. That's literally how I got.

ELLEN GEORGE:

I felt more exhausted. But it was labelled postnatal depression. The sister, and everyone else picked it up, and said yes: that's postnatal depression. I said to the sister, Piccadilly Circus is more restful than this place. Oh it was so bad, I had one hour's sleep for three nights running, and no sleep during the day. I recognised that I might have broken down.

I think with the loss of the blood and the manual removal of the placenta which was pretty ghastly really, although I was knocked out for it, I felt terrible just after the birth. Finally I got in such a state that I rang my mother [a GP] at four o'clock in the morning which I've *never* done . . . because I was having problems with the doctors and sisters not getting the rest, and someone who's lost a lot of blood has got to have a lot of rest and a high protein diet, neither of which I was getting. The diet was appalling and the rest was non-existent. Routine was what mattered. If you'd fed the baby at five in the morning, you still had to get up at six to join the band. I just wasn't sleeping, and I thought you've just got to get out of this place or you'll go mad. I thought if I have to go one more night in this place, I'll go crazy. I'm feeling I'm going crazy anyway. My mother realised this and she said well I'll ring the doctor in the morning. So she rang, she got hold of the registrar and he said I was obviously having a postnatal depression. . . .

In other words, this kind of 'depression' is situational: a symptom of hospitalisation. Studies of childbirth in other kinds of societies where childbirth is still a family affair do not mention depression as an after-effect.[5] As Nancy Carter, Hilary Jackson and Ellen George describe it, feeling 'depressed' is feeling exhausted, bereft of the skills needed to comfort a crying baby, powerless to change the bondage of remorseless hospital routine. Any man subjected to major surgery and then told to start a new job immediately for which he has had no training and in similarly rigorous conditions would probably also react negatively (at the very least).

Perhaps I was tired, I don't know, feeling a bit sensitive. I don't *think* it was depression – I was upset. I felt in a dream. But I don't think it was postnatal depression. I mean *I probably would have felt like that if I'd had an operation or something.* (*Jane Tarrant*)

Asked to unfold the short-hand term 'postnatal depression' as applied to feelings during the hospital stay, most women give causes other than hormones for feeling blue.

My depression came on the eighth day when I rang Robert up at work to tell him what to bring for me to wear, and he hadn't been at work that day. I was terribly upset. His secretary wouldn't tell me where he was, she said he's working out of the office. And it really sounded as though she was covering up for him having an affair with some other woman. And I got *terribly* upset – I burst into tears in the phone booth. And then I rang here and he answered the phone – and he'd been out for a booze-up the night before with his best man and of course he'd been sick the next morning. So that started me off. But I think it was really tiredness. I didn't cry because I was depressed; that's the wrong word. *It was being pure overwhelmed with emotion at the whole thing.* I wasn't depressed; I was delighted. But you don't realise how much it's taken out of you.(*Elizabeth Farrell*)

Oh one day I wept and wept, I just couldn't stop. I just prayed that nobody would come and visit me because I don't know how I could have coped. But I mean they do say that nearly everybody has one day. I was just surprised at how weepy I was because I'm not the kind of person that gets depressed. Mind you, I wasn't actually depressed, it was funny, I just felt terribly terribly *worried* about the baby and I just couldn't stop crying you know for a whole day. And so that night, that was about the fifth day, that night they took him off to the nursery and they bottlefed him for that night, and they gave me some sleeping tablets, because they said I was so tired and I was so tensed up I wouldn't have been able to sleep . . . and the next day I was as right as rain again. (*Rosalind Kimber*)

I wasn't weepy or anything, I was just very tired. I don't think I got weepy at all apart from the day I was crying with the piles and that was the fourth day but it wasn't depression: I was in pain. (*Caroline Saunders*)

You feel really happy and hospital is the last place you want to be, because it's really like being in jail. (*Sue Johnson*)

The sentence of hospital confinement is a lonely one. Husbands may have acquired a place in the delivery room, but they are still merely visitors in the postnatal wards. Many women having a first baby will never have been separated from their husbands before. It is ironic, and a further reason for depressed feelings, that the occasion when the couple becomes a family also drives husband and wife apart.

ANNE BLOOMFIELD:
I cried every time he come in the door, it was getting on his nerves. I was crying *all* the time. Because I missed him so much. I don't think it was hormones: I'm not crying now, am I?

DEBORAH SMYTH:
Two days it was. One day Patrick turned up late – it was the trains. First when he didn't come at ten past eight I went and sat outside and had a cigarette and there was a lady out there having contractions and talking about her baby and I couldn't concentrate. I was worried, I wondered where he'd gone. I thought it's not like you to be late. Then I went down the end and waited. I cried at the slightest thing, feeling fed up really, not depressed as such. Because in the day I was fine.

Then Patrick'd come and after he'd gone I'd get upset and I'd go and have a bath and sit in the bath and cry.

The average length of time the sample women stayed in hospital was just under nine days. Louise Thompson was the only one who stayed only forty-eight hours:
Oh God, there was a woman opposite, she had a premature baby, it was in an incubator. And one night, the second night I guess, the woman next to me, she says she's crying. I said let her cry. And then I heard this awful sobbing. And I went over, the social worker bit, I said what's wrong? I mean I didn't know what to say. And she said she's premature, I hate her, I never wanted her. I'm sure I was the only person she ever confessed this to. And I felt so bad. I said oh that happens to everyone: I didn't want a baby, either. I didn't know what to say. But that was sort of the atmosphere of the hospital, in the hospital everyone was depressed. It was much more like leaving a mental hospital than this happy maternity hospital. And it was just incredible. I thought no wonder everyone is so crazy when they grow up, because the mothers are so crazy.

But in the hospital, everyone is in the same boat. Strangers become confidantes, pooling the most intimate details of their lives, and united by common concerns: breast versus bottle, bowel movements, baths, beating the system.

Mothers united

CHRISTINA LYNCH:
They were very short on baby linen – sheets, wraps and gowns. And of course, the boys, they wet everything straight through, every time. So we'd traipse off, have you got a sheet, a gown and a wrap? And they'd say no. Some of the nurses would say stick it over a radiator to dry it and then another nurse would say what's that on the radiator? . . . We all got told off for doing something wrong. We felt there should be a list of dos and don'ts. Especially don'ts, like you mustn't change the baby on the bed because they can pick up cross infection where you've been lying. You mustn't walk around without shoes on because you might pick up splinters of glass. It wasn't until you did something wrong that you realised it *was* wrong. We felt there should have been a list up in the ward. So of course we all changed our babies on the bed: we said who's going to get a nice bit of cross infection, then?

DEIRDRE JAMES:
The girl in the next bed to me flooded the corridor. We had a system

whereby if we had a bath we'd run it for the next girl in the ward. Our
method was we'd leave the plug in and run it. Well, this girl had put
the plug in and, Sue, her name was, had just washed her hair and
someone said Sue have you had a bath yet? She said no and she looked
outside the ward and saw the water up to here. So she took her
slippers off and she was wading up to the bathroom and Dr Allan
came along and said what are you doing? You're not on Brighton
beach, you know! He said will you come back to bed, then? And I was
laying in bed and I had the hysterics. He said you'll do yourself a
mischief if you have the hysterics like that. Oh dear: we did have some
laughs!

FELICITY CHAMBERS:
One night we sat up until about, it was the last night I was in, we sat
up till about twelve o'clock laughing with the nurses. And one of the
girls sat there and she was laughing so much, she was eight-and-a-half
months pregnant and her baby slipped down she was laughing so
much. And in the middle of the night she got up to go to the loo and as
she was climbing back into the bed her waters broke . . . we had such a
laugh that night. And she came down the next morning lying on the
trolley: well, it's a girl. . . .

LEARNING TO CARE

*This spirit of sisterhood enlivens the two tasks of getting better and learning to
look after the baby. Establishing a satisfactory feeding routine, bathing the baby,
dealing calmly and efficiently with all the appalling messes babies make; these
are signals that the new mother is ready to take her place amongst all mothers.
From their first encounter on the delivery table, mother and baby, so inseparably
joined for so long, must now bridge their separateness with interlocking love and
need. Face to face (or mouth to breast) they must 'bond' so that the emotional
adhesions become the way mothers and babies feel and behave in our culture.*

GRACE BOWER:
I had to ask to see him; they didn't bring him round to me. I didn't
even know where to go or anything. All the other girls were going to
get their babies – in the end I said: where are they? Can we see them?

VERA ABBATT:
When I was lying in bed they came over and said that I could go down

and see him in the nursery. Of course I went down there and there was me picking up all the name tabs. I'd seen him for about two minutes, and I just hadn't a clue – I mean he was covered in all the blood. And when I eventually found the cot that had my name on it I just stood there and cried.

JUNE HATCHARD:
I had to walk up and down looking at the names to see which was mine. They all looked the same and had the same wraps on and were laying in the same sort of cot. You're a bit unsure, you don't want to take the wrong one. It doesn't say very much for the maternal instinct, does it?

Angela King's and Deirdre James's babies both went to the special care unit. Angela had a caesarean and Deirdre's baby was an awkward instrumental delivery; he had a badly bruised head.

ANGELA KING:
The baby had a bad infection and I didn't see her for two days. It was horrible, going through all of that and then not seeing her, because I started to think maybe something was badly wrong with her because they said she's got an infection, and she was in an incubator just for a day and she was on antibiotics, she was on them for about six days afterwards. They said she's on antibiotics and she's in an incubator and she's just got a small infection, but I thought it was something really bad because I wasn't able to see her. And in the end I really pestered sister because she kept on saying we'll take you down, we'll take you down, but she never did. I kept on and on and in the end they got a wheelchair and took me down. It's nothing when you can't hold them. I didn't really enjoy the beginning of her life. I felt like I'd been *cheated* I suppose – that I wasn't given her.

DEIRDRE JAMES:
I didn't want to see the baby. I was frightened because I hadn't seen him since they first showed him to me. The sister came down after I was in the ward and said he was alright; he had three chins. She said he's getting on fine, don't worry. But seeing his head like that I thought if he's got brain damage and all these things . . . I didn't want to go and see him. He was still in the prem unit. My husband took me down on the Saturday night. Sister said take your wife down. So they put me in a wheelchair and off we went down the corridor. And I got in this gown. And I cried and I said I don't want to see him. He said

he's alright. I said his head, I don't want to see him, I was frightened. Then I saw him and I held him; it was lovely, although the black bit on his head was still there. He was half asleep. He opened one eye and then the other eye. I said oh he *is* mine. He's lovely, I don't want to put him down.

Becoming emotionally involved with the baby means worrying about the baby. At first there is a need to establish that the baby is 'all there'.

FELICITY CHAMBERS:
I held him the next morning before breakfast. I was so pleased. I counted his fingers and toes. When I was pregnant I had an obsession that he was going to have six fingers on one hand and four on the other. So as soon as they gave him to me I unwrapped him and counted his fingers and toes. Silly, but you know, the nurse said a lot of women do this.

During this period it seems that even trivial incidents can spark off terrific anxiety in the mother that the baby is not healthy and normal. Separation after the birth for some hours, a hospital 'rule', is an opportunity for all sorts of fantasies to take hold.

RACHEL SHARPE:
After he'd stitched me up they brought me down to the recovery room and I'd just dropped off to sleep, and then they woke me up for breakfast. And then I got this horrible feeling that there was something wrong with the baby; I kept thinking oh I'm *sure* they're not telling me, I'm sure there's something wrong with him. And when the medical student came I think I asked him is the baby . . . oh yes, yes, he's alright. And then I asked if I could see it and they said no, it was in the nursery or something. And that just *convinced* me that there was something wrong with it. And I know Dr Allan came in and went to see the girl in the bed next to me and I thought oh thank God I'm going to see him, at least he's somebody I know and I'm *sure* he would tell me. And when he'd finished with her he just walked out. God I thought, I was just about hysterical at that point.

I still didn't see him because when they moved me to the ward I got to the point where I didn't *want* to see him, I didn't want to have anything to do with him. The sister came in, she came in and said to me why are you crying? And I said I'm sure there's something wrong with my baby and they're not telling me. Well she said, everybody feels like that she said, there's nothing wrong with your baby. She said you can go and get him if you like. And of course I couldn't get out of bed. So I said no I didn't want to see him but I wanted to know if he was alright. Oh yes she said. And then she just sort of walked away. There was another one there, a Ceylonese girl, and she was fantastic. She said I'll bring him down to you and *show* you that there's nothing wrong with him.

But even assured that her baby is normal, the new mother is prone to all sorts of anxieties: these express a desire to care, a developing commitment. Rachel Sharpe again:

It was his left hand, when I went to get him from the nursery on the second day he had this big red blister on his hand. So I asked them what had happened to him and they sort of – one of them asked the other one and then the other one asked the other one and then they said to me oh he was sucking his finger you see, and he got this blister. Well I reckoned that somebody was smoking and dropped ash on him. It was a blister, so it was obviously a burn, a nasty-looking thing. I mean even I couldn't get one from sucking mine you know, and I've got teeth! So I never left him in the nursery after that.

It was just one of those days. I think it started off when I was in the nursery having his cord done, and he was being weighed or something, and he'd been sick once or twice and while I was in there he was sort of screaming and I thought it was because of the pain in his finger because it was an awful-looking thing. And I thought oh God what am I going to do for him, he keeps vomiting and his poor finger! And I'd been changing him and this great stream of urine just sort of shot up and went right in his face dripping in his eyes and his mouth and then he started to cry again. . . . I spent most of my time *weeping* over him.

KATE PRINCE:

I cried because I thought she was going to *die* one night. She had terrible diarrhoea the fourth night, it was just coming out non stop and it got worse and worse as the night went on and I couldn't be consoled at all. I was just hysterical and the sister said look I'll take her off to the nursery; I really did think she was going to die, and that they weren't telling me she was. First of all that staff nurse tried to deal with me and then the sister but I thought she was pulling the wool over my eyes. I was crying and crying and the baby was lying there and it was just coming out all the time. And I had visions of this little coffin and funerals . . . she was just so tiny and so apparently sick. Silly really, but it was a tremendous worry at the time.

PAULINE DIGGORY:
I thought she was going to contract all sorts of illnesses. Every time she had a snuffly nose or sneezed – I kept thinking she was going to die. I didn't *really* think she was going to die. But I thought she *might* die.

SUE JOHNSON:
I had terrible nightmares. Have you had anyone else who had that? One night I dreamed that these people turned their doberman pinscher on her and they thought I'd done something to this girl's boyfriend, so they turned their dog onto the baby. I was really crying. I had to go outside and the night nurse took me into her office. And I'd also dreamed that I dropped the baby on her head, that the same people had made me drop the baby on her head. In my dream it was the same floor as in the hospital. She said you must be careful with the baby, sometimes these things are a warning. She was a black nurse. I didn't mind, because the way she said it it was as if she was a gypsy fortune teller. It kind of appealed to me.

The lack of interest most mothers feel when they first see their babies is truly shocking to them. But reassurance soon follows as protective feelings develop and signal the arrival of maternal love.

JO INGRAM:
That was awful actually. When they gave me the baby I wasn't interested a bit. I thought oh fucking hell, I've just done all this work, and they've handed me this thing and I'm supposed to do something with it.

I got upset afterwards, they took him away and the nurse said oh poor little thing, your mum doesn't want you, or something like that. And I suddenly realised – this poor little fucker's got to spend the night, this poor little fucker's just been born and he's got to go off all on his own yelling to the nursery. And I suddenly got really upset and the nurse said what's the matter with you? I said I just feel awful because I can't look after the baby. And she said don't be silly everyone has their babies taken away for the first night, so they can get a rest.

I felt the separation thing really a couple of days later because he was ill. He did funny shits for a day so they carted him off to the isolation room. And that was awful: I was being really silly about it. I felt really down. When he was taken away I really was upset then: I realised I really did like him.

BARBARA HOOD:
Some silly nurse said, I was feeding and he wouldn't get on, so she sort of picked him up and said now come on John you bad-tempered old thing. And I went – he's not a *bit* bad-tempered, which he wasn't at the time: well, I felt like giving her a thump, talking to *my* son like that, picking him up like that rather sharply. And I think that's when I started to feel it. . . .

NINA BRADY:
I got to like him about the fourth or fifth day. I got a feeling that I wanted him to be with me in the bed. I took him into bed with me a few times and I was caught. I began to get very fond of him, you know? And the sister came in and there was no baby in the cot, and she came and took him off me. She said don't you *ever* do that, you could get very weak or fall asleep and fall on top of him, like roll over on him. I had him laid beside me in the bed . . .

MOTHER KNOWS BEST

Along with feelings of protectiveness comes a sudden burst of confidence in one's ability to mother: this is my *baby, I* know *best. Mother repossesses baby, baby is ceded by hospital to be mother's possession after all; maternal expertise and 'professional' expertise have some uncomfortable encounters, and in the wards mothers scrutinise each clash of opinion, staking out the logistics of their claim to be the best and proper guardians of their children.*

GRACE BOWER:
I found a couple of times when I was in the nursery they used to let them scream and scream, and they didn't used to do anything to them. And I felt so sorry for all the babies screaming. And I remember the third night in particular he was very bad, and I was up from ten till three, and at half past three I just gave up and went to bed. And apparently he didn't stop at all until about four o'clock: the nurses just didn't know what to do with him; they gave him milk and he went to sleep. Another time I was with him and they just wouldn't let me pick him up. They didn't do anything to stop him in his cot so in the end I just said I'm going to pick him up whether you like it or not. She said you can't sit here all night with him: I said yes I can and I will.

PAULINE DIGGORY:
We had terrible ructions towards the end. This doctor kept taking
blood from the baby. I think it was to do with the epidural. And one
day I'd just gone to sleep and the nurse came in and said can I borrow
your baby? I said well I don't really want her disturbed now. She was
asleep and I said she always comes back from you screaming. So she
went away and then this doctor came in and he said can we borrow
your baby? When they ask you it doesn't really *mean* anything – they
don't take no for an answer, do they? So I said yes, alright, but I don't
want her back all awake and screaming. So anyway he took her away
and she was away an awfully long time and I said to the other women
in the ward I bet they're giving her milk, and just at that moment he
walked in with her and she was all quiet and I said what have you
done to her? He said we've given her some milk. And I – I had tears
running down my face, I was so angry. I said what did you do that for?
Breastfed babies aren't *supposed* to have bottled milk.

*Such clashes between mothers and staff are bound to happen. Mothers are in
hospital to be looked after, but they are also very much left to do the routine
changing and washing and feeding of their babies: indeed achieving competence in
these tasks is the main rationale behind the hospital's official policy of booking all
new mothers for a ten-day hospital stay.*

What did it feel like when you first started looking after the baby?

JO INGRAM:
I didn't know what the fuck to do. There was this kid crying in the cot
and I just sort of stood there and then started rocking the cot – shut
up, shut up. Then I looked at the woman in the next bed and said well,
what do I do? She said well try picking him up. Oh can I?

DEBORAH SMYTH:
When they first gave him to me I thought God, what do I do with this?
When they gave him to me for breastfeeding I held him, I was so
careful you know – how am I going to dress him and that?

PAT JENKINS:
I was a bit, you know, frightened at first that I was doing it all wrong
and I didn't like people watching me, you know, all the other mothers.
But then as time went on you just did it automatically. But the first
time, oh dear me, he was really black and it was everywhere, he'd got

it on his sides, and it was halfway up his back, on his legs and on the sheets and blanket, but he was covered! And I went to change him and one of the girls said oh you should get a nurse to do that. And I said oh no, *I want to do it myself.* Well, I was going to have to do it sometime. But you know, she said, oh I'd get the nurse if I were you, because he really was messy. So anyway they called the nurse and she washed and dried him and I put his nappy on.

NANCY CARTER:
I was more or less dropped in at the deep end. I can't really remember very much about the first few days after I'd had her. She was put in a cot at the foot of the bed, and a nurse came round and showed me how to feed her. She spent about five or six minutes showing me, then you are more or less left on your own. The other girls in there showed me how to change her and all that kind of thing, where to get the linen from and where to get the feeds from and all that kind of thing. I thought that was very bad actually; nobody showed me how to top and tail her, another girl in the ward showed me that. I was only doing like her face. I didn't realise that you had to do under her arms. I was doing her bottom as well, but I didn't realise you had to do under her arms!

First-time mothers may be strongly motivated by the novelty of the experience, others less so.

HILARY JACKSON:
There was one girl there, it was her fourth and she laid in bed *all* day long and I thought to myself well obviously she is such an old hand at this. . . . She *refused* to have the baby in with her at night. She said she didn't mind being woken up to feed it but she refused to have it in the ward. She was obviously an old hand. I mean everyone was horrified at her because she laid in bed all day. But obviously she knew . . .

FELICITY CHAMBERS:
I couldn't believe he was mine, you know: you have him beside the bed. And the nurses say that you can tell who's a first-time mother because first-time mothers put them beside the bed and keep watching them. And second-time mothers put them at the end of the bed and forget about them.
I: Where was yours?
FELICITY: Beside the bed!

GETTING OUT

As the days go by, getting out of hospital becomes the major goal. Like prisoners whose sentences are under review, the mothers await the decisions of higher authorities, feeling dependent, vulnerable, anxious; some more determined than others.

PAULINE DIGGORY:
I did agitate a bit. I said I'm going home tomorrow, you know. The sister said oh yes, are you?

HELEN FOWLER:
I had a fight for it. It started on the Tuesday, the fifth day, just saying when can I go? I was getting bored, when can I go? It was Dr Howard I was dealing with. I was persistent, every time he set foot on the floor I grabbed his coat. He kept saying don't worry, don't worry. He had ward rounds about half past ten at night on the Tuesday night. And he kept putting me off – we'll see, we'll see. And I was really getting frustrated and I wanted to get home because I felt fine and fit. Wednesday he came round with the consultant, they were going through everyone. And they said fine, glad to see you doing so well, and started going on to the next bed. And I said oh and Dr Howard said just a minute, I'll come back, I'll come back and talk to you later. And I went down to the end of the corridor and I was sitting there. And Mrs Jackson the social worker that I'd seen the very first visit was there and I said hello: she said I'm glad everything's okay. So I said I wonder if you can help me, and she was there to see another mother in my ward, I said I've got a problem: they won't let me out and she said who's they? I said the doctors. And she went down to talk to Dr Howard. And that's when he came and said okay fine, we'll let you go. He made some joke about outside pressures.

Leaving hospital marks the end of an era. The ward is not a microcosm of the outside world but a protected medical environment. In it, mothers are connected by the lifeline of their patienthood to a whole army of experts; outside it this lifeline is severed and they are on their own.

CHAPTER 7

Learning the Language of the Child

It's so difficult to analyse what you feel. Occasionally I sit there and say what can I do? Why won't she go to sleep? And my husband says this is what you've always wanted. . . .

I used to think how can these people do these things to babies? But you know when you've had about ten minutes sleep in two weeks or something like this . . . because all the time you're not sleeping, when you go to bed you're still listening, you're always listening. And I was always rocking. I used to walk down the street and Mum used to say to me, Hilary you're rocking. And I was! I'd stand in a shop waiting in the queue and I'd be rocking.

HOMECOMING

Coming out of hospital may feel like leaving prison, but prison is also security and being free means feeling trapped.

In *hospital, biological motherhood is achieved, but the social role of mother is only rehearsed; the stage is set with uniformed figures whose job it is to care for mother and baby: motherhood is unreal when it is acted out in an institution away from ringing doorbells, hungry husbands, well-meaning mothers-in-law and dirty carpets.*

So the day comes . . .
It was an extraordinary feeling driving home, a peculiar feeling . . . I sat on the sofa and I felt very happy to be home and very very disoriented. I felt as if I'd been abroad and come back after a summer holiday . . . (*Ellen George*)

I don't know, the whole house felt strange to me. And *I* felt strange. I thought I was going to a new place I'd never been before. (*Grace Bower*)

At home the baby is finally the mother's possession.
When I first held the baby I couldn't believe it actually. I don't think I believed it all the time I was in hospital. I kept saying that it felt as if at the end of the stay there they were going to say right, we'll take it back now. It's not until you get home that you feel they are *yours* I don't think. Because everything is hospital property. Everything belongs to them while you're in there. (*June Hatchard*)

And if the birth was traumatic, a shock to the system, so is coming home. Most mothers describe a terrible sense of responsibility that dawns when there is no longer a hospital nursery to wheel the baby into, or a nurse to consult about the colour of a dirty nappy. Responsibility breeds anxiety, a state in which the mother is perpetually on edge, her nerves like a fine wire stretched taut. In many cases this anxiety is shortlived, being quickly overcome by a growing feeling of confidence, encouraged perhaps by a baby that instils confidence, being readily comforted with milk or love, sleeping for acceptable stretches of time. But a miserable baby makes its mother more anxious, taxing her nerves and powers of recovery with apparently limitless crying.

CHRISTINA LYNCH and ADRIAN, six weeks:
It was the same day I came home, I wondered what had hit me. I thought I shouldn't feel like this . . . it seemed to me that he was always crying, and I lived in a permanent *haze* . . . I can't really remember what I did the first day. All I can remember is crying. I was and he was. It was always feed, change, and the first few days I couldn't *eat* anything; my stomach was just a knot. And every time he cried my stomach just *churned* – you know how you get that kind of *butterfly* feeling in your stomach? Well every time he made a noise my stomach went into a knot like that. I wanted to cry. If it was between feeds I said what are you crying for? And *I* burst into tears. I was alert all the time. I couldn't *rest:* in the afternoons Keith said lie down, and have a rest, but of course he, the baby, was in the same room, he would whimper in his sleep or make a noise and I would be up like this! It seemed that he was always crying and I was always crying.

SANDY WRIGHT and SARAH, five weeks:
I'm finding it quite hectic. Well I suppose being a first one you're just lacking in confidence and you're nervous the whole time. I'm not nervous about *handling* her: she's quite big. It's knowing what to do and the right thing to do – I suppose there *isn't* a right thing to do.
This is the problem of coming home. In the hospital you always

knew you could wheel her down to the nursery and somebody would look after her for a few hours if she was difficult. The first evening we got her home she was due for a feed and I fed her: she started crying. I was pretty depressed those first few days. I hadn't got any depression in hospital; I seemed to get on quite well. There were friendly people in the ward and everyone seemed nice: at home I found myself suddenly *responsible*, and I started to get a bit upset about it all. I still do. Like in the night, oh, you think it's never going to end. You think she's *never* going to go to sleep – she'll go on all night. She wakes up sometimes after a couple of hours, and I think basically *she's* not taking enough – I think it's *her*; she goes to sleep, it's impossible to wake her up, she's right out. I expected her to have a feed and be awake for up to an hour with the feed and changing her and then go back to sleep again.

I suppose all the time I'm thinking, I'm going about doing bits of housework and thinking am I going to have time to do this before she wakes up? Is she going to wake up now? You know because if she *does* cry, there's isn't anyone else who can go and see to her, you've got to stop what you're doing. I haven't taken to motherhood very well, I don't think. I don't know if it's a general feeling. Sometimes I think: why did I bother? I'm sure it will get better. I *think* she's more of a problem than she is really. . . .

WHAT HAVE I DONE?

It does get better of course, almost always, but meanwhile there can be some very black moods. Knowing that life can never be the same again inspires a nostalgic longing for the past, the time before the baby, and the baby, stating its existence and demands day and night, innocently becomes the target at which maternal anger is guiltily but helplessly directed.

KATE PRINCE and GILLIAN, six weeks:
I sometimes think she's a cow. I *hated* her at first, not so much in hospital, but the first week or two here: I just wished she'd never been born, couldn't *bear* her. It was a mixture really, half and half, I'd be either madly in love with her, she's ever so good, dear little baby, terribly protective and all that, and then sometimes I'd think oh: I'd wake up and remember that there was a child there.

I think I was terribly affected by the whole thing. I was really surprised at that – the whole thing about adjusting. I was just miserable, tearful, crying at everything, at the slightest thing. When you're in pain you cry about that, and you cry when the baby cries, but apart from that I just felt *so* miserable and at night she wouldn't go back to sleep and I just was beside myself. I just wanted to die. I would happily have committed suicide. I just didn't know what I was letting myself in for. I thought oh God: I've got her till I die – it was this attitude – even when she's away and married and all the rest of it I'll still worry about her. What have I done? Why have I got this baby? What am I going to do? Why can't it be like it was before – just the two of us?

These feelings are not the 'baby blues' of the hospital stay. This kind of 'postnatal depression' is a deep-rooted anxiety state, expressing terror and panic, devotion and despair, helplessness in the face of power. For most of the 71 per cent of women who experience it, it passes within days, two or three weeks at most, but for some it becomes a chronic problem, a feeling that one simply will never be able to cope.

Perhaps the question should be not, why do some mothers get depressed, but why do some mothers not *get depressed? Should we not express surprise at easy satisfaction with the maternal role (the experience of the minority) rather than at anxious despair (the fate of the majority)? Again, the metaphor of masculinity[1] helps to highlight the problem. Sent to a socially isolated environment to perform, untrained and ill-experienced, a complex twenty-four-hour-a-day job (unpaid, uninsured, perhaps altogether unrewarded) what worker would not fall prey to anxious feelings? Adding those who reported 'baby blues' in hospital to those who described an anxiety state on coming home produces a figure of 91 per cent. Nearly a quarter of the sample women were also overcome by more enduring depressed feelings (though only three of these had drug treatment).[2]*

Postnatal depression	
'Blues' in hospital	84%
Anxiety state on coming home	71%
Other depression	24%

Ellen George and Maureen Paterson are two of the three women treated by their GPs with drugs for postnatal depression. Both had 'difficult' births: Ellen had a manual removal of the placenta with a general anaesthetic and a postpartum haemorrhage; Maureen had a protracted labour and a forceps delivery under general anaesthetic. While they mention the possibility of some connection between these experiences and feeling depressed, it seems that what they describe is truly an exacerbation of the normal tensions first-time mothers feel when they first become sole guardians of their children.

MAUREEN PATERSON, ex-library assistant:
Oh terrible I was, really. I came out of hospital on the Friday, came home here and I was fine. And the Friday night he was very unsettled, because he wasn't feeding properly and it just – I just kept *crying* all the time. Poor Henry, he didn't know what to do. So we were going up my Mum's for Christmas anyway, so he rang her up and she came down. She said look, you come up with me now, just bring everything up she said and you stay with me. I just got worse. I felt awful. I felt I could never – I would never be able to cope, you know. And in the end, the Saturday after Christmas, they had to get the doctor in because I was so bad. I didn't even *like* the baby and I was so *tired* all the time. Anyway, he came round and he said it was acute postnatal depression and he said I wasn't to do *anything* for the baby. He said if somebody can look after you and the baby, or else he said you'll have to go into hospital. Of course my Mum said she's not going back into hospital; you can stay here. So me Mum and Henry looked after him.

But it was terrible. I felt really awful. I've never *ever* felt like that in me life. I thought I was going mad, I thought I was going peculiar. I said to Henry I'm sure I'm going . . . I kept thinking that I'd never be able to cope with him and do anything else at all, because when the doctor came round he told me exactly what I was going to tell him. He said you're useless, he said, and he said you'll never be able to manage. But he said probably what it is, he said, you had a bad time, and it's just taking it out of you like that: it's just a shock to your system.

I mean I'd heard about baby blues – I mean postnatal depression, I thought that was it in hospital, those few tears, that was it. I never *dreamt* that you could get . . . and I mean I thought it was *me*, but when the doctor said it *is* quite common . . . but to feel that bad with it, I don't think I've ever cried so much in all me life. That's something I *never* want to go through again: that couple of weeks, it was a terrible feeling. I don't *know* whether it was reaction because I'd had a rough time and I was still probably tired. I don't know. But everybody was very good. If I hadn't had anyone to help me, I mean these girls that *do* turn against their babies, I think it would be quite easy to do it. If you didn't have somebody there and if you felt the way I *did* feel. I mean I think if I'd been on my own I would have just *left* him, I think. I wouldn't have seen to him, I felt that bad. . . .

ELLEN GEORGE, ex-health visitor:
I blame it on childbirth, the whole thing. I mean I may have been

waiting to have a depression all these years and it took childbirth to trigger it off, but I don't think so. I think it was the whole childbirth.

In hospital everybody expected to cry on the third day. I mean I laughed about it beforehand and said well if you come to see me on the third day I'll be having my crying day! But that's all you're warned about, and I think you should be warned that the whole thing is much more of a trauma than perhaps you expect – to your physical and emotional state.

There didn't seem to be any *reason* for me to be depressed. And Emma was a good baby, which was another thing – she never really got on my nerves. I just felt so *drained* myself, I got feelings of panic, I felt so uptight in my stomach and I looked around me and I thought gosh: there's no one here who can cope with her. I felt uptight to the extent that I've had the runs, and I remember when I did exams I used to get exam nerves and I would get the runs, and it's exactly the same. And it's counter-productive because I knew I was meant to be eating well to get the iron up and resting a lot to get back to normal as well as for breastfeeding, and I felt I was just losing the battle. It was a sort of battle. I felt *so* desperate. I mean I've done all this academically, which I don't think helps at all, having to go out to people who are breaking down. I'm worried about breaking down.

My GP put me on Valium which didn't make any difference. I had several little crises, big crises. I went home to Ireland suddenly; one day my mother came over and collected me. I just felt so desperate and I couldn't cope and Andrew couldn't take any more time off work. I felt gradually more desperate. I stayed there three weeks, and Andrew came over and collected us both; I felt terrific at home. But when I came back I was sick, I think it was food poisoning, but I don't know – I associated it with nervousness. And gradually the week after I came back from Ireland I went downhill. And that weekend I just started to cry nearly all the time for no reason. I just couldn't stop, and I think Andrew was reluctant to accept that I really needed help. He *felt* that I just didn't have enough confidence in myself, that I *could* cope, but it was a question of confidence. Fortunately my social worker friend visited that weekend and she saw that I was very down. And I rang her up on the Sunday evening and said that I really couldn't face the next day. And she said see your doctor, and she came before Andrew left the next day, she was fantastic. She said I know *just* how you're feeling because I've been through depression myself. And when she arrived that morning she said you can either go to the Maudesley – they have an emergency department – or contact your

GP if you think you have faith in her. I said well I think I do. And sure enough she came, I rang her up that morning and she came pretty promptly, prescribed the tryptizol and explained all the side-effects. And at the same time as prescribing that, she put me in touch with her sister-in-law who was a doctor's wife, also a social worker, who'd also been very depressed, and she came round that afternoon, and she kept in touch with me practically every day for a week. She was really fantastic, and she described the whole thing, she'd had practically the same experience. That was lovely, it was good of my doctor, wasn't it? She offered me psychiatric help and I said see how we go over the next twenty-four hours: I was resisting that a bit. And she said well you *may* have to go into hospital, that might be the best thing for you. And Andrew said she wouldn't want to be stuck with the baby all the time. She said arrange this week that you've *always* got somebody with you, and I did: Mrs Lewis sat down and arranged the whole week. Andrew stayed home one day, and Mrs Lewis came another . . . and the week went by. Although I found it so humiliating; the day I went to Mrs Scott down the road I had to be down there at eight o'clock in the morning before Andrew left. And I found that terrible at my age with a baby. But once the drug had settled down I felt much better; she said it'd take about three days to work: it actually took about six to seven. I didn't feel depressed then but I felt terribly peculiar – I felt there was a sort of veil between me and the rest of the world – which was slightly better than being depressed, but still pretty ghastly. And then gradually the side-effects wore off. . . .

MOTHERS AND OTHERS

The way we live now most women have only their husbands to turn to when they feel like this. Yet the strain is too much for the nuclear family to take; mothers, mothers-in-law, sisters, aunts, can be saving graces. Would Ellen George have been depressed at home in Ireland with her mother, the rest of her (large) family and her childhood friends? It is clear from these accounts that sometimes 'depression' is nipped in the bud when someone else steps in to relieve the mother's isolation.

SASHA MORRIS:
When I actually came home with her and put her down I thought

good God, what if something's wrong: what am I going to do? It was the coldest day of the year, it was the worst time I could have picked to have the baby. I came out of that hospital and it was *freezing* – it was like being in the open: I was *terrified.* . . . I felt like sending her back because it was so cold. I stayed up on Friday night and they gave the long-range weather forecast, and it couldn't have been worse; they said there's going to be snow and sleet and temperatures won't go over freezing point. Oh God what am I going to do? I was in floods of tears, I cried for two whole days. It was everything.

She went to stay with her aunt, an ex-midwife, who lived next door to the hospital.

I think we've settled down very nicely. I think moving here and being able to go from room to room without freezing to death and being so close to the hospital I was reassured: I had this marvellous feeling – I could *see* the hospital out of the window. And having somebody to ask: my aunt really is very useful. She's got some good sound advice. She says stop worrying, stop panicking about things . . .

But the advice is only the tip of the iceberg. It is the solid emotional support and the practical help that count. Homecoming is a time for mothers and daughters: nearly three-quarters of mothers gave practical help to their daughters at this time.

ELIZABETH FARRELL:
I couldn't have managed without my mother, I couldn't have coped at all. I was so shocked, I couldn't *do* anything. I mean Mummy did all the cooking, shopping, cleaning: for two days I just had tears rolling down my cheeks all the time.

LOIS MANSON:
Honestly I don't know how I would have got through that first week if my mother hadn't been here. I really did need someone, because when I came home that Saturday, I didn't think I was ever going to go out again, I thought I was not going to be able to cope with normal life. And David mentioned the possibility of us having a meal, and I thought Christ am I expected to cook *and* have a baby? You know I just didn't think I was going to be able to cope with everyday things. She was super, in fact I did the cooking and she did absolutely everything else. She did all the washing and ironing and nursing the baby inbetween feeds and calming me down and gradually getting me back into normal life.

In some cases the transition to motherhood is smooth because the new mother's mother acts as scriptwriter, director, stage-manager and producer all in one. Nina Brady was very worried before Joseph's birth about how she would adjust to motherhood. She saw herself as a worker, not a mother (see pp. 64–5), and was concerned about the loss of independence and money that full-time domesticity would bring. But in the event . . .

I: Did you feel at all depressed?

NINA: No: I had my mother, that's why!*

I: Did the nurses give you advice about how to look after the baby?

NINA: Yes. About how to hold the baby and how to feed it. One nurse'd say one thing and another nurse'd say another. It didn't worry me because the only advice I took was from my own mother. She had eleven in poor times back in Ireland and they were all lovely. There was no such thing as sterilising but she always said she used to boil her bottles. Make sure everything was spotlessly clean. She said do that . . .

I've got four teats but them teats I found was too fast. It was my mother who told me: he started vomiting and I got scared when he used to throw up his feed. And my Mum said this teat is far too fast for the child . . . I had spare bottles, three spare bottles, with Cannon teats, so Mummy took one of those. She said your child won't vomit any more. She said the slower he takes his food, the better he digests it. If he takes it too quick, and gulps it, he'll bring it all up. And that was what was happening.

My mother says use your commonsense. If the child is roaring crying, he's obviously hungry or else thirsty. If you have fed him and he wakes up after one or two hours then the child is thirsty.

She used to leave here about eleven or twelve at night, when I'd given him the last feed. And she used to nurse him so long and rub his back and she'd say now he'll sleep all night, you wait and see. And he did. She used to nurse him, hold him differently from the way they do in hospital: she used to hold him like that [horizontally across her lap] and let him rest on her arms that way. She said that's very good for the baby; she said don't sit him up like this and hold him up. Rub his back: that's very comforting to the child. That's how I do it now. He brings up his wind real quick. And he falls asleep in your arms.

He cries when he's hungry. I always let him cry for about ten

---

*Her mother came over from Ireland for a few weeks and stayed with Nina's sister (a more capacious household) who had her fifth child at about the same time. She appears to have spent most of her daytime hours with Nina, instructing her in motherhood.

minutes. I think it's good for his lungs. Mummy said they must cry to exercise their lungs, because he doesn't cry at all, so he must cry sometimes, so let him cry for his feed. It's nice being a mother. It's nice looking after him. It's nice when he's awake and you can talk to him. I love talking to him. And when I'm feeding him I sing to him because Mummy always sang to us.

Mothers who have brought up children are the only people who really know what looking after a little baby is like. They do not have to be told about the appalling loneliness of nights spent with a baby crying.

ANGELA KING:

In the beginning she wouldn't go to sleep from about nine o'clock till about three o'clock; she just wouldn't go to sleep. She wasn't really crying, it was just sort of whining. It really gets you in the end. But I was lucky in a way because when she got too much my mother-in-law would take her. If she went on crying, she'd come in and take her out of the room. Because she said I know what it's like – she's had four – in the end she said it really gets you. She told me afterwards: that's why I used to come and take her from you when you'd had enough.

HILARY JACKSON:

In the night my mother gets out of bed as soon as she hears her. She gets up and I get up: we both get up. And I say to her: now what are we going to do? So she says well, I'll feed her – I'll warm the bottle and she feeds her, and I go down and make a cup of tea. So we sit there, we do a joint thing. It's quite good. I said to my husband well if I'd been on my own, and you'd been at work, I said you'd have come home and I wouldn't have been here and the baby wouldn't have been here. I would just have gone, literally.

Four months later, she reflects on the role her mother played:

Actually it was just being with me, being in the room with me while she was awake. And we both took it in turns to rock her off at night, to get her off. Or if I got up and went in and I just couldn't get her back I'd go into Mum and say I just can't get her back to sleep. Oh don't worry about it; you go back to bed, and I'll get her off! I mean she says *now* – I say to her now: were you tired? Oh she says I wouldn't admit it at the time but she said I was *really* tired. Much as you were. But she said I knew there would be a time when it wouldn't happen. She said of course you never believed that there would be a time because you'd never known it. She said I knew it wouldn't be for ever.

CRY BABIES

Everybody knows that babies cry but nobody knows how much they cry until they have one to look after. Crying time averages just over two hours a day at one month, and night sleeping under six hours.[3] *In the end, and even with the most patient of mothers, the baby makes its mother cross. Seventy per cent of the women said they sometimes felt angry towards the baby.*

Do you ever get cross with the baby?

RACHEL SHARPE:
Oh yes. I've threatened to drop him on his head. A couple of times I've really *hollered* at him and felt really terrible afterwards; I really wanted to shake him. He'd wakened up and I'd just got to sleep or something: I hadn't heard him, that was it; Francis woke me up and said I think he wants some food. And I had a *splitting* headache. And what he did, he took him out of his pram, and put him next to me so he was screaming in my ear and Francis was saying aren't you going to get up and feed him? I got up and ripped all the blankets off him – I was horrible!

JANET STREETER:
Yes, furious. Two o'clock at night, then it really makes me cross. In the beginning I felt like shaking him. I mean when I'm cross in the middle of the night I'm cross because I've got to get up: when I actually see him I'm not cross at all. But in the beginning I think we both felt like shaking him. I mean I did get hold of the basket thing and go like this [gestures] several times – only because you don't know *why* they're crying. I don't feel guilty at all because I realise it's normal and all my sisters have said they felt like that.

DEBORAH SMYTH:
Sometimes I did in the night, I used to shout at him. I feel sometimes like giving him a shake, but not a smack. He does make me cross when you're trying to go to sleep and he starts, I shout at him but as soon as you see his little face . . .

CHRISTINA LYNCH:
Not really. I think I did the first week. I was very tired and it was the

last night feed, half past twelve, and he wet his nappy as soon as I put it on him, and he started crying. I said shut up you stupid little bugger . . .

GILLIAN HARTLEY:
Oh yes. I wanted to stuff the dummy down his throat.

MAX: He'd got himself into a cycle which must be fairly typical I'm sure, when he would cry, I'd get out of bed and I'd lift him up, give him a couple of pats on the back, get him down again, make sure he was dry, wrap him up warm, rock him back and forth or bump him up and down until he subsided, get back into bed, put the clothes round me, switch the light off, and as soon as I'd done that he'd start again. And when I'd done that sort of six times in succession I really felt like thrusting his dummy so far into his gullet that it would stop. But I didn't, of course not. I did realise before that people come up to you and say silly things like how can anybody ever batter children? I would say that it must be the easiest thing in the world.

GILLIAN: He's not a *bad* baby.

NANCY CARTER:
I: And now you've got your own baby, can you understand how people can hit them?
NANCY: Yes.
I: I remember you saying before you had Joanna you couldn't understand it at all.
NANCY: Mmm. Yes.
I: What did you feel about being able to understand? Did it worry you or frighten you?
NANCY: I just felt I'd misjudged a lot of people. It was a revelation!

JULIET MORLEY:
I occasionally get cross with him when I'm trying to wind him and I *know* he's got wind, and he keeps sort of stretching and arching his back and won't sit forward. I sometimes feel like *grabbing* him and making him, quite roughly, because I know that's what he needs, and he won't do it. But I can understand how people feel – particularly in bad housing conditions, what it must be like in two rooms I dread to think.

Dawn O'Hara lives in one room with her husband and baby Simon.
I have to admit I have felt like that. It was one of those days when he wouldn't settle down all day and he would sit quiet on the bed if I'd

play with him on the bed, but the minute I put him in his cot he started. I gave him this hard knuckle, I didn't really hit him, don't think I hit him: I *tapped* him. You feel guilty then afterwards. I knew he was just being cranky. My husband says you're spoiling the child sometimes, that gets me really mad. I mean it's alright for people to say that, but when you're in one room listening to the baby crying you have to do something to please them. We're stuck in the one room. My husband comes in at night, the television's on. It's not fair really, when he comes in from work to have to keep the telly down low and the baby's crying and crying and crying, you know. And I know my husband can't get to sleep. And he gets up at half past five the next morning and he doesn't know where he's going. I can't live with him in one room, you see. I feel that I'm not pleasing Kevin and I'm not pleasing the baby. I just go out and I slam the door and I go into the kitchen and have a good old cry. Stupid. But I feel like that sometimes: I feel sometimes that he doesn't understand, yet he does. He's at work all day, I know he does a day's work and it's a hard job; and then when he comes in at night I'll give him his dinner and I mean I have the baby all day, you know what I mean?

Again, perhaps the right question to ask is not why some parents batter their children but why most parents refrain from doing so. If 70 per cent feel angry it is, after all, the minority who do not. And although feeling angry and expressing it in violence towards the child are in theory separate, in practice the feeling precedes and (in appropriate circumstances) provokes the action.[4]

One answer to the problem of crying is a dummy. Now out of fashion amongst the middle classes, a dummy can pose quite an ideological dilemma. Kate Prince swallowed her principles for the sake of peace:

It was last week, I was busy, I wanted to get on with something. A kid, at a school I've been doing some articles about, gave me a dummy along with some other presents and I'd stuck it in the steriliser and Mark said but we're not using *that:* he was absolutely going *crazy* about it: he said don't give it to her during the day, I can't bear the *look* of it. So I didn't and I didn't and I wanted to get on with this bit of sewing and she was going on and on and I thought hell, he doesn't have to *sit* with her all day screaming, I've *got* to get on with this job. So I gave it to her and she was quite happy, she seemed so contented, she wasn't all red and crying, she went all nice and pale and dozed off. I thought it *can't* be bad for her . . . She's happy and I'm happy. The funniest thing was, when I was ill just after that and I was miserable and Mark virtually had flu too, I mean he was really feeling bad, sore throat, cold, the lot, and he came in from work and she started to cry, and I mean I quite value the time we have together, our meal and so on, and I try to make it so that she's more or less asleep and quiet when he comes in: then she started, and we'd just sat down. And I thought oh hell, he was so snuffly and tired, so I thought well, and I crept upstairs and gave her the dummy and she shut up and he said what have you done? I said I gave her the dummy. He was so sick he didn't really complain very much; he was quite pleased. And the next day we were going somewhere and she was down here and she was crying and crying and crying in her carrycot. And suddenly she went quiet and *he'd* given her this dummy. And now he advocates the dummy! I do like her so much more since the dummy. It's changed our lives!

A REWARD IS OFFERED

Such problems may predominate in the early weeks, but they nevertheless coexist with tremendous feelings of love and commitment, delight, reward and pride. The baby is the mother's creation and possession. Through her labours she sustains it, and before her eyes the baby finds its toes, its fingers, its capacity to smile: comfort, happiness, excitement, laughter. Like those speeded up films of flowers blooming, babies almost visibly grow and prosper. Gradually the crying that seemed to have no cause or cure lessens, the baby begins to show by its behaviour that mother will become the needed and preferred person.

What do you like about looking after the baby?

I love the feeds and holding him, he looks up at me. He smiled last night, it wasn't wind; his whole face lit up. (*Deirdre James*)

The whole thing really, I enjoy sort of feeding him and that and holding him – I'd cuddle him all day I think if I didn't have anything else to do. (*Maureen Paterson*)

I mean it is a marvellous thing that one can actually *feed* this little thing and see these double chins growing and it's all from your body. (*Alison Mountjoy*)

This stage when he's falling asleep: I like just after a feed when he's a bit dozy and he wants to fall asleep. He's lovely. (*Grace Bower*)

I like doing her bath – I like washing her hair actually because she loves it so much. She's been yelling and screaming while you undress her and then there's absolute silence when you wash her hair: she loves it. (*Emma Buckingham*)

It's so satisfying when she's screaming her head off and you pick her up and she immediately stops. (*Catherine Andrews*)

He's just nice to have. (*Mary Rosen*)

Now I enjoy looking after her. I like to see her looking comfortable and clean and relaxed. And she seems a very confident little baby. She never seems to be fretful or whiny. And she instills confidence into me. (*Sasha Morris*)

I think that's why I don't want him to grow up. I think knowing that he's mine and no one can take him away from me. (*Michelle Craig*)

I *particularly* like breastfeeding her. I don't know whether I like the sensation, but I tell you what I *do* enjoy: I can be miles away from her and you suddenly think about her and you can feel it sort of beginning to come. And I enjoy the feeling that she's dependent on me. She smiles tremendously and she's started to make noises now. I'll never forget seeing a documentary on television about a monkey , and the mother had had every single muscle in her face cut so she couldn't move her face at all, and the baby monkey was sort of clutching onto her body but would look anywhere except at her face: he got no response from the mother's face, it was *terrible*. (*Elizabeth Farrell*)

She does smile, but that's wind isn't it? I always smile back, and I think what a fool you are Lois, smiling at her, she's not smiling at *you* but I mean I *respond* to the smile. (*Lois Manson*)

Do you feel you have a relationship with your baby?

Yes I think so. She always takes a whole bottle with me but with no one else, not even Barry. She leaves the last ounce. (*Anne Bloomfield*)

He's beginning to follow me with his eyes. I think he laughs more to me. I wouldn't say it in front of my husband, but I think he does. He has more of a hearty laugh; he laughs more often. (*Dawn O'Hara*)

Well no, I think it's developing. I think she knows who I am now. I think she responds to me but I wouldn't say that there's a real relationship yet. (*Clare Dawson*)

I'm beginning now, at first she was my every waking thought if you see what I mean, but now I do actually try to read a book when I'm feeding her or listen to the radio or think. . . . It's a natural process, you begin to turn your eyes out a little bit. (*Sophy Fisher*)

While the baby is learning who its mother is, the mother is learning to be a mother. First birth is a momentous event in a society that assigns the child-rearing role to women. From being secretaries, factory workers, schoolteachers, women become Mothers.

ARE YOU AWARE OF BEING A MOTHER?

LOUISE THOMPSON, law student, 1 month after Polly's birth:
That's funny because a friend of mine asked me the same thing and I said you have this *image* of mothers, it's a different person from being just a woman who has a baby. I mean that's all it is really. I mean *being a mother*, I don't know.
  I feel stuck in a way, stuck to her. I mean I really feel much less free. I said to Oliver you know *your* life is really the same. You just come home and there's a baby; that's the only difference. It's funny because *he* was the one who wanted a baby.

ANNE BLOOMFIELD, ex-barmaid:
No, not really. I don't really feel any different. I think when you feel like a mother you're supposed to feel different aren't you? I don't feel any different.

DEIRDRE JAMES, ex-jewellery assembler:
I forget it sometimes. Especially in the afternoons, he's gone off to sleep, I've thought, I'm free. Then I've heard a little noise on the intercom and I've thought I mustn't forget the baby. I feel *proud*. Especially when people say he's a nice baby, isn't he lovely?

JO INGRAM, further education teacher:
I don't feel I've changed that much really. I just feel I've got another thing to do – to fit in.

JANET STREETER, ex-dance instructor:
I suppose one will be when he gets older but at the moment you're a *machine* more than anything else.

NINA BRADY, ex-shop assistant:
I don't feel like I'm a mother. Until he starts talking and calling me Mum. I was making his bottle the other day; who was holding him? It wasn't Tom, it was my sister, and I said never mind Auntie Nina's coming with your bottle – this is what me sister's kids call me. And they started to laugh!

I still have the feeling that I'd like to be at work. I haven't got much to do. I think it's boring if you haven't got a lot to do. If you have three or four children you wouldn't have time to be bored. Now, if you hadn't come in, I would have sat down and read that paper, or written a letter. Nothing to do.

GRACE BOWER, switchboard operator:
At times I still don't think he's mine. Lying in bed yesterday I heard him crying and I thought what's that? I still haven't quite realised that we've got a baby and it is *ours* – no one else's. I still think he's a stranger at times. I still can't think of myself as a mother. When Bob talks to the baby about 'your mother' I think who's that? A lot of times when I'm downstairs, I'm not with him, I forget *completely* that I've got a baby.

CATHERINE ANDREWS, ex-receptionist:
I'm very conscious of her being upstairs all the time, my thoughts keep going up there. My mother said I kept referring to her as 'she' – I never used her name, and I suddenly would say something about 'she' – oh 'she' did such and such today or something; and Mummy said it was incredible, nobody else would know what I was talking about. I expected everyone else to click immediately. A one track mind.

ELIZABETH FARRELL, ex-publisher's assistant:
I went to Queensway shopping, and I looked round at all the mothers pushing prams and felt a great *empathy* towards them: I've got a baby, too.

JANE TARRANT, ex-librarian:
You *do* feel different once you've had a baby. I remember going round the shops – I was doing my Christmas shopping – and seeing other mothers and thinking I'd been through the same thing as they had. I think you feel a shared experience with other mothers. It was quite a nice feeling.

If I go out somewhere I take a lot more trouble over my appearance now. People have said ooh you look very nice and I've said yes, because I don't want people to think of me as a frumpy old mother. And yet when I was at work I didn't bother at all.

SARAH MOORE, ex-civil servant:
Yes I think I am. I feel older; I feel much older. I think maybe I feel more satisfied in a way. I wasn't uptight before and I've always been quite calm, but now I feel even calmer. Maybe it's because I'm still breastfeeding – there are still hormones surging around. We'll see what I feel like in six months' time! I do feel much more satisfied and calm is certainly the word at the moment: nothing ruffles me.

LOIS MANSON, research worker:
I told the greengrocer I'd had a baby. I sort of generally bring it into the conversation. I feel that it's very important being a mother and people don't appreciate it very much, unmarried people, people without children. I don't think they *begin* to realise all the changes it makes to people's lives. And I think they don't appreciate the *importance* of being a mother.

DAWN O'HARA, ex-packer:
Yes I think you feel, it makes you feel different, sort of, doesn't it? I think it makes you kind of – not *better*, but you feel a better person. I like it. I wish I could give him more, though. I wish I had a place of my own, a nice little house. With his own little bedroom.

SASHA MORRIS, was an air-hostess, but gave up work after marriage:
Actually I feel more *useful* now. Before I had her I did feel I was a bit useless – I *did* nothing; I never bothered to work. I feel *better* for having things to do. I often felt at a loss for things to do before.

JULIET MORLEY, ex-rebate officer:
I don't know quite what you mean by that. I don't really feel that I've got an identity at the moment. So I suppose I do feel different, yes. I spend far less time thinking about myself and what I want to do and how I feel.

CHRISTINA LYNCH, ex-traffic warden:
Even if we're just the two of us on our own I keep thinking, I'm a Mum. It's nice. I've always wanted to have a baby.

MAUREEN PATERSON, ex-library assistant:
Yes, now. It's a nice feeling, sort of proud, we sort of take him out and think he's *ours* . . .

Some women welcome the label 'mother' for what it represents in the feminine image and in ideas about family life. Babies are symbols. The line of nappies in the garden, the pram in the hall, the toys on the carpet – these impedimenta of babyhood proudly announce the full achievement of femininity, the making of a family. Others, less taken in by the notion that being a woman means being a mother, may nevertheless find recognisably maternal feelings overtaking them. Motherhood may also mean a loss of identity, the self becoming submerged in the needs of this other person, so that it apparently has no separate existence. But most of all at this stage, it is simply difficult to comprehend what has happened. The feeling of motherhood will only begin to fit comfortably when time eases the shock of birth.

LITTLE PEOPLE

Babies are born individuals. Of course they are moulded by their social settings, but they have ready-made personalities as well.[5] To the first-time mother this may come as a surprise, particularly if her only learning experiences have been with the plasticity of dolls and with the easy admonitions of babycare books, which read as though a baby can be guided into any pattern of behaviour. In the descriptions that follow, babies appear as immensely capable from an early age of making their needs known in no uncertain fashion. It is clear that their characters are partly assessed in terms of behaviour – a 'good' baby is quiet and regular (predictable) in its habits. A 'bad' baby cries and is more difficult to comfort.

What sort of person is your baby?

A cry baby! What sort of person? Very bad-tempered, very bad-tempered. (*Grace Bower*)

I don't really know. I think he's going to be *strong-willed* really. When he makes up his mind he wants to do something, he sort of keeps on. (*Deirdre James*)

He's stubborn. He has a temper. When he's pleased – he's just like us actually, when he's content and happy he's a perfectly wonderful person to have around and when he's out of sorts he's absolutely a monster man. (*Gillian Hartley*)

I know that my feelings about his personality aren't right, I just feel that he's a wilful minded little fucker. He wants his food. But I know that's ridiculous. I know that he's just a little animal that needs feeding. (*Jo Ingram*)

I suppose babies are a bit schizophrenic. When they're good, they're very very good. Most of the time he's calm and happy. I think he's quite good – I think he needs to be handled just by one person. (*Jane Tarrant*)

Oh she's got quite a lot of personality. She's very alert, and she's not a crier really. She's got quite a temper – when she really wants to, she's one of these babies that doesn't *breathe*. (*Alison Mountjoy*)

I think she's getting rather spoilt. She seems to cry and then as soon as we pick her up she stops. She's quite contented. (*Catherine Andrews*)

I'll tell you something – he's a good baby. There's no night feed. Never. He's not a four-hourly baby, you know. (*Nina Brady*)

An angel! No, he's good. (*Dawn O'Hara*)

Oh dear. Demanding. Loving. That's all really. (*Nicola Bell*)

I think it's incredible that they can do all these human things like fart and shit. I don't know: a baby. A cry baby. (*Louise Thompson*)

She's marvellous – I praise her to everybody. Everybody says how lucky I am to have such a quiet baby. (*Sasha Morris*)

Some mothers feel that their babies lack personality because five weeks is too early for it to have developed: they have much more to say about the characters of their children at five months. Yet one aspect of a baby's character is evident from birth: its sex. Ideas about the different behaviour of boys and girls abound in our culture. Thirty per cent of mothers thought (before they had their own babies) that even as babies boys and girls behave differently. Hence it is not surprising to find that in these personality descriptions of babies certain terms are associated more with femaleness and others with maleness (see table).

This awareness of a baby's sex may be quite unconscious. Asked if they thought the baby's sex affected their relationship with her or him, 34 per cent of the mothers said yes. But it is not an easy question to answer:

I wondered about that. I wondered how I would be feeling if I had a boy. I don't know. I can't imagine it really – what it would have been like if I had a boy, whether it would have been any different or not. I mean a baby is a baby really isn't it? There's definitely nothing boyish about her. (*Catherine Andrews*)

I suppose it must do. It's difficult to say really because with little boys I think their mothers have a sort of sexual relationship with them. . . . The first week I thought she was me; it was really strange: such a strong feeling. I could just see myself, and it was as if I was feeding myself. (*Sue Johnson*)

That's another difficult one. Certainly to start with I didn't take his

Terms used to describe the personality of babies at one month

Girls	Boys
A little gannet	A little devil
Very nice	A mind of his own
Quite good	Crafty
Loving	A bit irritable
Niggly	Stubborn
A thinker	A little animal
Like her mother	Like his father
Very good temperament	A monster man
Very alert	Got a temper
Smiles really easily	He's going to lead the union
A cry baby	Bloody minded
Pretty	Very strong
Responsive	A two-legged pig
Placid	A nuisance
Self-possessed	Nosy
Very independent	Dead cheeky
Interested in what's going on	Very inquisitive
She knows what she wants	Wants attention
Wakeful	An artful little thing
Quiet	An angel
Rather spoilt	Greedy
Quite cute	A straightforward personality
Marvellous	Very bad-tempered

sex into account at all, I don't think. But recently sometimes I wonder if I feel differently about him because he's a boy. Particularly when it comes to, I start wondering if he's going to get an Oedipus complex, you know when you're sort of changing his nappy and breastfeeding him, you know you start wondering. I'm always particularly careful to see that he's dry before I put the new nappy on and you're sort of patting him round and virtually caressing him: you start wondering if he's going to be scarred for life! (*Juliet Morley*)

He *looks* just like a little boy. But I can't tell whether it's my conditioning. He's got Steve's hands. Steve's hands are really broad, he's got a worker's hands. He's an advanced builder's labourer. He's going to lead the union. (*Jo Ingram*)

I'm aware of him as a boy. He's quite violent now, he scratched my face the other day. And he's always kicking – you can't get his legs down when you change his nappy and he's got his arms up here under his bib when you take the bottle out to see how much he's had: his arms go straight up; try and take them down – he won't let you! (*Janette Watson*)

I think he's a *cuddly* baby. He likes to be cuddled and a lot of people have said little boys are more affectionate than little girls. But no, I don't, I couldn't imagine really *having* a little girl. I think you get used to what you've got. (*Maureen Paterson*)

I didn't want a boy so I suppose so. I don't really know: I suppose it's a terrible thing to admit, but I think they're nicer to dress. Little dolls. That's one reason. I think they're more fun. I quite like the idea of a daughter, giving it motherly advice when I'm fifty. It's a terrible thing to admit but because she's a girl I think I don't mind what she does in life. If it were a boy I'd think oh he's got to be a doctor or a brain surgeon. But I think so long as she's nice and pleasant to everyone . . . which is *bad*, that attitude. But she won't necessarily have to be a breadwinner. I said to Mark I'm sure if she'd been a boy baby, one of these ten pound lumps, I would have hated her guts, because in the first two or three weeks I hated her anyway. On and off. (*Kate Prince*)

I think I do slightly. I think I feel a bit closer to her. I always wanted a daughter. (*Nicola Bell*)

Yes. I'm really glad she's a girl. What's the opposite of a misogynist? (*Loise Thompson*)

I think if I didn't have a husband it wouldn't make any difference. But it's rather nice in a way still to be the only woman around. I mean it's a bit stupid really, because there's nothing sexual in it. But you might think oh they're going to dote on their daughter . . . I think it's only insofar as *other* people react to him. (*Jane Tarrant*)

THE OTHER SIDE OF MOTHERHOOD

Looking after a baby twenty-four hours a day is an experience that cannot be imagined in advance. Ninety one per cent of the sample mothers said it differed from their expectations – motherhood is

Is looking after the baby anything like you thought it would be?	
Yes	9%
No	91%

more exhausting, even if it is also more rewarding, than the rosy pictures in the books. Images of how people thought it would be come more sharply into focus when viewed through the lens of reality: a full-time job, a responsibility for life. . . .

SARAH MOORE, ex-civil servant:
It takes up so much time. I honestly didn't realise how much time it would take up. I mean I *didn't* realise I'd be feeding for an hour – and that's how long a feeding takes, you know breastfeeding and bottle-feeding . . . then water, then changing the nappy. So I mean I don't have much time. I'm amazed how I managed to go to work before and run this place.

ELIZABETH FARRELL, ex-publisher's assistant:
I think you have to learn several things, or at least I've had to. The first is that she's not a machine – that's just there to be fed and watered and changed and bathed and so on: that she's a person, that's one thing. And another thing that I've had to learn is that you don't need to take any notice *every* time she cries.

SOPHY FISHER, television producer:
I don't think I'd really prepared myself for quite how restricting she would be. I mean I hadn't actually thought about it, about just how much planning it takes to have a haircut or go out and buy a loaf of bread – or think of going to see a play, that sort of thing. I mean even taking her to see friends or something, not only do you have to pack up a bag of nappies and spare babygros and all that sort of thing – which I wouldn't have known – but you have to time it very carefully so she's not going to want feeding on the journey or on the way back. It's not something that *worries* me, but it wasn't something that I particularly *anticipated.*

CHRISTINA LYNCH, ex-traffic warden:
It's about twice as bad. It's not really hard work, it's *extra* work, extra washing. Obviously from a purely selfish point of view your time is not your own. If I feel like it I can't just sit and read a book all day. I can't just go out to the shops when I feel like it. You're tied. I used to say to Keith, you wait till you have to get up in the night and do night feeds, but I never realised, it was very stupid of me, exactly what was involved. You can read about it but. . . . The fact that it *is* so restricting. I mean obviously you can get babysitters and so on, but it never occurred to me that I wouldn't be able to go down to the shops,

or I couldn't even just slip out to post a letter. I mean I *could* do but I don't fancy leaving him. All they've got to do is be sick and inhale it and you'd never forgive yourself. It *is* difficult, because although you read it, they don't actually tell you *all* the aspects. They tell you about the feeding and changing and clothing – they don't tell you about the other side, it is not until you have the baby that you know what's involved.

LOIS MANSON, research worker:
I wasn't in the *least* bit prepared for any of it. When I spoke to you before I wasn't the *least* bit worried about it, I was going to cope with it. But honestly, I was absolutely shattered at the terrific demands she made upon me and the total change it made to my life. I hadn't thought in terms of the three-hourly or four-hourly commitment at all. And I suppose in a way you can't *really* appreciate it until it actually happens. People say to you rest now, because you won't be able to when you have the baby, and you just don't take it in: you say, oh yes.

How much difference do you think having a baby has made to your life?

It's really changed my whole life. That's the truth. What an awful thought. (*Louise Thompson*)

I don't go anywhere now. (*Anne Bloomfield*)

Everything is absolutely completely different. I mean I look at the news and there could be a third world war and it's really not important at the moment. (*José Bryce*)

I used to drink cups of tea all day long; now I don't drink any tea. I can't make it or I can't drink it. [To baby] I can't do anything, can I? (*Diana Meade*)

Oh a lot. Turned it upside down. She has changed it completely. I used to be self-centred and I'm not any more; I haven't got the time to be. I'm thinking of her all the time. What time she'll be waking up, what I must do. I don't think about myself any more. (*Sasha Morris*)

He's turned it upside down, if that's any sort of difference. I mean everything just centres round him, the whole day and night, it all depends on his whims and needs. (*Rachel Sharpe*)

Well I can't imagine life without him now, I suppose. When I came home from hospital I said to Simon can you imagine life without him? And Simon said oh yes quite easily. I was *horrified*. I said *I* can't. But that's automatically a woman . . . (*Mary Rosen*)

He's changed my life completely. My actual *way* of life, and also to being a different person. It's really the feeling of being a family. Before you're just two people who are together. And afterwards you're a family. You've got this real interest in common with your husband. I think that's probably the biggest difference. (*Jane Tarrant*)

I was thinking the other day this is probably the most important single thing that has ever happened in my life up to now. And probably ever will happen. And it is *totally* possessing isn't it? (*Sophy Fisher*)

It's changed my life completely because I'm not working now. I had to give up work. That's the biggest change of the lot. For nine, ten years I've always been working. I've always been out at work, I've never missed a day. It's different altogether. Very strange. I suppose you get used to it just like you got used to going to work. . . . (*Nina Brady*)

CHAPTER 8

Menus

I used to think breastfeeding was like falling off a log, and then I found out otherwise.

. . . the first principle of infant feeding is, after all, to feed the infant.[1]

A major theme of the early weeks is feeding. Indeed, for months the mother's concern for the baby tends to be focused on what, how much and how often it eats. A baby that is feeding and growing 'well' is a prize for the mother's efforts, a tangible token of her love and work. Conversely, a baby who gains weight more slowly than it 'should', and who perhaps cries a lot and seems unsatisfied, is a thorn in the mother's flesh, a sign of maternal failure. Of course such an attitude is fanned by the professional advisers of baby feeding – paediatricians, health visitors and so forth – who take it as axiomatic that the baby's growth and happiness must depend on a mother's care.

A new mother listens to these advisers, but she also listens to those who have reared babies without the benefits of professional training: mothers, mothers-in-law, sisters, friends. And she listens to her baby, who may have ideas of its own. What goes into the mouths of babies is a mix of all these ingredients, a compromise between the different messages. The baby (its size, sleeping habits, contentment, bowel movements) becomes the only valid arbiter of success.

BREAST IS BEST?

Before a first baby is born, breast versus bottle is a theoretical question only. Classes may be attended, books read, friends and relations talked to, but any decision made is apt to be challenged by the reality of a screaming infant with gums like an iron clamp, a bottomless stomach and a rage of quite unimaginable proportions. Similarly, notions about when 'solid' food should become part of the infant's diet may be thrown out with the baby's bathwater once a real baby's real appetite becomes a factor to be reckoned with; the way to a baby's heart is, after all, through its stomach. One result of this conflict is that nearly a third of mothers do not feed their babies on the kind of milk (human, cows') they intended, and more than half introduce solids earlier than they planned to.

Intention and practice in baby feeding	
Breastfed or bottlefed:	
as planned	70%
not as planned	30%
Solids introduced:	
when planned	45%
not when planned	55%

Professional opinion today strongly supports breastfeeding. Like natural childbirth, natural infant feeding has to become fashionable in a society that is technological 'by nature'. But the impetus for a return to the old ways – prolonged breastfeeding, late introduction of solid food – is scientific, not sentimental; medical research has shown that these ways are simply better for the child.[2] Most mothers pick up this conclusion; why then do they not all follow it? As with questions about postnatal depression and baby battering, common sense should perhaps lead this question to be rephrased. Given all the obstacles prevailing in today's technological culture to 'natural' behaviour, why is it, for example, that some mothers choose breastfeeding?

Why do you want to breastfeed?

I automatically think of babies as being breastfed. It's natural. So many people say ugh, I couldn't bear that – my friend's got four and she's bottlefed all of them. I can't understand her attitude, it's not as if she's a gadabout, going out to the theatre and dinner and that, so that feeding it herself would interfere with that. To me it's not natural, to my mind every woman should want to breastfeed. Whether I'll be able to, or not, I don't know. (*Christina Lynch, breastfed for 3 weeks*)

Before I was pregnant I always found it repulsive, I never wanted to. Since I've been pregnant I've felt differently about it. As soon as I got pregnant and started reading books about it I felt it was my responsibility. (*Nicola Bell, still breastfeeding at 5 months*)

Well purely because it's a natural thing . . . I just feel that it's a natural thing and God intended it to be that way and it should be that way. (*Josephine Lloyd, breastfed for 9 days*)

I don't feel incredibly religious about breastfeeding. I'd like to do it because I'd like the sensations of it and because it's supposed to be better for the baby. They're also supposed to crap less which I was thrilled about. (*Alison Mountjoy, still breastfeeding at 5 months*)

My mother's always done it, to me it seems more natural. That's what breasts are made for really. (*Pat Jenkins, breastfed for 11 weeks*)

I probably will, given that anything's going to be a hassle I think it'll be less of a hassle than bottlefeeding . . . I'm lazy, that's the only reason. I'm not breastfeeding for emotional reasons – that I want to be close or anything. Just because it's convenient. (*Jo Ingram, breastfed for 4½ months*)

Women who want to bottlefeed put some of these arguments in reverse: bottlefeeding can be seen as more convenient than breastfeeding for example. But the superiority of bottlefeeding for the baby's health is not cited as a reason. Many of those who say they want to bottlefeed also say they are unclear about their reasons.

Why do you want to bottlefeed?

HILARY JACKSON:

Because I don't want it so dependent. I don't want to be there every single time that it needs to be fed. And I think that my husband would like the idea of taking over and feeding it himself. I think he likes the idea of it. I think he would think I was too protective towards it if I was breastfeeding it, I'd *have* to be there every single time. I know they're supposed to get on better being breastfed, well fair enough, I was bottlefed and I survived. The disadvantages of breastfeeding are enormous. I've been out with people for a meal and it's all leaked and you know friends have been really distressed over it. They've walked down the road and seen a kiddie, and it's started, this is the type of thing. I wouldn't like to put myself through *that*.

RACHEL SHARPE:

I think probably for health reasons more than anything. Probably I'll become anaemic and I just feel I'll probably have a lot of trouble.

JANET STREETER:

I'm not at all keen to breastfeed, it sounds quite ridiculous but it really almost turns my stomach. Doesn't it sound stupid; I can't explain why. It embarrasses me to see other people breastfeeding in public; this girlfriend who's just had a baby, she would come to dinner and do it, I'd have to ask her not to. I don't know why: I can't understand the feeling, but it is there. And my husband's very keen that I should breastfeed. But I really think that if I don't want to, there's no point in doing it, because half the reason for doing it is the feeling, isn't it? So that you can give it the nearness thing. I *know* it's better for the baby, and all that. It's a very difficult feeling to overcome; one feels a bit guilty, because it *is* better for the baby. And there is such a lot about it now, and I get the impression that the hospital are going to do their best to push one to breastfeed if they can.

And the hospital does; VERA ABBATT:
Well I wasn't sure at the time but at the hospital, the midwife advised me that I should breastfeed, she just said I should, so I said I would probably do it in hospital but I didn't really believe in it, so I wouldn't do it at home. She said that's entirely up to you Mrs Abbatt, she said, but we would rather you did it in the hospital. So I thought well, fair enough. But to me it's a stupid idea altogether, well, you can't see what the baby's having, you don't know whether it's being fed properly. To me, if you're feeding it out of a bottle you can tell exactly what he's having, whether he's had enough, you know that he's well fed. But I can't see how you can possibly know he's well fed if you're feeding him with the breast.
I: Have you ever seen anyone breastfeed?
VERA: Yes, my aunt. I saw my aunt breastfeed. I didn't really think about it at the time, I was a bit young at the time. I thought my mother would *never* do something like that.
I: So your mother didn't breastfeed you?
VERA: I don't know; I've never asked her. I don't think she'd approve of me asking really.

KIRSTY MILLER:
I: What did you say when the doctor asked you if you wanted to breastfeed?
KIRSTY: Said no. He said why? So I said I didn't want to.
I: What did he say about that?
KIRSTY: Nothing . . . he just said that there was a sister or somebody that you could, you know, if I wanted to go and see her about it.
I: Did you?
KIRSTY: No.
I: Have you ever seen anyone breastfeeding?
KIRSTY: No. My sister never sort of believed in it. None of my family did.
I: Did your mother breastfeed you?
KIRSTY: No. Well my mother never agreed with it actually. Don't

know why. She just, you know, I remember when my sister came back to her and she was expecting her first and somebody had told her about breastfeeding, she, mother, said don't. She never gave any reason. . . .

The hospital's admonitions in favour of breastfeeding simply come too late for most women, whose attitudes are already shaped by the intimate influence of 'mother knows best'. And if a woman has never seen anyone else breastfeed, she may come to the conclusion that breasts are not to be used for feeding babies.

Mothers and breastfeeding		
Mother:	% of women who want to breastfeed	% of women who did breastfeed
Breastfed	83%	88%
Didn't breastfeed	50%	36%

People say are you going to feed her? Shall I take the children away? No, what the hell! They don't know what they're there for, do they? They just think they're some sort of ornament. One little boy, he was watching someone do it, and when she changed sides he said what's wrong with that side? Is that its first course and that its afters? (*Sandy Wright*)

Decision and indecision

Of those women who eventually bottlefeed, many remain 'don't knows' throughout pregnancy. Responding in part to outside pressures in favour of breastfeeding, they continue to feel that breastfeeding is somehow not 'nice', i.e. it is sexual or 'animal'.

DAWN O'HARA:

9 weeks pregnant:
I hear some people breastfeed, some people, they can't breastfeed, they have to bottlefeed. I think my mother always gave us the bottle. I can't remember really. I think she did, or maybe she did breastfeed and I didn't know. Do you have to breastfeed a baby? Is it nice? I don't know which is best.

32 weeks pregnant:
Some other girls was telling me if you don't breastfeed your baby they take the milk from you. Is that true? They don't take it for other babies, do they? Could I do it just in the hospital, and then . . . the baby wouldn't get sick? Because people say it's better for your womb and everything. Last time you came I was definitely going to bottle-

feed but now I'm definitely going to breastfeed. I would like to breastfeed my baby but I can't.

I: Why not?

DAWN: Well I'll tell you now, when the baby's born his sister wants to come over just to be with him while I'm in hospital, right? Now we've only got one room, you see, and the television – we actually *live* in that room, and I don't know the way I'd feel. But I feel embarrassed now. I just couldn't be sitting down . . . I really couldn't, you know. And everyone is telling me oh you should breastfeed your baby and I feel *guilty*, you know what I mean?

I: Does the thought of breastfeeding upset you?

DAWN: You see I don't really know when it's *your* baby, you're not used to things like that, are you? I would love to if I had my own private little room and I was with the baby myself. You know what I mean? But I wouldn't like to be doing it in front of my husband or anyone else. I just couldn't you know. I don't know whether other people feel that they don't want to, because I never really speak to anyone else about it. . . . [She bottlefed in the end.]

NINA BRADY:

20 weeks pregnant:

I have one sister who breastfeeds, she's in America. The one over here doesn't; I don't know why. I think she breastfeeds while she's in hospital – they really make you do that for a few days. But as soon as she gets it home she puts it on the bottle. I think it was because it hurted her or something: she couldn't do it. There's a lot of people who can't breastfeed.

I: There's a lot who can.

NINA: And don't do it, I know.

I: What about your mother?

NINA: No. I don't know why, she didn't feed any of us. And it wasn't a sterilised bottle, it was a Guinness bottle, if you don't mind. I remember her giving it to Timmy, the Guinness bottle, the one that's at home now. In Ireland they couldn't get these bottles. They're miles away from the shops, darling, you're in the country and the bottle might fall into the fire, an open fire, and it's plastic, and you mightn't have too many of them. And the child is crying: you've got to feed it.

I: At the hospital did they ask you how you wanted to feed the baby?

NINA: Yes, three of them asked me, two nurses and the doctor. I said I didn't know and he said have you talked it over with your husband,

and I said no, which we hadn't. And they said we've got classes here on breastfeeding which we'd like you to come to. I don't know: but they persuade you a lot in the hospital to breastfeed. The way they talked yesterday – they said it's a natural thing, it's more natural than anything else in the world to breastfeed your baby. I don't think they're wrong, I think they're right, I know it's natural. And they explained that your baby doesn't get as many colds or flus . . . I wouldn't mind. I'd be scared, like I said to the doctor, that I may not be able to do it. He said you've got two breasts, haven't you?

35 weeks pregnant:
I'm going to bottlefeed. My husband doesn't like breastfeeding, I don't know why. It took him a long time to tell me as well. I think the reason is, he thinks of it – and I'll be quite honest with you, because some Irish people are very ignorant and they laugh about it and they think it's wrong – and himself, he was brought up that way. My husband was breastfed, but he's brought up like your body is dirty, this is it. He thinks it's an animal thing to do.

In this sample of women having their first baby, antenatal education seems ineffective in its declared objective – to raise the breastfeeding rate.[3] Women who originally wanted to breastfeed were confirmed in their views that breastfeeding is best, but those who chose bottlefeeding had to carry a heavier burden of guilt.

In all, 77 per cent of the women did breastfeed their babies at least once. By five weeks, the proportion was down to 59 per cent and by five months 38 per cent were still breastfeeding.[4]

Bottlefeeding, a technological act, should be difficult but in fact seems easy. Modern paraphernalia (plastic bottles, sterilising tablets, ready-prepared easy-to-mix milk formulae) mean that the elementary rules can be readily grasped and followed. The bottles are transparent with the ounces or millilitres clearly marked, so that the mother always knows how much food the baby has had. Bottlefeeding involves no complicated physical sensations, no management of clothing; supply and demand can be instantly equated.

I'm so tempted to go over to total bottlefeeding. It's so straight-forward, you mix up the feed, you know how much you're giving and it's all so clean cut. I mean, for instance, if I don't rest during the day I dry up slightly, and stuff like this. So therefore when you're bottlefeeding it's so much easier, and also the babies I'm sure thrive on it because it's so much easier. They don't have to work so hard . . .
(Cary Wimborne)

A CONFIDENCE TRICK

*On the other hand, because breastfeeding is 'natural' it is expected to be easy.
'You think because it's natural you ought just to be able to do it.' But culture
affects nature, and, like childbirth, uncomplicated delivery (of baby or milk) is
uncommon. The mother does not instinctively know how to position the baby at the
breast and even if the baby does there may be too much or not enough milk. The
baby has not read the baby books and may not know that it is supposed to take its
required rations in exactly ten minutes or whatever each side, then fall into a
contented sleep for three hours forty minutes until the next feed is due. The mother
has never fed a baby before and the baby has never been fed. Like skate-boarding
or piano-playing, only practice makes perfect.*

LOIS MANSON and JANE:
I can understand why they give up; it's *confidence*, isn't it? You really
did have to persevere; the obstacles were incredible. I suppose I spoke
in terms of I want to *try* and breastfeed, and I just thought of it being
initially a problem for the first two or three days, and if you got over
the first two or three days and established breastfeeding that was it. I
wasn't aware of the fact that the really traumatic time was the few
days afterwards when sometimes you *aren't* producing enough, and
it's quite natural that you aren't perhaps producing enough to start
with, and you've got to work out some kind of compromise between
the baby and yourself.

The first six or seven days it was fine: I was producing a terrific
amount of milk, they're test-weighing her and she was putting on
weight, she was getting ninety mills or what have you just from one
breast, and I was terrifically pleased. And then suddenly it all seemed
to go wrong. I'm sure it was all tied up with my emotional state; but
this was the worrying thing, I hadn't thought about that possibility,
that everything would be fine at first and *then* you'd start to get
problems. About day eight or so I got a bit worried because she was
waking up quite often and I thought that I wasn't producing enough
milk and foolishly I said this to them. I said perhaps I'm not
producing enough milk because she's waking up quite often. And in
fact it was quite normal that she should wake up quite often – and it
wasn't *that* often, a couple of hours, two and a half to three hours,
which isn't bad. And apparently on day five or six they can be fed up
to eleven times, breastfed babies. But they didn't appear to be aware
of that at all. And their *automatic* reaction without any question was

well supplement the feed with the bottle. And I *knew* that this would
be wrong. That if I gave a bottle I would automatically stop stimulat-
ing the breasts to produce the milk and it would be a vicious circle.
They said well, alright, put her on the pump, you see, just to see. And
they put me on this bloody pump which was the most pornographic
thing, have you seen it? Oh God, it was awful. It was just like being
milked, it was awful. And the amount of milk I produced was
absolutely *nominal*, and I'm sure it was because I was so worried about
being put on this bloody machine anyway – it was totally emotional. I
think the idea was to reassure me in a way, that I had enough milk,
but of course it had the completely contradictory effect. The fact that I
produced so little convinced me that I was running out. I realised for
that particular feed I wasn't producing enough, and it might just have
been my emotional state or perhaps at that particular time of day I
just wasn't producing enough, I don't know, but they said right,
you're not producing enough, give her a bottle. The very day they put
me on the pump they weighed her again and she'd gone down – I
mean it was only a fraction, but it was enough. They showed me the
graph and there wasn't any question that it was a minute amount but
it was 'she's gone down in weight' and *that* on top of the fact that I'd
produced so little milk on this bloody machine, I mean I was just in a
terrible state.

And from that point on I was absolutely worried sick; I got really
miserable and tense. In fact I've never felt so bad since I did my finals,
I was in a real state over my finals, it affected everything – the way I
felt, I lost my appetite and I felt *exactly* like that. I was *so* keen to
breastfeed and I wanted to be able to do it at home for David – I knew
that David wanted me to do it as well and I think that was terribly
important. And when I was so worried about it, I was dreaming about
breasts and what have you, the thought of David not being able to see
me breastfeeding and *sharing* it. . . . . They kept *trying* to reassure me
but they did it in the wrong way. They just kept saying don't worry
about it; just get a good night's sleep and we'll give her a bottle
tonight, and everything'll be alright in the morning. I knew darn well
that was the worst thing that I could do, and yet they insisted on doing
that.

And once they lied to to me; they said no they hadn't given her any
food, and she was on this special food, this soya bean stuff, because I
said I didn't want her fed on cows' milk [because of the theory that
with a family history of allergy – which David Manson had – cows'

milk is better avoided in the early months] – and I went along to the fridge to check whether they'd actually used any and they had. And it turned out they had fed her and they'd lied. I made a fuss about it, I was terribly emotional about the whole thing – but they continued to say well you know you can't starve your baby. If she's not getting enough milk you've got to give her a complementary bottle. And they gave me some stuff to bring home *just in case* you know, and the very first feed I gave her when I came home I was in a state and I did give her some and she took great amounts from the bottle. But I had a few cigarettes and a drink and David was reassuring, and we read Dr Spock together and that made a lot of difference. We had a pretty traumatic weekend, but I *refused* to give her a bottle and I fed her on demand which was sometimes every couple of hours. And then I spoke to the health visitor on Monday and she was super. She was very anti the idea of supplementary feeds, and she told me to persevere. She was really first rate, she told me to control myself and sat me down and spoke to me as if I was a five-year-old which was just what I needed, and from then on it was fine. And now I'm producing loads of milk. I took her to the clinic last week to be weighed and I was praying that she'd put on some weight, because I was so worried: anything, just half an ounce, *anything* to prove she'd gone up in weight. And she'd put on fourteen ounces, she'd gone from eight four to nine two and in fact she's overweight now, she's enormous!

The official policy of this and most hospitals is now in favour of breastfeeding. But the amount of help a mother actually gets is dependent on the particular attitudes of the particular staff she meets. Neither test-weighing nor supplementary bottlefeeding is conducive to successful breastfeeding and many women feel that they are allowed – or encouraged – to give up too easily. It is a modern myth that breastfeeding can be properly established by the time (nine or ten days) a mother leaves hospital. This is far from being the case.

SARAH MOORE and JONATHAN:
The first week I was home my Mum stayed here and I had all these problems feeding him. I was told don't let him go more than four or five hours, and I tell you the first night I was home he was supposed to wake up at one and he didn't. I lay awake for an hour and a half and he kept sleeping, sleeping, sleeping. I thought this is ridiculous. I picked him up and fed him. I was doing that for ages. My Mum found out and said it was ridiculous and Dick said well I said that to her but she wouldn't listen. And they were ganging up on me.

It wasn't till I came home that I realised he wasn't getting enough to eat. He wasn't test-weighed in hospital, but on my way out they said he was *just* starting to pick up weight. The doctor saw me the night before I went home and said he's slow to pick up weight, but then big babies are; they lose a lot. So I didn't worry. Came home, fed him, great, lovely. He was always very good at night, he'd only ever wake up once at night, and he'd go longer than four hours between feeds at night: he was fine. I came out on the Monday morning and my health visitor arrived on the Tuesday or Wednesday and they asked me on my way out of the hospital to take the baby in the following Friday to be weighed to see that he was picking up weight. I explained this to the health visitor and she said well if you want you can do a test-weigh yourself before you go in or afterwards, and you can see how much he's put on. She brought me the scales on Friday morning and I went to the hospital on Friday afternoon, he'd only put on an ounce in the whole week! I came home and I test-weighed him and he'd only taken one and a half ounces from me, so I put him back to the breast, and my nipples were then very sore because I was giving him twenty minutes each side and that really was exhausting me and him. And I realised then that he was getting chronic wind as well.

On the Friday I carried on giving him breastmilk, breastmilk, whenever it was there and on the Saturday a problem arose when there was just nothing there to give him. So I phoned up the hospital and I spoke to the sister and she said I could supplement the feed, that he probably needed to take four ounces altogether. So I then weighed him again and he was one and a half ounces short, so I made up one and a half ounces of SMA which I promptly sent my mother up the High Street to go and get in the middle of feeding him, and she came rushing back, and he ate all that up. And he promptly threw it up all over the place, the whole feed, everything. All over me, all over the floor, the settee, my mother, just like a fountain. My mother said don't worry, just don't panic, don't panic, it'll be alright. Let him settle down and either he'll want more or he'll go to sleep. Just don't worry, don't worry. So she sat at my side and we rocked him and rocked him, and I was rocking him like this [gestures] and when I put him down he started to retch; oh my God, that was it: I wouldn't listen to my mother, Dick was out playing rugby, I phoned up my mother-in-law to find out which doctor was on and it was the emergency service; it wasn't my doctor, it was the young doctor. Anyway he said don't panic, everything's alright. He told me just to feed the baby on breastmilk and glucose and water for the weekend and indeed it worked out alright. Having cursed for about five minutes solidly on the telephone saying that I was panicking and that I was probably overfeeding him and he was too hot and everything, he really calmed me down which was very good.

Eventually after this traumatic weekend I went to see my own doctor. I went in and explained what was happening. I said for example last night he slept for longer than four hours and I had to wake him up. He said you did what? I said I had to wake him up. He said you've always appeared to be very sensible to me – you are *stupid!* God, he cursed me. He said if that baby wants food, he'll soon wake you up. He said when we had our children the book was just thrown immediately out of the window; he said I told my wife to fill those kids up at eleven o'clock so full, they were as full as eggs, and they didn't wake up till seven. We did that with all our children and our grandchildren and they've never woken us up. He said don't you *dare* wake your baby up!

He told me to supplement and my own milk would gradually come back, because apparently this often happens when you come out of hospital – the milk is reduced and then gradually it comes back. I'm still doing that, I give him SMA not at every feed, but when I think he needs it. I went to the clinic last week and had him weighed and the doctor there seemed to think that I could give up breastfeeding altogether. I was quite surprised. And I said I'd like to try for another fortnight or three weeks, if I've got the milk there he might as well have it. I don't want to give up. I don't mind doing both, people say oh what a terrible bind. Well granted you've got the disadvantages of both and the advantages of neither, but. . . . [Sarah was still breastfeeding Jonathan at five months.]

Determination is clearly the key word here. A woman's motivation must be strong and unwavering:

ALISON MOUNTJOY:
Having had an epidural, I thought right: there is only one thing left to do naturally and that is breastfeed. And I think if I'd had a natural childbirth, a more natural, unmechanised childbirth, I just wonder if I'd still be breastfeeding. Because I mean there are times, I mean it *is* difficult, some days it's bloody awful; at this stage I'm still scared that she'll sleep extra long one night and then my breasts'll get engorged and then there'll be another painful day for me and a difficult day for

her. I mean I don't mind the pain of engorged breasts but every time I use the teat to help her I think maybe she won't go back to the breast. [She has an inverted nipple which is difficult for the baby to grasp and an artificial nipple placed over the top of it sometimes helps.] I'm surprised when I think she's a month old. Each time I think we've settled down something will go a bit wrong and it feels like going back to square one. But I certainly won't give up. My milk would have to dry up. I mean even if I had to use that teat on both breasts at every feed I'd go on. I'm pretty determined because I *know* it's so much better. I feel emotionally satisfied insofar as I do feel quite proud of myself because I am still doing it at four weeks and I know a lot of people would have given up.

The pain *and the* difficulty *that many women experience with breastfeeding at first conflicts with the rosy romantic image of the 'nursing couple'.*

What did feeding the baby feel like at first?

Well I expected to feel more than I did. I thought I'd feel much more. It just sort of seemed rather a novelty more than anything else. I expected to feel this sort of tender moment between mother and baby and I didn't really. But as I say, they were trying to sort of clamp him on and I was at such an awkward angle so it all seemed rather funny. It was really when I was on my own with him later on and he was feeding properly that it began to feel more special I suppose. (*Rosalind Kimber*)

Nothing really. I was expecting this elation, or whatever you are supposed to get – this feeling that only mothers can feel – and I felt absolutely nothing, and I thought ooh it hurts when she first started . . . (*Mandy Green*)

I didn't really feel sort of anything in particular. I still felt a bit tired. And maybe it was just the effect of the drugs, I remember feeling particularly sort of cut off and a bit, not disinterested, but I remember thinking to myself oh I expected to sort of treat this moment far more seriously than I am. (*Cary Wimborne*)

It felt strange. I thought you were supposed to feel things, but I didn't really feel anything. I thought you were supposed to feel the milk going but I didn't . . . (*Grace Bower*)

The very first time I found it quite painful, but then of course after a few sucks you don't feel it any more. And then I liked it. But I wasn't prepared for it to be so painful. (*Juliet Morley*)

I wasn't shown how to put him to the breast and so consequently I thought he just had to suck the nipple and not the whole, what do you call it, the brown part? I didn't realise he had to get the whole of that in his mouth. (*Polly Field*)

None of the breastfeeding mothers said they found it a sexual experience. Not only is the breast a sexual object in our culture, but for physiological reasons the stimulation of the nipples by the baby can in theory be sexually arousing.[5] *In natural childbirth literature this is certainly presented as a bonus of breastfeeding,*[6] *but it is not one reported by any of the survey women. Instead, reasons for enjoying breastfeeding have to do with feelings of physical and emotional closeness with the baby. Pride in nourishing the baby with one's own body may be one factor, doing what is best for the baby another. But breastfeeding can also be addictive for some women, a habit that it becomes difficult to kick.*

HABITS AND VICES

When do you intend to give up breastfeeding?

LOIS MANSON:
When she's about five. Years old. No, seriously, I think about six or seven months, then she can go straight on to a cup. But I don't look forward to the end of breastfeeding at all. Not because of any erotic sensation I get from it, I don't, I feel I've missed out there because so many people say to me that they get some kind of sexual sensation. I don't think of it in terms of any *physical* sensation. It's nice and convenient and nice to be close to Jane and you know I just feel that she's getting so much from it, that it's just a nice thing to do.

SANDY WRIGHT:
At 5 weeks:
I've got a friend who really raved about it, I don't feel as strongly as that about it, I don't want to give it up so I suppose I must feel strongly about it. I think you feel closer to the baby. When she looks at me when I try and stick a bottle in her mouth, it's really amazing: what on earth. . . ?
At 5 months:
One of the health visitors said of *course* you won't want to breastfeed

for more than two or three months. I said I'll breastfeed as long as I want to, as long as I can.

ELLEN GEORGE:
My mother said you'll feel much better once you've stopped breast-feeding. In fact when I had the breast abscess at one stage I said I'll give in, stop breastfeeding, put her onto the old bottle. But it really went against the grain. I thought I've got this far: why don't I go on? I'm almost doing it for myself now. I get so much enjoyment from it. I feel really when I do stop it'll be almost like leaving home. I feel *dependent* on it.

LOUISE THOMPSON:
I'm just too lazy to give her the cup. I mean she *likes* the cup, but she just won't drink enough to satisfy her. Like it's a *game* for her. But then when she's really hungry she'll start crying . . . I think it's so *nice*.
I: So if she continues like this until she's a year old, you'll go on breastfeeding?
LOUISE: Oh come on, is that possible? Oh please! No; another couple of months'll be enough. [Still breastfeeding at 2½ years!]

SARAH MOORE:
At 8 weeks:
If I can carry on for say three or four months that'll be fine. I'm enjoying feeding him tremendously. The girl down the road, she was feeding her baby every half an hour. I think that's carrying it a bit far. That I find quite *animal* actually.
At 5 months:
People have said how can you go on this long? A few girls I know to chat to in the High Street have said oh I would never go on longer than two or three months. Oh no! It's *animal* . . . They look at me as though. . . . No: I am *so* determined that he can have the milk as long as he wants it.'

Breastfeeding for two or three months is regarded as one's duty; after that social attitudes become a little ambivalent. Why are you still breastfeeding? Who are you doing it for – the baby or yourself? What are you trying to prove?

I find a lot of people are surprised. I've got a neighbour who lives a couple of doors away, she's about 65, and she can't stop praising me for breastfeeding. She's so surprised that a young mother these days does breastfeed. There was another girl I know she just didn't *know*

you could breastfeed for so long; she thought you could only breastfeed for about six weeks! (*Nicola Bell*)

Juliet Morley's baby has 'breast with everything' at five months:
People express surprise. The health visitor said are you breastfeeding? I said yes. Are you *totally* breastfeeding? No bottles? No. That's
very good, with a first baby.

Apparently my sister-in-law used to go to the clinic and there used
to be all these girls there she was at primary school with and hadn't
seen since, with their third or fourth child, and the health visitor used
to sort of boom down the cubicle hallo Mrs Crow, are you still
breastfeeding? All you mothers should be breastfeeding like Mrs
Crow. They all thought she was incredibly stuck up for having gone to
grammar school anyway!

It is funny. People say when are you giving it up? As though it's a
vice that you must kick. If it was a bottle they wouldn't – kids go
round with bottles for ages. People think it's *unusual* to be breastfeeding. I find if you mention it people think you're clever somehow. They
say oh that's *very* good, when I had a child my milk dried up or I
couldn't feed: they all say that they *couldn't* feed – never that they
didn't want to. That's always the reason. (*José Bryce*)

Reluctant breastfeeders

Perhaps there are set excuses that hide an underlying reluctance to breastfeed.
People who find it distasteful cite a long list of reasons why it is also difficult;
those who describe it as difficult may also be saying they found it unpleasant.
Reasons for giving up breastfeeding include: not liking it, having sore or cracked
nipples, not having enough milk, exhaustion, an unsatisfied baby.

ANNE BLOOMFIELD, breastfed for 4 days:
I tried breastfeeding and I *hated* it. And I was so determined to
breastfeed. The minute I saw her hanging off my boob it made me feel
sick.
I: Why?
ANNE: I haven't the faintest idea. I thought I'd love it. It hurt; I don't
like pain. I don't know why. I mean look, she's really got a strong suck
and that on the end of my boob was really horrible. I just didn't like it.
It was making me ever so frustrated. So I did it for four days, and I
was *really* getting frustrated and I kept sort of crying . . . I didn't know

how much she was taking and she sort of kept slipping off it and I kept having to put it back in her mouth, you know, and I really hated it, so I stopped it. She had the colostrum so that's alright, you know, they say that's a good thing.

MAUREEN PATERSON, breastfed for 2 weeks:
Well you see I'm not feeding him now. I was, but it wasn't enough, you know. For two weeks, well really over the time I was in hospital. When I came out I was doing both really because when I was in hospital I was feeding him but they were topping him up with a bottle and I didn't have him all the time at night because sister said I needed the rest. And of course he was having a bottle as well and when we got home I was feeding him, I was giving him a quarter of an hour each side and he was still screaming. You could tell he was hungry. And of course then we had to make up a bottle and it was *terrible*, it was taking ages and ages you know, and then once I got home I was *exhausted*; it was just taking it right out of me, so we went to see the doctor and she said no, wean him off gradually; give him five minutes and then some bottle. But it was making him so unsettled because he didn't know – I mean he'd be going to me and then it'd be the bottle, so my sister said express your own milk off. She said I'll help you do it. . . . She brought this great big basin, and I think there was about one drop in there. It was just going. My Mum had the same trouble with my sister and with me. She only breastfed for a couple of weeks. With my sister she was underfeeding her; she didn't know at the time. It was her first baby and she had nobody to help her, but my sister was really not getting enough. So perhaps I take after me Mum.

SHARON WARRINGTON, breastfed for 10 days:
I: You are feeding him just on the bottle at the moment, aren't you?
SHARON: Yes.
I: But you started to breastfeed when you had him?
SHARON: Yes.
I: You wanted to breastfeed?
SHARON: Yes.
I: Are you happy about bottlefeeding him now?
SHARON: Well I dried up . . . I brought him home on the Friday and in the early hours of the Friday morning when I got up to feed him and I fed him, what I thought was feeding him, and he was screaming his head off, my Mum come and said what's wrong with him and I said I don't know, he's got no wind. She said he's hungry, and I said I've

just fed him. Anyway I sat up all night feeding him to satisfy him. And then I went up to my Mum's doctor and he said to me take three tablets, one today and one tomorrow, you are drying up, you've hardly got anything left. So I was broken hearted, and he had to go on the bottle. But he's been alright.

CHRISTINA LYNCH, breastfed for 3 weeks:
I definitely wasn't very happy about breastfeeding, not afterwards. I mean I wanted to so much at the time because I thought this is good, this is natural. I suppose I was trying too hard. I'm on bottlefeeding now, I've done it gradually, but last Sunday was – I went right over to bottlefeeding on the advice of the health visitor because I was still you know, depressed. And she said you'll feel much better if you come off breastfeeding. I wasn't really happy about it: it wasn't *enjoyable*. I kept thinking oh God I've got to feed him, I've got to undo everything: I had to wear something that buttons up the front, and I couldn't wear a full length petticoat, selfish really. It was a bit of a nuisance. But I didn't feel as beautiful if you like breastfeeding as I thought I would. I feel happier bottlefeeding because I'm more relaxed. I'm not tensed up: how much is he getting? Will he bite me or hurt me?

I went to see her at the beginning of last week. I was just talking to her and I started to cry. Oh she said, I hadn't realised you were still so depressed. She said right, you must put him straight onto the bottle. All bottlefeeding. So that by the time you come next week he'll be all bottlefed. And I was rather relieved to hear her say it. I do notice the difference – not overnight. I mean Sunday night, Monday night, I was very ratty, irritable: I didn't shout and bawl and scream but I felt *irritable*, and then Tuesday I felt fine, as I do now. It's the hormones switching over – they switched off very quickly. She said the longer you breastfeed the longer the hormones are still in your body and the longer you'll feel depressed, she said.

GRACE BOWER:
At 5 weeks:
I: Are you happy about breastfeeding?
GRACE: Yes, the only thing is I'd like to know how much he's taking. They say ten minutes, but how do you know how much he's taken in ten minutes? He might be mucking about, and taking nothing, or he might be taking a lot. I think I'd like to really know. If there was a pump that you could buy I think I'd put it all in a bottle and give it to him that way, then I'd know. Because I did it one time in the hospital

because I had cracked nipples and I did it that way; they said to me that I had to express myself. That was a bit tiring. But one night one of the sisters said look you can use a pump. That was okay – it was all out in five minutes. And then I knew what he was taking, and I felt a lot happier. I'd feel a lot happier if I knew what he was taking because when he wakes up in between I wonder if he's hungry.

At 5 months:

I've stopped breastfeeding now. I stopped when he was two months old because I was having such trouble with him. We didn't know what was wrong with him, he was forever eating. They put him on solids at two months as well, I know it was a bit early, but I was getting a bit desperate. I just didn't know what to do with him, and when they suggested it I thought anything, anything, just to keep him quiet. He was absolutely terrible, he just kept crying and crying and eating and eating and he wouldn't stop, so I decided that was it. I gave up breastfeeding slowly and I introduced solids as well, at the same time. Like I gave up breastfeeding, say I started on a Monday, by the following Monday for one of the feeds I was giving him apple or something. But once he got onto solids he was much better. I decreased the bottled milk when I gave him solids. He was drinking twelve ounces of milk at one time. I gave him a whole bottle – nine ounces – and my aunt was here and she said the poor baby's hungry, you're starving him. I said he's had nine ounces. She made up another bottle and he drunk it. I thought oh Christ he's a pig.

I: So why did you give up really?

GRACE: Because he was crying all the time. I didn't know what to do with him. I just didn't know. He wouldn't sleep and he wouldn't let us sleep. I just didn't know: I was desperate. I thought I'd try anything just to get him to stop crying. I don't know if it was right but I think if I had another child I'd try to persevere a bit more. I don't think it's done him any harm: I hope it hasn't anyway. But I wish I could have persevered a bit more, but at the time I was so exhausted and so fed up I thought: anything!

MARY ROSEN, breastfed for 5 months:

I wanted him to have something else at lunchtime on holiday so I could leave him during the day. . . . My father-in-law said well you'll want to be leaving him during the day and I thought well I *can't* if I'm feeding him. I couldn't leave him for more than three hours and it seemed pointless going on holiday really unless I could leave him. I mean I really did it mostly because of the holiday. But also I was getting a bit tired of feeding him. I do think it's the best thing for him and everything but I think it was dragging me down a bit.

Jane Tarrant was really quite determined to breastfeed her baby, and the account she gives of her subsequent 'failure' to do so highlights the great emotional sensitivity many women feel about breastfeeding. There is no doubt that being a successful breastfeeder is an aspect of what some people in our society mean by womanhood – it is one among many elements in the cultural construction of femininity.

JANE TARRANT, seven weeks after Christian's birth:
Well, I did have the attitude that oh well you know I would try it and if it worked it would be great and if it didn't work I've seen so many people getting neurotic about it and having terrible feeding problems later on, you know. And I don't know, I got awfully *upset* in the hospital, and in the end it wasn't going very well, and then they said ooh that's a challenge and you can't give up and I was just dying to give him a bottle. I was having all these nightmares that he was dying because he was losing weight, I was waking up sort of sweating and things. And then in the end they said oh well alright have a bottle. I didn't keep asking them you know, but by that time I felt terribly tense about it. When people mentioned breastfeeding I began to feel a terrible failure that I hadn't done it, you know, I got very upset about it. Since I've been home I've begun to see it a bit more in proportion you know, that it's not the be all and end all of life: he's sort of healthy and everything else, that's the main thing.

I didn't have much milk you see. He'd suck a little bit and they'd test-weigh him and I don't know, he'd taken a few grams, and I was getting really worried . . . The ducts were a bit blocked and he had jaundice for two or three days and he was asleep most of the time: all these things contributed. If he'd had a bottle for a couple of days I wouldn't have felt so worried, but they wouldn't give me a bottle. They said oh it'll come tomorrow, and I felt that it *wouldn't* come tomorrow, and it was only about the sixth day I went and had a bath and it started to come out – I said it's started now. But by then they'd said oh you haven't got enough milk, give up, and by then I'd been at the weeps so many times. Two days before I was going home I thought I can't be expressing bits of milk at home and then doing bits of bottles and things; I thought I'd go up the pole if I was doing that. So I stopped. This friend of mine who'd had trouble breastfeeding herself, hadn't had much milk, I told her and she was the greatest help I had, because she said oh she'd gone through this complementary feeding, she said give it up. She didn't force me to give it up or anything, but she was the only person who *understood* what I was going through. Because my mother didn't. And I don't think Neil understood either because he was sort of saying the baby's crying, oh he wants the breast, you know, I'd think oh I'm failing . . . because I felt in a way that he was very keen for me to do it and that he was going to think I was a failure as well, I was letting *him* down. . . .

I'll tell you something I have felt – it's all to do with this sensitivity about breastfeeding. It's that everything you read claims the advantages of breastfeeding. It makes you feel very *sad* somehow. You keep hearing and reading about it and they never have any sympathy for people who've *failed*. I think it's more or less the attitude that if you haven't breastfed you haven't *tried* or you couldn't care less, and I think people who have handicapped children must feel terrible; how they keep being *reminded* of things all the time. I mean I'm probably being sensitive about it, the worst thing is that everybody keeps asking you: even your next door neighbour will ask; I think, well mind your own business. I *do* feel like saying to people well mind your own business: it's not that it's anything private, but it's *personal* and I don't think anybody realises how *personal* it is. It seemed that everywhere I went people were talking about breasts. It must be like people who want to get pregnant and everywhere they go people are having babies. I said to Neil it's like admitting every time yes I've failed, people always ask you if you're breastfeeding. I don't know why, I've never asked anybody except my best friend. But if somebody has a baby I don't say are you breastfeeding?

I still *do* feel bad about it but I think well it's better that I'm sort of coping with life now than if I were really weeping over him. I think he's better off as he is. I think there's no point brooding about it now: it makes it worse. Another time I think I'd probably do it differently. I'd do it on demand if I was doing it again. You had to do it every four hours in the hospital.

I'll tell you what I think part of the problem was. I think if I'd been on my *own* a bit more. They come round and they think they're being awfully helpful, sort of manipulating you. You don't mind at the time but I think inside it is sort of tensing you up. I think probably if you're left on your own with the baby it's better. If I had been say in a room on my own and just sort of picked him up every time he made a sound

I'm sure it would be alright.

Women are not like cows and even cows are known to have emotional reactions that interfere with the milk supply. Bottlefeeding may have its problems, but they are perhaps less obvious. While some women complain about the disadvantages of breastfeeding, none who bottlefeed from the beginning recite its difficulties.

HILARY JACKSON:

At 4 weeks:

I was thrilled I was bottlefeeding. It convinced me even more when I was seeing these cows, it was like cowsheds, the girls in their little cubicles. And I used to say when can you lot open the curtains? Because I was the only one that could sit there and . . . and as I say they were having great problems and great difficulties over it and they were getting very worried about it, and they weren't getting a lot of advice. You know, I'm thrilled now that I decided to bottlefeed because the thought of that – I mean they are literally on demand for twenty-four hours.

At 5 months:

I: Have you ever regretted not breastfeeding?

HILARY: Never, never in a million years, you're joking. My sister-in-law, she thought I was the world's worst because I didn't breastfeed. She kept saying to me: well what are they *for*? I said if you didn't have any children, they wouldn't be for it anyway. She thought I was *terrible*. So I said to her how was she doing – she said oh he's getting enormous, and they said it's because she's breastfeeding. I said I don't think it's that, he's probably just a big baby. Anyway she said they keep saying to me at the clinic I must be giving him bottles on the sly. So I said well, I wouldn't go. Anyway she rang me up the other day and she said he's having bottles. So I said oh is he living? He's alright then? He's surviving? Oh she said, he's thriving on it. So I said I bet you're surprised aren't you? She lost her milk, her milk dried up or something. She hoped to do it until six months but she didn't have enough so she's giving him SMA and he's thriving. It's a wonder, but he is!

MENUS – FIVE WEEKS

In the early weeks most (91 per cent) babies are just fed on milk. Their menus may vary from breast on demand to a strictly scheduled system.

ANNETTE BELL, birthweight 8lbs 8ozs:

5.45am   Breast
10am   Breast
2pm   Breast
6pm   Breast
10pm   Breast

THOMAS PATERSON, birthweight 6lbs 7ozs:

6am   4½ozs Cow and Gate Babymilk Plus*
10am   4½ozs Cow and Gate Babymilk Plus
2pm   4½ozs Cow and Gate Babymilk Plus
6pm   4½ozs Cow and Gate Babymilk Plus
11pm   4½ozs Cow and Gate Babymilk Plus

TERESA KING, birthweight 8lbs 12ozs:

10am   Breast
12pm   Breast plus 2ozs SMA
4pm   Breast plus 5ozs SMA
8pm   Breast plus 5ozs SMA
12pm   Breast plus 2ozs SMA

But some are already having 'solid' food.

SIMON O'HARA, birthweight 8lbs:

6am   7ozs Cow and Gate Babymilk Plus and half a Farley's rusk
10am   7ozs Cow and Gate Babymilk Plus and half a Farley's rusk
2pm   7ozs Cow and Gate Babymilk Plus and half a Farley's rusk
6pm   7ozs Cow and Gate Babymilk Plus and half a Farley's rusk
11pm   7ozs Cow and Gate Babymilk Plus and half a Farley's rusk.

A baby fed entirely on milk must eventually become a child whose eating habits approximate to the adult cultural pattern: three meals a day. Some time in the first year the transition is begun. So-called 'solid' food (it may in fact be very runny) is heaped onto a spoon or put in a bottle and the infant persuaded to swallow it – he or she is on 'mixed feeding'. A mother may choose as the first food a cereal, fruit or vegetable or meat purée. She may concoct her own or serve the baby commercially prepared infant food – packet (dehydrated), jar or tin. She may be in a hurry to start it, feeling that the introduction of solids signals an important developmental stage (and makes motherhood more interesting). She may delay solid food out of a conviction that it is healthier to start at five or six months than at six or eight weeks – or she may just feel lazy and disinclined to create more work for herself.

* *This is the brand of milk used in the hospital – a powerful influence; 54 per cent of the bottlefeeding mothers subsequently used it (86 per cent of those who left the hospital bottlefeeding).*

The breast versus bottle debate is one that most women have strong feelings about, even though they may find translating the decision into practice difficult for some reason or another. When and how to start solid food is another kind of dilemma altogether. In the first place few women, in imagining themselves as mothers, see past the milk stage. Tiny babies are fed on milk and although they eventually become children who eat off plates the move from one to the other is, at best, hazy. Secondly, feeding a baby solid food may be seen as an important maternal duty but it does not arouse the depth of feeling that the breastfeeding dilemma does: mammary glands are not involved. Partly for this reason, the new mother is relatively open to the influence of health visitors, doctors and her own friends and relations. She may feel torn between the various kinds of advice, and in the end the whim of the moment decides (what she feels like one morning, the packet or tin that first catches her eye on the chemist's shelves). In the long run the new mother's task is to develop confidence in her own ability to be her own baby's menu-planner.

Clinic conversations

I: What advice do you give about solid foods these days?
HEALTH VISITOR: Well I try if I can and keep to the three months. This seems to be the pattern now. I recommend soup, the strained soup and broths at lunch time. If it's at all possible leave the cereals alone. But of course nine times out of ten they put them on cereals.

This battle cry of modern professional advice marks many encounters between mothers and experts. The following encounter between a first-time mother and a health visitor was recorded at a baby clinic that some of the sample mothers attended and is fairly typical of the kind of advice mothers report. It illustrates well the attention to detail, the spelling-out of what should be done exactly how and when, that seems to be an intrinsic part of the social construction of motherhood today. The mother is 24, an ex-nurse.

HEALTH VISITOR: Twelve two, that's not bad, is it?
MOTHER: Not bad at all, for thirteen weeks.
HV: Are you still breastfeeding?
M: No, I've finished. She's having Cow and Gate Two. The other health visitor last time told me that she was going to start her on broth this week, at her midday feed.
HV: Um, full cream Cow and Gate. She's what, three months, isn't she? She's on orange juice?

M: No, she told me to stop that. I keep her on the vitamins and she said to give her the Cow and Gate Two.

HV: She ought to have orange juice, because in all fairness, in the Cow and Gate you've got A and D so you don't need the vitamin drops, but you haven't got any C. I would complement and give the C – I think it's better if you could give the orange juice. She quite likes it, does she?

M: Yes, well, I put a spoon of glucose with it.

HV: Okay then, that's fine. Start the soups at lunchtime. I suggest you use the broths. I think you'll find the Heinz is going over more to mixed dinners now, so if you can get the plain broth, preferably do so. If not, you'll have to get what you can in the strained foods. And what you do is you put about four teaspoons in a cup, heat it up, and start off with two – no more. Preferably before her bottle. But it's not easy, because she gets annoyed and frustrated because it comes so slowly. So give her half the bottle, then the spoon, then the remainder of the bottle. And as she gets used to it, so you can bring it to the foreground. Now I would leave her on two teaspoons for a week and then increase it sort of every couple of days until you come to a third of a tin, then come to a halt for a week or two. Then cut down the bottle.

M: Right.

HV: At least an ounce, or a couple of ounces, she'll be a better judge than you.

M: Well she only takes 4½ ounces anyway of the bottle, she doesn't take that much.

HV: She won't take any more?

M: No. She will not take any more.

HV: Yes, well, I wouldn't be surprised then if she's not keen on that, she might be keen on the soups.

M: Yes.

HV: But the only thing is, it's a case of getting used to flavour, so don't worry, just see how you go. Buy the tins – don't buy the packets. I know the tins aren't economical, but you can leave them in the fridge for two days. Then discard that; a new tin, a different flavour. And then you can start her on the yolk of an egg.

M: Right.

HV: It doesn't really matter when it is – who's going to finish it? Only one teaspoon of the egg, lightly boiled.

M: Lightly boiled.

HV: Some like it, some don't, so see how you go. About twice a week, and if she likes it, build it up and let her have all the yolk. If she doesn't, then leave it alone for a few weeks and just see what happens. The ideal thing is to start the soups first. Not the sweet things, because otherwise they get a liking for sweet things, and you'll have difficulty – and if possible no cereals, because it's all anti-cereal at the moment. Doesn't matter if it's the rusks or what it is – it's all cereal.

M: Right. Also I want to put her on cows' milk.

HV: Not yet.

M: Why not? She's too fat.

HV: No she's not.

M: Yes she is.

HV: No she's not.

M: I don't like Cow and Gate.

HV: Well, in all seriousness, the theory is don't start cows' milk too early. About six months.

M: Oh dear. I'll never agree with this! [laughs]

HV: It's a battle, isn't it? Absolute battle. Why are you keen on going onto cows' milk? Because you think she's putting on too much weight? Well, look, put it this way, she's now how old? Three months? Thirteen weeks – she's five four kilos, I agree she's double her birth weight, I'm not going to dispute that, but then she's only five four. I think you'll find personally, that when you turn round and start introducing the solids and then start reducing the milk, she'll simmer down a bit. But cows' milk isn't going to be the answer. I don't think you'll find it's the answer in the sense of reducing weight. I think six months is about the earliest you should start. You see, you've got your added vitamins in dried milk. It's easier for digestion because the casein is broken down more easily than it is in cows' milk, so she might get a bit more indigestion with cows' milk. I'm not saying if she was having anything you could mix with milk, I don't say no, you couldn't start using cows' milk then, but she's not having anything at the moment that you could mix with milk. Because you're not giving her cereals.

M: I give her some Farex at night time.

HV: Do you? Well, try to avoid that. That's where the weight comes in. I think you'll find, once you get her on the soup, and then you get her, as I say to about a third of a tin, reduce the milk by at least an ounce, if not more. See how you go, then start on the puddings in the evening. Then when you've got her up to a third of a tin of pudding, cut that cereal last thing at night out. Because she'll be having something solid twice a day and it's going to fill her up more. But the important thing is once you've got them up to X amount of solids, then reduce the milk. Some will just take it: the more you give them the more they'll take. But that's when you're going to put on masses of weight. . . . But otherwise, as I say, I think she's doing very well.

It is in anecdotes about clinic encounters that mothers express a growing confidence in their own ability to decide what is best for the baby.

I: When did Christian first have solid food?
JANE TARRANT: There's quite a tale about that. He wasn't putting on weight properly, and I really was worried about that. I could see he wasn't putting on much weight. And he lost interest in his bottle. Although there didn't seem to be anything *wrong* with him. And then I mentioned that I'd put him on solid food in a while and they said oh no you *mustn't* do that. Anyway in a fortnight he'd only put on two ounces which seemed *dreadful* to me. And the previous fortnight he'd only put on perhaps five, so he really wasn't doing very well. So I really panicked then.

I went to see the clinic doctor and he said, well he hasn't got a cotside manner, he comes on a motor bike, he's a middle-aged man, a middle-aged ton-up kid, he's really awful, and he said oh nothing to worry about, sort of thing. And I said well shall I change his milk? Perhaps? Don't do that! He shouted at me. Well he was very busy I suppose. But I was really in a worried state. One of the district nurses, I suppose that's what she was, she's young, actually she's very nice: she could see that I was worried. And while I was waiting for the doctor she came up to me and said well have a bit of this – have a free sample; and why don't you put up some liver and potatoes and things; but she was very sweet to me really, she was very nice. . . . And suddenly I felt so *pleased* that there was something that I could *do* about it because in a way they were sort of saying you mustn't do this and you mustn't do that, when every baby is different! So I started on this and of course I didn't take it the way you're supposed to at all, starting with half a teaspoonful: I thought *I must get some weight on him.* And I was getting neurotic; I had this spoon, and every time he opened his mouth to cry I shoved it in his mouth. This lasted about a week, he got used to it: he took to it very quickly. And he put on half a pound in that week. So I thought oh he's alright, and I began to calm down about it.

I talked to a friend of mine and she said oh she never paid any attention to the clinic. She was determined that her babies were going to put on a certain amount, the standard amount every week, and she had them on – I think she was putting cereal in their milk by the time they were a certain age. Well in a way she was quite sensible because she didn't go through all these terrible worries about what you should and shouldn't do. And so now I don't ask them very much. I think I'm just as sensible as them. I can make up my own mind. I can read the books as well.

MANDY GREEN:
Oh yes, we talked about her food and said me with my big mouth that I happened to be giving her some Farex at night time because it had been suggested that it would help settle her, because that was the worst time of the day. And she said, oh no, you want to keep her off cereals, you know, she shouldn't be on cereals, it makes them fat and you don't want a fat baby, etc, etc. And she gave me all these bits of information and I stopped the cereals, and it [evening crying] had been improving and then she went absolutely haywire. She was up all the time crying and wanted bottles and things. And the next week I went, I said you know [pause] that she had this colic very badly. And she said perhaps she's one of these babies that needs cereals. Now the week previously she told me on no account was I to give cereals. So I thought rhubarb, rhubarb, or words to that effect.

MAUREEN PATERSON:
They said at the clinic, they tell you to give him yoghurt and stuff like that, bits of this and bits of that, but she said don't give him cereal because it makes them fat. But I mean he was only small to start with [6lbs 7ozs] and I started him on different bits out of the little tins and I think that upset him, trying too many. So I stuck to the cereals for a while and he loves them now.

I think you really find out by your mistakes, well not by your mistakes, but as you go along really. I think at first I used to listen to everything they said at the clinic and take it all as *gospel*. But now I think to myself I'll take that with a pinch of salt. I mean I know they *mean* well most of them, but a lot of them haven't got children – I think they just read books!

The expert mother

One person who has invariably had experience in infant feeding is one's mother.

Some mothers openly proclaim themselves as experts, others only give advice when asked for it. Nicola Bell has not yet given five-month-old Annette any solid food:
I have a very good health visitor so I just took her advice. She said not to introduce them till five or six months, the longer you left it the better. My Mum, she thinks I ought to give her little bits and pieces and bits of chocolate. She thinks that. At one time they used to think you should put them on solids at six weeks and now the longer you leave it the better. This health visitor told me to stay away from cereals and rusks because they're fattening, and to give puréed vegetables and fruit, this sort of thing. The health visitor said don't give her anything until she needs it.

While Kate Prince, who when pregnant refused to listen to her mother's tales about birth, is now beginning to wonder whether her mother might not be right after all:
I don't really go by the health visitor, she seems to say the same thing to everybody. And yet she's really the only source of information I've got really. I mean she says give her this, give her this, give her that. I wanted to give her my own food that I made myself, our dinner, and she said oh don't give her that, it might upset her, wait till she's a little bit older. It's too fiddly to make yourself. And I don't think it's fiddly at all. I'd much sooner give her food that *tastes*, instead of all this bland stuff. I really think she should start to have proper food. My Mum says we always had bits of their dinner, peas mashed up, and we loved it. I gave her some carrot and potato *before* I'd asked the health visitor and she loved it, she really enjoyed it. I feel *instinctively* that she should have more solid food and stuff that we eat because she's getting on now. She's not just a little baby.

And some first-time mothers have, of course, never doubted the value of their own mother's advice; in all, 63 per cent listened to their mothers:

PAT JENKINS:
Well, Mum told me not to listen to what they said at the clinic, because she said they're not at home with your baby all the time and they don't realise, they're not living with them, and every baby's an individual.

I went to the clinic you see, and I think he was about three months old, and she told me off because he was too fat. Because I had this little woolly thing on him and it did make him look big, and of course mothers don't admit it, do they, and I said he's not fat. I said it's only that little woolly thing that's making him look fat. And she said well look at him, look at his face, she said. And, do you know, I've never gone back since I saw her! She said leave him another month before you start on the solids and cut his bottle down. Anyway I listened to her, I cut his bottle down. And then I put up with him for a week. I thought I won't listen to her, I'll just do it my way. And I put it up and he was more content, because he wasn't getting enough when I cut it down.

SHARON WARRINGTON:
I: Whose advice do you think you take most notice of?
SHARON: My Mum.
I: What do you think of the clinic's advice?
SHARON: If I took notice of what they said the other week I'd be starving him.
I: How?
SHARON: Give him a yoghurt for his dinner. And no pudding. Then give him cereal for tea. I thought that would be too heavy. So I didn't do it. He's okay. He's putting on weight well.

Sharon had been giving her baby rusks in his bottle since he was four weeks old.

Milk plus

Putting rusks or other cereal food in the bottle to make the baby sleep at night is part of the folklore of motherhood. This is not considered by mothers to be mixed feeding proper; rather the cereal is seen as a supplement to the milk feed.[7]

VERA ABBATT and DARREN, aged 5 months:
He took solid food at first, he was alright at first, but since he started teething he won't have a spoon or anything in his mouth.
I: So he doesn't have any solid food?
VERA: No.
I: Nothing apart from milk?
VERA: Well I do put a rusk in his bottle because I tried it out one night and it knocked him out in the night and I thought oh that's ideal, I'll use that. So first of all I only used it at night time to make him sleep. But then when he went off the solids I thought well he's got to have *something* so I started putting a rusk in all his bottles. . . . .

The number of mothers who start solid food early with rusks and cereals of various kinds is counterbalanced by those who delay till three months or later. Two of the sample had not introduced solids by five months: the rest had, and the average time was just under twelve weeks.[8] More than two-thirds did choose a cereal food as the first solid food – Farex or Farlene were the most popular.

First solid food	
Cereal	70%
Fruit	15%
Egg or meat	9%
Vegetables	6%

Another early addition to the milk feed is paracetamol syrup, available over the counter at any chemist and the modern version of the opiates with which many babies were sedated in the eighteenth and nineteenth centuries.[9]

He was going through a bad patch. I think it's teeth. We gave him some medicine [Panadol Elixir]. My sister said it knocked them out. About a month he's been having it. Every day, four times a day in his milk because it says *not more* than four times a day on the bottle, so he was having it at every feed. But now we've stopped, we got another one didn't we? Pink [Calpol]. It says half a teaspoon not more than four times a day. In milk. I went to the chemist to buy Panadol and they didn't have any. They said we've got one similar. But we don't put it in his milk now, we just put it in his little feeder with some boiled water whenever he screams. (*Deborah Smyth*)

MENUS – FIVE MONTHS

JOSEPH BRADY:

9am Tin of apple in a bottle.* 9ozs Cow and Gate Babymilk Plus. 4ozs water.

1pm Tin strained chicken dinner in a bottle. 9ozs Cow and Gate Babymilk Plus. 4ozs water.

6pm Rusk in 9ozs Cow and Gate Babymilk Plus. 4ozs water plus one teaspoon of Calpol.

JONATHAN MOORE:

7.30am Breast

9.30am One Weetabix mixed with cows' milk and glucose. Breast.

1pm Plate of minced roast lamb, roast potatoes, gravy and sprouts. Plate of minced apple pie and custard. Breast.

4pm Bottle 8ozs diluted cows' milk.

*Nina Brady put all her baby's solid food in a bottle to avoid the mess of spoon feeding.

6pm   Plate of stewed apple mixed with one ounce of grated cheese
           and cows' milk. Breast.

JANE MANSON:

4am   Breast
8am   Breast
11.30am   Breast
4.45pm   Breast
10.30pm   Breast

MARTIN MILLER:

8am   Tin egg and bacon breakfast. 8ozs National Dried milk.
1pm   Jar vegetables and ham. 8ozs National Dried milk. Tin
           bananas.
6pm   Tin egg and ham. 8ozs National Dried Milk.
10pm   Rusk in 8ozs National Dried Milk.

*Beginning solid food is one milestone. The path is quite adequately (too
adequately) mapped out and the signposts of advice not hard to find. But after
that the new mother, despite expert advice, may find it difficult to decide on the
balance of solid versus liquid food, and bewildering to choose the 'right' brand of
food from among the many on the chemist's or supermarket's shelves. Jo and Steve
Ingram share their puzzlement at this problem, as they share the care of their baby
(Steve looks after the baby during the day while Jo goes out to work).*

I: Are you having any problems with feeding at the moment?
JO INGRAM: Yes. We're worried about solid food.
STEVE: About the amount of milk he's taking.
JO: About whether he should be progressing on solid food more than
he is. I mean we didn't start forcing anything down him before he
really wanted it. We introduced one meal a day and I didn't give him
any more than one meal a day for about six weeks.
STEVE: She, the health visitor, didn't say you've got to give him this
one. She gave me a list. She said he can have this one or this one or this
one. And I just went in there and looked on the shelf and saw baby
foods. I brought cans home to start with and that was the wrong stuff
['junior' as opposed to strained foods]. So I went back and got
packets, but I got number two [for older babies] so I had to go back
and get number one.
JO: Difficult, really. For all I know he ought to be having those lumpy
foods. How much food should he be having? Because we decided it
was time to cut down his milk. Almost arbitrary: right, we must cut

down his milk. And it just doesn't fucking work. They yell or they're not satisfied. So what the fuck do you do? *I find the feeding difficult, the most worrying thing.*

But looking back over the first five months of infant feeding, anxiety and lack of confidence tend to fall into place as necessary steps in the learning of motherhood. Common sense or instinct or whatever you choose to call it triumphs; the autocratic reign of the expert gives way to a more democratic order. It is easy to be wise after the event.

If you were advising a new mother about feeding, is there any particular piece of advice you would give her?

Go by your own intuition. If the baby seems happy enough with the food you are giving him, then, fine. (*Mandy Green*)

Be guided by your baby. (*Ellen George*)

I think I would say that you ought to give a baby what you think a baby needs. And not to worry. I would say go by the baby and not by what they tell you. (*Jane Tarrant*)

Listen to your instinct. That's the one thing I wish I'd done right from the beginning. But obviously you don't, especially with a first baby. I think I'd know next time to be a bit more instinctive – not instinctive, but to trust yourself, because there are so many times when I've thought I'm *sure* that's what she needs, but so and so says you can't do that and you shouldn't do that: or maybe it isn't. I'd start using logic. I mean the health visitor would be shocked if I'd told her that Lily had her jar of whatever it was at twelve o'clock and then I gave her a bit of me two hours later. I mean I shouldn't have done that! But I'd rather do that if it keeps her quiet. I think it is here, it's mine, I can give it to her if I feel like it! (*Alison Mountjoy*)

CHAPTER 9

Domestic Politics

After I'd been going out with him for a year he said, oh I'd love to walk down the road with you, be married to you and have a little baby. It's like a dream come true.

It's not really what I hoped it would be, the marriage thing. Being a mother you have to stay in, somebody's got to stay in to look after the baby. And the man still gets out as much as he used to, he's really just like a single man. He comes home and sees the baby when he wants to, and he can get away when he wants to . . .

It takes two to make a baby. After that fathers are, biologically speaking, unnecessary. The meaning of 'fathering' is insemination; 'mothering' means child-rearing. But if biology makes fathers dispensable, society carves out particular roles for them. These roles are shaped by history and circumstance, so that fatherhood in pre-industrial France differs from fatherhood in the African Congo, and both appear foreign to an English urban businessman fathering his first child in the 1970s.

Yet in a sense the problem for every society is the same. If men are to feel involved with (or at least responsible for) their children, they must be impressed by a sense of indispensability: they must feel necessary. Our industrialised culture achieves this end via a logic of economic dependence: women and children must be supported by men. The logic is reinforced by an appeal to a set of ideas about the nature of both men and family life. A proper man fathers children, who are then visible confirmation of his sexual and social normality. A proper family is made up of a male and female parent and their children: a 'family man', a 'housewife' and the patter of tiny feet (or 'may all your troubles be little ones').

Looked at another way, the problem for men is how to share the experience. The seed that started it off is lost inside a foreign body and the long months that preface its re-emergence can often be a kind of limbo.

FATHERS-TO-BE

JANE TARRANT:
He's thinking of himself more as a family man, I suppose he feels he's going to be a father. He talks a lot about the baby. He talks about, you know, is the baby moving? And if a plane goes over can the baby hear the noise? And he's very very *involved* with it. He wants to come and feel the baby moving and all the rest of it. He thinks of being the father of a family, and when will we have the next one? And things like this. He often comments on my stomach and things and I say don't keep commenting, and he says but it's nice. And he thinks of me as a mother.

LOUISE THOMPSON:
He's more interested than me. He says let's have a girl, I'd like to see how a girl turns out. We've always had this quarrel on psychotherapy. I say to him if I thought everything you said was the word of God, wouldn't it be boring for you? It's true. We have these incredible arguments about penis envy. I say it's incredible that a man should think a woman wants a penis. Don't you think that's compensation for not being able to give birth? Only a man could dream it up and only a man would believe it.

LOIS MANSON:
David's read the hospital booklet: he's really quite involved and he keeps saying things like I'm eating too much and I should put my feet up.
DAVID: I just think it's interesting; obviously I feel it's my child as well as Lois's; it might be growing inside her but I still find the whole process very interesting, although I'm not such a direct part of it as she is. I like to know what's going on. . . .

JOSÉ BRYCE:
He's read the books I have. Sometimes he does it of his own accord and sometimes I say *now read this*. And participate in this pregnancy!

IAN HATCHARD to JUNE: It's difficult for me, because apart from when you take your clothes off and you look a bit bigger round there . . . I think it's something you gradually become more aware of. I mean I think about it occasionally, but I don't think about it that often. I think that again is something that increases.

JUNE: Yes, I think it comes to me in flashes sometimes, you've got something inside you.

IAN: I think to a large extent you really do have to take it as it comes anyway. Physically I'm helpless, there's nothing I can do. Like you've been saying that you feel you get wind a lot: all I can say is have an Alka Seltzer.

I: Do you think of yourself as a father?

IAN: Very rarely. I don't think I've thought about that side of it very much at all. I mean that side of it is nice, isn't it? That's the optimistic side, when you sort of think of yourself as a parent, having a daughter or a son. The thought of saying 'my son' sounds really fabulous, really nice . . .

NINA BRADY:

He's worried, he goes down here on his knees every night praying. Now you might think he's some kind of fanatic, he's not. He's worried that something might happen to me or the baby – that it might not be normal or something. . . . He talks about it: he says everything will be alright with God's help and praying. . . .

JEAN CLARK:

I think up odd names and he says yuk. Stupid names: Mark, Fleur, Paulo, which is Italian for Paul which he doesn't like. He doesn't like Fleur. I said oh we'll call it after your friend Benito Mussolini, or Ho Chi Minh. I said what about Karl Marx? What about Lenin or Trotsky?

Through such discussions the baby may acquire an advance personality. But the problem for fathers-to-be is that they cannot 'conceive' the baby.

I: Do you think about the baby as a separate person?

ELIZABETH FARRELL: I suppose I think about it more inside me. When it kicks and makes a fuss I suppose I must think of it as a personality actually . . . I asked Robert: I said, have you any feelings about it at all? He said no. I couldn't understand this. He said, well, I've never *seen* it – I don't know what it's like.

JULIET MORLEY: That was one thing that I particularly noticed when we were talking to some friends about this business of whether the husband should be at the birth. This chap had been at his wife's birth and he was saying how wonderful it was to be there when this new thing came into the world. Well, I found that almost discordant because I think it's here already. I don't think of it starting when it's born.

Some fathers-to-be, like Jane Tarrant's husband, are keen to feel the baby's movements in the womb. Others are less so, finding the whole business curiously distasteful.

I: Does he like feeling it move?
TANYA KEMP: No, he doesn't like it.
I: Why not?
TANYA: He says it's like a frog. He doesn't like it at all.

LOIS MANSON: David says it gives him a funny sensation: it gives him a queasy kind of odd sensation. He wants to feel it and he does feel it but I feel sometimes that it's out of obligation to me: that he feels he ought to show he wants to feel it. And he does say that it makes him feel odd. He says that it definitely affects the way he feels sexually. Because I don't think he finds it offputting – it's not that; but he doesn't want to hurt me in any way, and I think that's something that's been in the back of his mind.

The vista of a pregnant abdomen may alter sexual appetites. Some men may be turned on, others turned off:
I think he looks at me in a different way from what he used to. . . . I don't suppose he finds me so sexy. Well, I don't suppose I look so sexy. No, I think, he thinks of me more as the mother of his child. (*Jane Tarrant*)
Nick's not very keen on it at the moment. I'm offputting by my shape at the moment. I wish he was one of these men that found me – you know, some men find it, we've got some friends and he found her so *lovely:* he said I kept *looking* at her. And I thought well. . . . I think you've got to *be* like that though: you're either that type or not. He doesn't find it *revolting* – he just laughs, especially when I walk around without any clothes on. He says you look like Guy the gorilla. (*José Bryce*)

I: Has the pregnancy affected your sex life?
JANETTE WATSON: No. I think in the last six weeks it starts changing round and the womb – does it open up? And the baby start to drop? I'm worried about that but he says . . .

DAN WATSON: Actually I'd like to get some advice on when is the best time to stop for a while from the safety point of view. I was reading one of the books that she has and it said it's alright to continue provided it doesn't become a bore for the woman. . . .

Growing size and tiredness do usually become disincentives from the woman's point of view.

I: Any problems with sex?
PAT JENKINS: No, sometimes, I think probably because I'm tired, I don't really feel like it.
I: Does that worry you?
PAT: It did at first, because you know I think Alex didn't understand: he just said did I really not love him? And I said I was just tired. . . . We always had a good sex life and he felt as if I rejected him. I think he didn't understand and I think I probably hurt his feelings.

Tiredness can be one of the most shattering aspects of pregnancy, and perhaps one of the most difficult for husbands to appreciate. To them their wives remain the people they married, not only sexual performers, but bringers-of-cups-of-tea.

EMMA BUCKINGHAM:
He finds it very difficult. For instance, if I burst into tears he doesn't understand that you get tired. He realises that I get tired but he doesn't make allowances. Sometimes I say I'd like a cup of tea in bed sometimes thank you very much. I have to be totally honest about it and say I'd like to stay in bed, will you bring me a cup of tea?

I: Has being pregnant affected your relationship?
JOSEPHINE LLOYD: I wouldn't say it's altered it in any way at the moment because I get the feeling sometimes that Howard forgets that I'm pregnant. Because he doesn't – sometimes I feel that, you know, he doesn't really show consideration for the fact that I *am* pregnant. . . . For example, first thing in the morning, as soon as he wakes up, he likes a cup of coffee in bed, and he says to me, he gets a bit ratty, if I don't get up and get him a cup of coffee straight away. But I don't always feel like getting up straight away and making coffee, especially when I've had a bad night and I've got these wind pains. I feel as if *he* should be getting up and getting *me* a cup of coffee, but he still expects his cup of coffee. . . .

I think we're further apart in the sense that I do get irritable and perhaps there's not the same amount of understanding between us that there used to be. Because if I'm feeling a bit ill or miserable or something, perhaps he doesn't always associate it with the fact that I'm pregnant although I know that that's probably the reason.

HOWARD: I know it's there but I'm still not – you know I look at you and I can't see it, you know.

A couple's reactions to pregnancy depend of course on the kind of relationship they have. The firmer the foundation the less disruptive pregnancy is likely to be. On the whole, women say that they and their husbands feel closer during pregnancy: there is a greater emotional, if not physcial, intimacy. The growing baby symbolises their joint love (and not yet sleepless nights and dirty nappies). The birth awaits them as a miraculous experience bringing that long expected sight of the new human being, arousing feelings not felt before, putting a seal on the success of their relationship.

PRESENT AT HIS OWN RISK

Should the father be at the birth? In the last ten years or so, it has become increasingly fashionable to admit husbands to the delivery room. What started out as a movement among middle-class couples has permeated downwards until it is now the rule rather than the exception in many hospitals that the father is present. The father's role is carefully prescribed, however, as indicated by this form the sample women's husbands had to sign if they wanted to attend the birth:

> I understand that whilst the husbands of patients are encouraged to be present during the first stage of labour – that is to say before their wives are taken to the delivery room – if I wish to be present during the delivery, in my wife's interest I will sit at the head end of the labour bed on the chair provided and I will leave the delivery room immediately if I am requested to do so. I agree that I shall be present at my own risk.

GILLIAN HARTLEY:

We asked questions about husbands being there during labour. The sister seemed quite pro-husbands being there. But she said that she didn't like them to look down at the bottom of the bed, some of them tended to be squeamish. She said they should keep up the head end where they belong. I think it's terrible, it is a male chauvinist thing, the idea that seeing your wife giving birth, seeing the blood and the placenta, will be repugnant to the husband and put him off you as a sex object. That seems to be in their minds somehow: that we don't want to see women doing these disgusting things. Even being sewn up if you have to be. I mean, why not?

You know about John Ruskin don't you? Oh well, his wife, the marriage was never consummated and she would have had it annulled, but the reason it was never consummated was that John, being a great lover of art, had seen all these naked statues of women, and of course they didn't have pubic hair. And on the wedding night when he confronted his wife, who was indeed hairy, as most women are, he was so put off by that that he couldn't consummate the marriage!

NICOLA BELL:
Well, I'd like him to be there but he won't. I just think for reassurance that it's nice for a husband to be there.
NIGEL: I'm a bit squeamish really. And I tend to feel it would put me off a bit.
I: Off what?
NIGEL: Off sex, I suppose.
NICOLA: I think it's something that you should both share, the birth really. You never know, he might change his mind.
And he did:
He was glad to be with me; he didn't want to be there, but he stayed; he got so tied up. And afterwards the nurse said to me he was pushing harder than you were. And all the time he said he wouldn't be there! He said he was squeamish and he said it would put him off me.
I: It didn't?
NICOLA: No. And in fact he was the first one to shout it's a girl. He was really pleased . . . I don't think I could have done it without him, really.

There are many reasons why people feel a father should or should not be there.

ALISON MOUNTJOY:
I feel that if I could go through it without him, then perhaps I would rather. He's quite old-fashioned, and I know it would be nice to say here's your baby, afterwards: aren't I a clever girl? He's still not sure how much he wants to retain the romantic image of it all. Like you say, don't you, that you don't know whether you want to be there when it's born because it's rather nice to be *presented* with it afterwards.
LUKE: I think I'd like to be there during the first stages really.

ALISON: Again, that's another thing that different people say different things about. Admittedly, I've never heard any man who's been present at the birth saying they wish they hadn't; but you do hear the fears of other men who haven't been there, or doctors who don't think it's such a brilliant idea.

LUKE: It's a very difficult thing. Part of my reasoning behind *not* wanting to be there is that if one is there it might be difficult to back out and it might be difficult to take an objective view of any problem that might arise.

ALISON: You mean it's healthy to be a bit disassociated from it for the health of the mother and baby?

LUKE: Yes.

ALISON: That's an interesting idea. But of course he's a doctor's son.

Margaret Samson's husband is a GP.

I: Will you be present at the birth?

JAMES SAMSON: No. No chance. Because I've seen too much obstetrics and I know from bitter experience that the *worst* thing ever is for the husband to be present when something goes wrong. The staff's on edge, the doctor's on edge. I've seen things *really* happen. When women haemorrhage in childbirth they *really* haemorrhage. I've had on wellington boots with it lapping round my ankles. There's just *no way* I'll be present.

MARGARET: He's said that right from the word go, as well.

JAMES: And the next thing that happens is of course that you're treating the husband because the husband faints. I worked in a place once, when I was in Australia, that handled the whole of New South Wales. I didn't know what a normal delivery looked like, because every delivery I did was abnormal – forceps, caesareans. . . . They just introduced this business of the husband being present as I started my senior year in obstetrics: it was dreadful. The sister would say the husband's going to be present and we would say something's going to happen for sure.

LOIS MANSON:

14 weeks pregnant:

I don't particularly want David to be there.

DAVID: If Lois were to say I want you there, then I would be there but if she says if you want to go you can, I've got a free choice, so I'm not sure. I'm not sure how I would react. If it was someone else having a baby, it wouldn't worry me, I think I could even help if necessary. But being Lois, the relationship's a bit different. If she were in pain I'm worried about whether I can cope with it being her. I mean I've seen films and things and it doesn't worry me from that point of view, it's the fact that it's *Lois* in that situation, not that it's *someone* in that situation.

LOIS: And I'm afraid that my attitude is totally selfish. It would be nice, idealistically, that we share this wonderful experience together, but it's not for that reason that I want David there. It's that I want someone to be there so that there'll be someone there I know who cares while I'm going through it, that's purely selfish.

I: So you *do* want him there?

LOIS: From that point of view, yes, but if it's going to be traumatic for David and upset him then I don't want him there because I don't want him to be upset.

Five months later:

He will be there. I'm much more definite than I was: that's something that's really developed over these last few months. I suppose it must be some kind of build-up of fear in me, a build-up of the obvious *need* I feel that he's got to be around. Not just to share in the experience and all that stuff, but so there's someone who can stand up for me when I'm not going to be in a position to stand up for myself. You know, I *really* want him to be there if they're going to do things like cut me without thinking about it: I want someone there who's generally going to look after my interests, if you like. And secondly, I think the more I do find out about it and the more I learn about childbirth, I think it would be nice to have someone there that you know very well, who's going to give you general comfort. So I feel much more strongly about it.

I: What about David?

LOIS: Well as far as he's concerned, if I want him there then he'll be there.

It was like seeing a good film

Women certainly find it easier than men to see the advantages of the father's presence at birth: 77 per cent of wives wanted their husbands there, while only 43 per cent of husbands wanted to be there. But, like Nicola Bell's husband, many find that in the excitement of the moment they simply forget to leave. Once drama takes over, the role sits more comfortably on their shoulders, and they become

necessary (and usually grateful) actors. Ian Hatchard and Francis Sharpe were
two husbands who were adamant that they would not be in the delivery room.

JUNE HATCHARD:
He was there in the end, yes.
I: Why did he stay?
JUNE: Well, they're in and out – they go out and come back·in, and
then he went out and had some lunch, and then he came back . . . so he
was just *there*, and I think I said to him well go out if you don't want to
watch. But he didn't. And he was really glad that he did stay.
IAN: It worked out very well.
I: Why didn't you leave?
IAN: I think the emotional side rather than the physical side, which is
what I thought I'd be more aware of. I mean obviously I thought I'd
be aware of the emotional side, but I thought the blood and stuff
would put me off. But when you've been standing around all day it
tends to get a bit boring and you get used to all the machines and
knives and stuff. . . . I suppose I just felt quite emotional at the time. It
was like seeing a good film: you want to see it again.
JUNE: All he said was you'll have to have another one, just about a
second after. That was his first reaction!

RACHEL SHARPE:
Francis stayed and watched, you know. Well you see he went down
into the waiting room and then after I'd been prepared and everything, and was taken to the delivery room, sister came down and said
to him have you signed the form? And of course he was in such a state,
he said oh no: so he signed it. And when he came in he told me what
had happened and I said do you know what the form was for? And he
said no. And when I told him, he went green. He said well when it gets
really heavy I'll just leave. So I said that was fine with me. So what
happened was when it got near the time for him to be born and things
were hotting up, it worked out that he was so enthused that he didn't
leave after all. He kept running down the other end and looking and
coming back and telling me what was happening, and giving me a
running commentary on the monitor. And he was *so* excited and I was
really glad he had stayed. Had I known in the first place what it would
be like I would have been really enthusiastic. I wouldn't do it again
without him. I thought it was great and he did as well. He said up
until then that he'd never really believed all these fellows who'd said
oh it's great, you know . . .

In every case, the 74 per cent of fathers who eventually stayed for the delivery were pleased to have done so. But most agreed that it was much more of an experience than they had anticipated.

JOSÉ BRYCE:

I was *amazed* that they let him stay in the end for the forceps. It was only because of the doctor, because every time the sister came in, she said could you leave Mr Bryce, and then he kept saying oh it's alright I've told him he can help. But Nick was worried for me especially when he thought I was having a haemorrhage, because he didn't know for sure . . . he just saw this blood, and he was frightened at that point. He said the only thing I could think about was never *ever* letting you have any more children. In fact even a couple of days after he told, I mean he doesn't know that I knew, he told a friend of ours that he was going to have a vasectomy later on and we weren't going to have any more children. He doesn't think that now. But I think he was in a bit of shock then: only because he didn't know what to expect. If I'd told him, or anyone else had told him beforehand what they were going to do he'd have said no I can't do it. If he'd seen a film of what was going to happen, he would have said no, there's no way I could stay there. But I think you get carried on from one stage to another. . . .

And of course there is always the legendary story:

DEIRDRE JAMES:

My husband said I've got to go outside, it's so hot . . . he goes outside and there was this noise. I thought oh no, he's passed out. Sister came in and said oh it's alright, your husband's just passed out. He passed out again down the corridor. They sat him in a wheelchair and he said next thing that he knew he was on the floor and his feet were in the wheelchair. . . .

Birth is literally shocking for fathers as well as mothers, physically wearing, emotionally draining, impossible to grasp. The front of common, everyday behaviour is breached, and feelings, normally inhibited by masculine reserve, flood out.

STEVE INGRAM:

It was a weird experience. My general attitude up to the point where I saw the head was I'll pretend I'm quite progressive about it and have a look. But I really couldn't face it. I thought I'll stand as far back as I possibly can. When it came out, once it's head was out, and it started looking like this [i.e., pink and human], this great emotional thing suddenly happened to me. I had this feeling all welling up inside me: nothing particular, it was just one of these things, I can't put it into words. Tearful, I suppose.

Because we were keen for a girl I noticed his balls. What it was in fact, when he came out, as I say I was expecting a girl, and I thought to myself – I rationalised to myself in such a way that I thought oh balls. Big balls. It's a traditional thing to say I suppose; I suppose I was thinking something like, it's a funny girl, it's got big balls. I was a bit disappointed actually, but the emotion that came over me, I was so charged from it. It sort of like builds up to the point where it's who cares? And that's how I feel about it now. It was a very emotional thing for me.

JO: He doesn't like being emotional. He doesn't like being moved.
STEVE: No, it freaked me out.

DAN WATSON:
It's unbelievable: it's quite an experience. Have you ever seen the birth of a baby? You have? And I was participating, because I was running around getting water for her and one thing and another, and trying to help out with the midwife. She asked me to do a couple of things, you know. And I was the first one to see he was a boy, even before the doctor. I think if I was sitting outside and the doctor came out and said here you are, that's your son, I'd be *pleased*, but seeing him come out, I mean I've known him from the actual *second* of birth, and I think that makes a lot of difference.

I: Was Kenneth there all the time during labour?
LILY MITCHELL: Well as I say he came back at half twelve and apart from lunch and coffee he was there from then on.
I: How did you feel about him being there?
LILY: Oh great.
I: How did he feel about being there?
LILY: He just can't get over the experience. He said you just feel so much closer to the baby. He said that he thinks that it would be the same sensation as a woman having a caesarean, someone giving a baby into your arms and saying that's yours – he said that he knows that in no way could it be anybody else's now, because he was there and he saw it. . . . It was two or three days before I actually got this out of him. I said to him, how do you feel about being there and he said oh

it was great; he said it was one of the most fantastic experiences he ever had in his life. He says that it was just something that you couldn't find words for. He said you just had to be there to understand.

SOPHY FISHER:
Oh he was overwhelmed by it. I think he'd decided that he would stay with me but he wouldn't *watch* too much. But when they offered to show him the foot [Sophy had a breech delivery and a foot was 'born' first] at five o'clock – after that he just couldn't believe it. He was very sweet because when I was holding my breath he was holding *his* breath – he wasn't actually pushing, but he was going as pink as I was. He was having her too! The next door neighbour – he came home, well obviously he had to come home and it was a terrible anti-climax for him, he didn't want to leave at all – I've got to go home to an empty house! Well, go to Susanna! And she says she had him till about three o'clock in the morning, getting fairly pissed, but apparently overwhelmed and in tears and telling her over and over again about it and how wonderful it was and how he saw the foot. So it was obviously an extraordinary experience for him. . . .

HELPING WITH BABY

There's no such thing as *fatherhood* really, except the initial day the baby's born. Fatherhood and that's it: he goes back to work the next day. *(Kate Prince)*

Birth is an extraordinary event. It breaks all the rules of ordinary existence. The difference between day and night ceases to matter, breakfast, lunch and supper become haphazard snacks in the interstices of disordered time: out-of-place emotions become curiously appropriate. In the ordinary course of a man's working life there will be few occasions such as this. But the moment is not sustained: time becomes tidy again, routines restrain him. He has become a parent but in everyday terms this has so much less meaning than it has for his wife, the course of whose life is altered for ever.

LILY MITCHELL, five months after the birth:
I: How does he feel about being a father do you think?
LILY: Oh I think he *likes* being a father. But I mean really he only sees

him in the evening and Saturday and Sunday. I think it's *easier* to be a father. This is a mother's twenty-four-hour-a-day job, whereas a father has an office job from whatever time he goes in the morning to whatever time he comes back. And that's it.

Our society defines fatherhood principally in economic terms. Father is breadwinner, mother is nursemaid. Social norms make the father's role within the family unit much less important than his role outside it; holding and keeping a job that produces enough money to provide for wife and child – this is his main duty. The only time that is available for fathers and children to be together is time left over from the job. One consequence of this is that a third of the sample fathers saw their five-month-old babies for an hour or less a day. But as families have become smaller and living standards have risen, the mother has more childcare work to do unaided and this is a strain for her that may overflow onto her husband. Evenings and weekends are liable to be laced with feeding and babyminding sessions, if only to free her to cook his *supper.*

In many cases it has *become more acceptable for a husband to 'help' his wife; provided he doesn't help too much, it is regarded as probable that his masculinity will survive. The concept of 'help' here is obviously political: because they 'help', fathers do not take the main responsibility for child care; or because theirs is not the responsibility, they must only 'help'. (The same is true of housework.)*

'Helping with baby' has thus become one index of a man's involvement with his children. The sample women were asked how much their husbands did for the baby at five weeks and five months, and what they (the mothers) felt about this. From their answers, it is clear that birth produces a peak of masculine domesticity; many fathers may be quite heavily involved in the early days, but this level of participation falls off as babies become older, life becomes more routine-like, and the novelty of fatherhood is eroded by time and sleepless nights. Parallel with this trend, mothers become less satisfied with father's role, expressing their resentment either directly (why won't you change a nappy/feed the baby/push the pram?) or indirectly, so that the domestic politics of baby care erupt into the emotional side of marriage. Wife nags at husband, husband moans at wife, and the rosy dream of the little family degenerates into a domestic nightmare.[1]

But, first of all, what do fathers do?

SOPHY FISHER, television producer, and MATTHEW FISHER, designer:
Tiffany, aged 5 weeks:
I don't think Matthew knows quite what to make of having her. She's less real to him than she is to me. I think he's slightly less involved

than I thought he would be.

I: Does he change nappies?

SOPHY: He's *watched* me change her nappy, but I haven't forced it. You see it's usually part of the feeding process [Tiffany is breastfed] so I mean I just do it. And I think he feels a bit unsure about *dressing* her, so he doesn't do that. Really the only thing he does is wind her: he's terribly good at winding her when she's got bad wind.

I: Does he get up in the night to her?

SOPHY: I take her into the bathroom to feed her in there. He slightly resents being woken in the night. I did try taking her into bed, and feeding her one night but he got very upset about that and said he had to live a normal life even if I could sit around all day and other such-like unjust things!

When Tiffany is five months old:

He gets more and more interested in her. But he is still on a fairly peripheral level with her. I mean he *plays* with her a lot and I think that's very important, but he doesn't *do* anything practical for her – that's not to say he *won't* but he *doesn't*, and I have the responsibility for feeding her and looking after her. And if he wanted to do more of that I wouldn't mind sharing it with him.

I: Does he change nappies?

SOPHY: He has done. I've gone to have my hair cut and if she's needed a nappy change he's done it. But it's probably not been half dozen times.

I: What about bathing?

SOPHY: He's never bathed her. I've shown him how to and said he ought to because it's such fun, but he never actually has. I think he's a little bit frightened, but he wouldn't admit it.

I: And feeding?

SOPHY: I've said do you want to give her her supper a couple of times but he's said no, you do it. [To Tiffany] We'll have to get him to, won't we darling?

I: Why doesn't he want to do these things?

SOPHY: I don't even know that it's really that he doesn't. I suppose it must be that he doesn't want to, or he probably would. I don't think he's particularly interested; I think he gets the pleasure from her from the playing times. He thinks I'm quite happy to look after her – as I am. He's got more involved with her personality-wise; he finds her much more interesting now; she responds to him, plays games and so on. I don't know; it doesn't worry me at the moment.

MAUREEN PATERSON, ex-library assistant, and HENRY PATERSON, shop manager:

Thomas, aged 6 weeks:

He's very good: he's *marvellous* with him. First of all he was a bit frightened to hold him; he kept saying, am I doing it right? Am I doing this right? But he's really good with him.

I: Does he feed him?

MAUREEN: He gives him a bottle. Only a couple of times he's done it. He usually does something else while I feed him. But he gets up, if I have to get up early in the morning, he'll get up with me. He gets up and he makes a cup of coffee. He's very good. He mixes all his feeds up, he mixes them all up for the day for me and puts them in the fridge.

I: Does he change nappies?

MAUREEN: Yes, he has done that. Only a couple of times. But he knows *how* to do it.

I: Does he bath Thomas?

MAUREEN: No. He's *helped* me sort of thing.

When Thomas is five months old:

He thinks the world of him. He's proud of him and that.

I: Does he feed him?

MAUREEN: Not very often, no. Not that he doesn't *want* to, it's just usually that I do it. But he will. He still mixes his milk, he always has done. And he changes the steriliser.

I: So how often does he feed him – once a week?

MAUREEN: Not that often. Normally I'll feed him and Henry'll probably get on, if it's tea time he'll get on with the tea while I see to him.

I: Do you prefer to feed him?

MAUREEN: It wouldn't worry me. I think it worries him a little but still, I mean he'd *do* it but I think he gets a bit panicky. And now especially you have to hold him down because he wants to put his hand in the dish.

I: What about nappies?

MAUREEN: Oh yes he'll do that. Sometimes if I'm doing something he'll start him off.

I: And washing his clothes?

MAUREEN: Sometimes if I've boiled the nappies he'll rinse them out for me. He doesn't *wash* anything, you know. The hand washing, I wouldn't like to see him standing there doing that anyway.

I: What do you feel about the amount he does for the baby?
MAUREEN: Oh he's good. Sometimes I think he does *too* much ... I don't know how some girls manage really if their husbands don't help them.

A mother's satisfaction with the amount of help her husband gives her with the baby depends in part on her own expectations of what he should do. Husbands, on the whole, should do so much and no more. Sometimes satisfaction is expressed in terms of the husband being 'very good' or 'marvellous' whereas in fact he does very little — Maureen Paterson's comments illustrate this well. What is important to some women may not be the amount of practical help given but the general attitude of interest and willingness: 'he'll do anything if I ask him'. In the two tables below, some figures are shown that give an idea of fathers' participation and mothers' satisfaction with this.

Fathers' help with babies*	
A lot	11%
Some	24%
A little/none	65%

Satisfaction with fathers' help	
Satisfied	54%
Dissatisfied	46%

* As described by their wives five months after the birth.

The most favoured paternal task, as Sophy Fisher's account makes clear, is playing with the baby. The least favoured task is changing a dirty nappy.

Dirty nappy stories

CATHERINE ANDREWS:
He *has* changed a nappy, although he tends to avoid that. If I go out and leave her and a bottle he'll change the nappy then, but otherwise he'll wait.
I: Why?
CATHERINE: I don't think he particularly likes the idea. He picks the nappy up and I say can you put that in the bucket; he goes ugh. He doesn't particularly rave about the idea of changing nappies. I think it is probably in case it's a dirty one.
I: So has he ever changed a dirty nappy?
CATHERINE: No. He'd never changed a nappy for quite a while and I said it's about time you did, just to show that you can. He said of course I can do it. I said show me. So he proceeds to undress her, to

the nappy, undid the pins and everything else, then he said oh it's dirty. I said well go on then. He said um ah well, do I *have* to? So I did it. . . .

MICHELLE CRAIG:
I mean we went swimming a long time ago, about two months ago, we was only out two hours and I told him where everything was and when I come back I said I bet you haven't changed his bum? He said well no I haven't changed his bum, I don't want to change his bum. He changes nappies unless they're messy ones, and then he won't, I'll have to do it. He'll undo it, then I'll have to take it off and clean up most of him and then he finishes cleaning him up and puts another nappy on.

JANE TARRANT:
He does moan about it sometimes if it's dirty. On Easter Sunday he took him upstairs and it was dirty and he called me up to see what he should do about it. He did know but I think he just wanted me to come and do it.

GRACE BOWER:
He has changed a wet one once, but he won't change a dirty one. I don't think he likes it to be honest.
I: Do you think that's reasonable?
GRACE: Yes and no. I mean *I* have to change it, why doesn't he? I keep saying to him what if I wasn't here? Oh then I'd change it – but if you're here you can change it.

Unlike most other couples, Jo Ingram and Steve are trying to share the work of bringing up the baby, who at three weeks is breastfed.

STEVE: All I ever do is wash and change him.
I: So do you do about half?
STEVE: No I think I probably do less than half.
JO: Right, right.
STEVE: I get all the shit work.
JO: That's the sad thing. He was changing nappies in the hospital, which made them quite cross.
STEVE: Especially when I stood at the end of the ward and shouted where do you put the shitty nappies, then?
JO: It was quite funny, because all the husbands in the hospital sat there with open mouths watching this one. I was *incensed*, one guy,

he'd come to collect his wife because she was going home that day and she kept saying 'packet'; she said he's just done a packet, and he went ugh and sort of backed off. I thought God! I just wanted to get up and hit him.

. . . At night Steve gets up and changes him so all I've got to do is just feed him. It really is helpful actually to have this baby handed to you. That's one of the biological myths, isn't it; it's very much a biological myth that's thrown at you isn't it, that if you breastfeed a baby you've got to do housework; all the nappy-changing and everything. You want someone who can perform the services of a lover *and* a nanny.

STEVE: I went to a benefit the other day and there was a play on and in the middle of it I had to go and change him, which meant I had to go down to the men's toilets. I started getting things out, and he'd really shitted and it was all at the back of his clothes as well. There wasn't an incinerator there or anything. So what I did was I took his pad off first and threw that into the toilet – the urinal part, not the other toilet; then I had to clean him up with these little cotton buds, and I started throwing them in all the sinks. And there was shit and everything all over the place. And I thought well fuck them, that'll show them!

A TYPICAL MAN

There are no facilities for changing babies in men's toilets because men are not supposed to change babies. (There are very few in women's toilets either, of course. This reflects a social double standard towards mothers and babies: women are expected to have children but on a practical level society is not baby-oriented.) Social norms define the proper and the improper and even those who reject such norms suffer from their consequences. In part, the issue is one of public versus private behaviour: what a man does in the privacy of his own home does not have to live up to the same standards of masculinity as what he does outside it.

ANNE BLOOMFIELD:
We had an argument last week, a really bad argument, and I stormed out. And I came back about an hour and a half later and she was screaming for food and I didn't have any clean nappies and I didn't have any disposables, I was going to buy them but I forgot, and he was just going out to buy some with her and he was going to push the

pram then. But he doesn't when I'm with him. He wouldn't do that because of his friends. I don't expect him too. I mean, you know, when he's in here and no one can see him he's lovely with her, but when he's out, he's a typical man.

Pram-pushing is a highly public act. It therefore stands as a cipher in the masculine–feminine code, a policy statement in the sexual politics of baby care, a delicate demarcation line between two countries: his and hers.

RACHEL SHARPE:
The only thing I don't like is the fact that he won't walk down the street with a pram. I mean he won't walk with me when I'm pushing it. When he saw the pushchair he said that's very nice. I don't know if it'll make any difference. He just says he hates prams. He just doesn't like to walk down the street with one. When we were at his parents at Christmas time his mother had a big pram she'd got from someone, and we were going into town one day, they live about a mile out of town, and there were three of us going, the two of us and his sister. He said you go ahead with Mary and I'll come later. It was just because he didn't want to walk with the pram.

DIANA MEADE:
32 weeks pregnant:
I: What do you think your husband'll do for the baby?
DIANA: I couldn't see him walking down the street pushing a pram.
I: Why not?
DIANA: I don't know. My brother never pushed a pram but would take the baby any place in his arms. He wouldn't push a pram but he'd take the baby wrapped up in his arms.
Seven months later:
He takes her off walking on a Sunday to the market. In his arms. He couldn't push a pram. Never would. That's a woman's job. He'll carry her any place!

KENNETH MITCHELL:
I wouldn't push the pram on my own, no way.
I: Why not?
KENNETH: I don't know. It's a stupid Irish thing. In Ireland you don't see men pushing prams at all. It's not that there's anything wrong. It's just like carrying a bloody handbag, isn't it? It's not that there's anything wrong with carrying a handbag for a woman you know but – I carry a shopping bag, no way I'd carry a handbag; if

she's loaded down I carry everything else but she has to carry the handbag.

TANYA KEMP:
Since we've got the buggy, he'll push that, whereas he wouldn't push the pram.

This liberated response to the buggy on the part of fathers was reported by many mothers – a case of technology bringing about social change?

THE POLITICS OF HOUSEWORK

Obstacles to change, to greater paternal involvement, are the ideas men and women hold about their roles. As Jo Ingram said, it is a biological myth that breastfeeding means housework. But it is a cultural attitude that a woman's place is in the home, and once this rationale is established it becomes 'logical' that all the domestic tasks should be heaped on her head. Measuring men's involvement in housework over the period from early pregnancy to five-month-old fatherhood, there is a clear trend towards men doing less and women doing more.

Caroline Saunders was a physiotherapist before she had Lesley:
He expects me to do more now I'm at home. He doesn't offer to hoover any more, which I don't blame him for. I mean there have been days when I've been occupied with her all day and I haven't got round to cleaning up and he's come home and complained about it.

Juliet Morley was a rebate officer before she became a housewife:
I've noticed that he's started to *expect* me to have done his washing and similar things. Which is fair enough really, I suppose. But I still find it going against the grain a little bit when he says something like what shall I do with this dirty sweater? Or something like this. A year ago he would have done something about it.

Rachel Sharpe, an ex-copywriter, has a similar complaint:
He doesn't take his shirts to the launderette any more. One day he said to me you never think about my shirts; I never have a clean one any more. But it's just, he's decided that he's going to let me do them now, but he didn't bother to tell me – he just sort of left them around and I just never pay any attention to them because I'm so used to him doing them himself. . . . I've done one or two but I still haven't got used to the idea that I have to do them and I still forget to do them.

Janette Watson, ex-factory machinist:
It's all my work, he says. It's my job.
I: Do you agree?
JANETTE: Sometimes I do, sometimes I say I'm not your slave. I suppose it *is* my job really, being a woman. That's what *he* thinks, anyway.

	During pregnancy	Five weeks after birth	Five months after birth
Husbands' help with housework			
A lot	22%	14%	6%
Some	30%	38%	33%
A little/none	48%	48%	61%

The division of labour begins to change when the woman gives up work in late pregnancy. From this point on the two roles become much more clearly divided; housewife at home, husband–father at work. And because housework is not 'work', all the work that has to be done might as well be done by her. Although the baby is the reason why a mother is not out at work full time, the walls of the home close in on her, as washing the floor becomes indistinguishable from washing the nappies, buying baby food no different from buying husband food. It is part of the housewife's oppression that ideologically housework and baby care are the same. There are very few marriages in which the politics of who does what are not, at times, a burning issue.

All the old dodges are dragged in: you do it better than me; we have different standards; I don't know how to do it; you won't let me do it; you go out and earn the money then.[2]

Louise Thompson admits to female chauvinism:
It was the Rapoports in the *Sunday Times*, I think they said that sometimes women really can't accept men's help and I think I'm like that. I mean I'm making him sound bad, but it's just as much me as him. Like if he washes the dishes I could wash the dishes in half the time: it drives me crazy!

Juliet Morley's husband never does it right:
I find that I have to be continually resisting the temptation to tell him what to do with David. He doesn't change nappies or anything; he does it occasionally if I'm doing something, and I have to make a

conscious effort not to say have you done this this way, have you done
this that way; you've done it wrong; don't do this – don't throw him
up, he'll be sick. He got nappy rash once after Paul had changed his
nappy. . . .

Keith Lynch hasn't learnt how to change a nappy:
Because you're at home all day you've got all day to do it. It's true, it's
quite true. He does say to me is there anything I can do? I did say to
him once can you go upstairs and get something or do something and
he says you've got all day to do that. So I said well don't ask, then, I'll
do it myself. He'll hold him, play with him, doesn't feed him or change
him. If I'm in a hurry and he's demanding his food I'll say alright you
feed the baby and that's it: he panics. He was on his changing pad and
I was doing something else: I said oh take his nappy off, will you? Oh
quick, quick, he's wet everything, he's wet everywhere, quick, quick. I
think actually if he were to change his nappies I think I'd have to
check up afterwards to make sure he'd done it right. He wouldn't stick
the pin in, but he'd probably do it too loose or stick the nappy out of
the plastic pant and of course that soaks everything. . . . (*Christina
Lynch*)

Vera Abbatt's husband draws the line at certain jobs:
When the baby was getting up in the night we were fighting like cat
and dog. I was tired and I was getting ratty and I was taking it out on
him and he was getting ratty and taking it out on me sort of thing. I
think about four times in one week he threatened to go. I wasn't much
help, I kept telling him to go. Lucky he didn't. I think probably
another couple of weeks and he probably would have gone. I couldn't
blame him, when I thought about it. But at the time I thought it's not
my fault I'm in a bad mood, it's all his fault.

Eventually I got to the stage where I thought why the hell should it
be me that gets up in the night? I thought why shouldn't he do a bit of
it? And then when he started to feed him he wouldn't change his
nappy. He used to put him down in the pram which meant he'd be
saturated right through by the time I got him up in the morning. And
of course that roused me, all this washing every morning, and he'd
end up with a chill. I usually get up now anyway. Anything for a quiet
life. I gave up arguing. By the time you've finished arguing you've
been up half the night as it is.

At times it annoys me. I get a bit fed up at times. I think it's all very

well his saying he's been at work all day, I've been working all day
and all with him. Other times I think well he'd probably make a mess
of it anyway. I might as well do it myself. Like when he feeds him in
the evening he'll sit and talk to him for about half an hour after and by
the time he's finished talking to him he's wide awake and he won't go
down, whereas if I feed him and put him down . . .

Neil Tarrant says 'you're better at it than me':
That's one thing I'm not very keen on – when I give him the ten
o'clock feed I'm in bed you see and then to have to get out of bed and
go into his room and change his nappy and put him in bed; I would
like him to do it. But he laughs and says oh no he wants his mother to
put him to bed, he'll sleep better then. (*Jane Tarrant*)

*Some couples, like the Hatchards, the Mansons and the Princes have extended
debates about the sexual politics of housework and baby care.*

I: Does he change nappies?
JUNE HATCHARD: He's put them on a couple of times but I usually
end up re-doing them because he's too gentle, they're all *flapping*. I
usually say I'll put it on, it's easier if I do because otherwise it does fall
off.
I: How do you feel about the amount he does?
JUNE: Sometimes I say you never do the nappies. He pretends: he says
I'll do it and then he says I don't know *how* to do it. I think he rinsed
the nappies through a couple of times. And like yesterday I said half
joking why don't you do the ironing? And he said oh I can't, I'll get all
creases in everything. I just don't know how to iron. I said if you did it
you'd learn how to. But again it's probably quicker if I do it, which is
wrong really.

I think sometimes I get a bit fed up and I say why don't you go and
do the washing up? But it's mainly because he doesn't *think*. I say to
him you'd walk over a pile of clothes. I think a lot of people are like
this. In the summer some friends of ours – Claire had a great thing
where Allan moaned at her at the weekends because she was washing
you see, and she said I've *got* to do it – because she works in the week.
She said it's *your* washing anyway. He sort of said well you don't have
to do it. So she said *right* – so there was this carrier bag of his washing.
I put the idea in her head because I did it to Ian when he moaned
about the ironing. I said alright, I won't do your ironing then, and he
had this pile and he's never moaned since about the ironing. So I said

you ought to do that and she did it with the washing, but she gave in and did it before the week was up. I said to him have you done the washing? And he said no I haven't – and you knew he hadn't because he was wearing the same shirt for about three days. But then she gave in on the Thursday, she only did it from the Sunday to the Thursday, so his carrier didn't get very full up, you see.

Lois and David Manson have been married seven years. Since they left university, they have both been working full time, and sharing the housework has been part of their view of marriage. A month after Jane's birth, Lois had not yet returned to work:

I: What about the division of labour?

LOIS MANSON: In that compartment David and I have had the odd ruction. Nothing more serious than that. David will jokingly come home and say oh Christ haven't you done *anything* today? You've been at home all day. And it will *only* be joking but nevertheless it riles me that he could even say that jokingly. We've never actually *rowed* about it but I know that when I'm at home and I'm dashing around doing the housework and all the miserable things that one has to do in the daytime and I get fed up and tired in the evening, and sometimes I say to David oh I'm so tired, go and make a cup of tea, nine times out of ten he will quite willingly, no question about it; but then sometimes he'll say oh come on, why are you so tired? And it only needs a little thing like that and I launch into a great, well, you don't know what it's like.

I: Does he change nappies?

LOIS: He has done, but he's not very keen on it. I normally change her nappy when I feed her or if she's made an enormous mess and she's got to be changed, so really the occasion doesn't arise when he comes in and says oh Lois she's all wet. But I think if it did, yes he might say she needs changing. In which case I would say to him change her then, and he would change her. But he would protest a bit. He's not as keen on changing nappies and that aspect of it as I thought he would be. But then that's because he's slow at it and he's just not very good at it. I'm much better and quicker.

KATE PRINCE:

Two friends of mine, their husbands have never once changed a nappy since the baby was born, and they say it's all because they don't know how to do it or they don't want to do it. I often think it's probably the wife who thinks oh he'll mess it up and won't do it properly. Well, I don't agree with that. They soon learn, don't they? Mark, when he first put the nappy on, the nappy was round her ankles; they seem to make the mistake of not doing it up tight enough. But now he's become quite a dab hand at it. He's as good as I am. Neither of us have done it in our lives before, so why these women are suddenly experts, pseudo-paediatricians – it gets on my nerves, I can tell you. I could lose a lot of friends through that business.

He rinses the nappies as well. He says he likes doing it – I don't like doing the nappies. He doesn't sometimes do them very well, he's got slightly lower standards than I've got; I go out and there are a couple of shitty nappies on the line: I say that's a bit stiff isn't it? And he says oh it'll do. And he's quite right. It's a terrible thing, but I think, God what are my neighbours going to think if I put shitty nappies out! I mean they've got a little brown stain on them, they're not sparkling white. He doesn't care.

There was a time when people said to him, he got a bit *rebellious*, we nearly had a revolution on our hands: he came home and said so-and-so said to me that they never do anything at home and they were amazed that I did. He said George doesn't do anything. And I thought hallo hallo and he was beginning to hear these stories, and everybody was praising him for the amount of work he did. He was beginning to think he was pretty wonderful. And he got a bit peeved one day and he was saying I think I do too much – I go out to work *and* I help you and all that. And he was in fact quite cross that day; I mean he *likes* joining in and it means we get the jobs done quickly and we can sit down and enjoy ourselves. And I thought oh God how am I going to handle this? Because he was really sort of *annoyed* . . . And I got cross, I snapped about something, I was fed up about something. It was late at night and we were both tired and he said I don't *mind* doing it, but you should say that it's very good of me to do it compared to other husbands. And I said no, and I refused to, and we had a row about it. I said no, I don't agree, I think *they* should do it. I don't think you're being particularly virtuous to help me with this baby. It's them being bastards and their wives letting them get away with murder. And he said oh no I know that's true, but you should *appreciate* it: you don't realise how *lucky* you are, and it was all this about how I should be *grateful*. Not that I don't *praise* him, but I don't feel that should be the case. And so we had a bit of a to-do about that. . . . I mean he *is* very good, but I still stuck to my guns. I'm not having any martyr on my hands carrying on like that about how terrific they are, would you?

Demarcation lines are re-negotiated; the map of domesticity is re-drawn. In such tales of domestic disharmony, the flavour of a relationship is conveyed. But it would be naive to measure the impact of parenthood entirely in terms of how many nappies are changed by whom and whose responsibility the dust on the carpet becomes. Nobody, after all, wants a baby so they can watch one another grapple with feeding bottles and the nappy bucket. Remember the reasons why people wanted a baby: to cement the relationship, to symbolise love, to create a family.

A PROPER FAMILY

Do you feel that the baby has affected your marriage?

We're a lot closer since I had him because we're one family of our own. (*Kirsty Miller*)

I think it's better, it's brought us closer as a unit. We're more caring and more loving. We show it to Mary and so we show it to each other. (*Clare Dawson*)

Yes, I think we're a bit closer. We've got a common interest in Annette. We haven't really got much in common – you know, the things I perhaps like to do he wouldn't like to do, whereas she's something we both take an interest in. (*Nicola Bell*)

I think we probably see one another – maybe it's made us three-dimensional, because you're seeing the person with another third person really, you know, which is a product of the two of you: this is something that we've cooked up between us. It's part of us, and it's quite nice to see how the other person is with our product. (*Lily Mitchell*)

We want a bigger family now. You're not *really* a family until there's another one – a baby – and one toddling around: then it'll feel like a *proper* family. (*Deborah Smyth*)

It hasn't *improved* it. It's still the same. But we're obviously not as selfish as we were. I mean now not only do we think of each other, but we think of one other person. ... But kids *do* put a strain on a marriage. I mean we've been particularly lucky, he hasn't put any strain on our marriage. We're lucky that we waited, we thought about having him so much before, and I think I am older than a lot of people who are having babies, especially their first ones, and I think that's helped. It's one of the reasons why he *hasn't* put a strain on the marriage. But I can quite understand how if they do this crying at night you rush around and things aren't ready, meals aren't ready when the old man gets home; it must be awful especially if you're married to that sort of bloke who gets *upset* about things like that. (*Sarah Moore*)

Janette and Dan Watson had been married just over a year when Peter was born; Janette is nineteen:

The baby's made a lot of difference. He hasn't changed us at all, but mind you we've been arguing a bit. Well we haven't *argued* really, because he starts arguing and I just laugh.

On Saturday he came in – because he didn't play football on Saturday – and he came home at five. So I cooked our dinner and he'd fallen asleep you see, because he wanted to feed the baby. So I went into the bedroom and he was asleep. So I came up and told him his dinner was on the table and he woke up; he must have been half asleep still and I didn't realise he went back to sleep again. So I came up and had my dinner and shouted at him. So he stormed out and ate it in the kitchen and what happened then? Oh he started shouting and swearing at me because I thought it was funny, he usually laughs. But he didn't laugh this time, and I did and that upset him. This was after his dinner. So he went out for about an hour, came back, picked up the baby and about half an hour later he came down to see me and he was alright again. I don't know why he was like that. I think he might have had a few pints in the afternoon. He's been like it before, before we had the baby. Mind you, it upset me; I didn't think he'd come home, but he did an hour later. I told him I didn't want this to happen. I didn't want the baby to muck up our marriage.

LOUISE THOMPSON:

There's just too much tension sometimes. This friend of ours who's been stripping the stairs, he says thirty points to Louise, forty to Oliver.

At first when Polly woke up a lot at night, he said she's a fucking pain in the arse – what a lousy crybaby. It was awful, it was like a caricature of men! He said I'm going to sleep in another room. I said I don't care where you sleep. He said I'm sleeping on the stairs: I said go ahead.

LUKE MOUNTJOY:

It's made problems in certain ways.

ALISON: What do you mean, it's made problems?

LUKE: Well things like lack of sleep some nights and things like that. But if you disregard those things it's been good for us.

ALISON: I think what Luke's trying to say is that it's made *technical* problems, like the *sleep* problem. As far as I can see that has been the biggest problem, the lack of sleep and what stems from it. Like for the first time since we got married there are occasions when I have to say I'm too tired, and it's not very nice to find you have to say it, and it's also not very nice for Luke to find that it's been said to him. Because there are the *classic* jokes: you remember that birthday card you sent me, it was really quite funny. It listed all the classic jokes one hears about old married couples – I'm too tired, I've got a headache, my mother's coming, which never happens until you have a baby and then you find that it's happening all the time, they're all real. [To Luke] I think you didn't understand to start with that I *was* so tired – you thought I'd gone off you, didn't you?

LUKE: There was one time, yes, and then I found out that a friend of mine's wife had gone off sex for a year, and I thought oh well . . .

ALISON: You thought you weren't doing too badly!

EMMA BUCKINGHAM:

We were discussing this last night actually. I know Lawrence feels a bit left out. Because I'm tired. I used to be an awfully happy, jolly person and I've just been so tired. Lawrence comes home and I flake: I don't *feel* like playing Scrabble at eleven o'clock at night and laughing when he gets angry, which I always used to do. I don't get angry, I just get *cross*. I'm crotchety and I feel emotionally drained: I get *terribly* tired. I just get perfectly horrid: I know I'm doing it, I can't do anything to stop it. No we don't have rows, we have discussions. We tell each other exactly what we think of each other. He can't understand how tired *I* get and he says I don't understand how tired *he* gets working in the office. I think I feel I get no relief during the day, and then Lawrence comes home and I'm feeding the baby, and I've got to get him tea. Deal with that. And then comes supper. You see he comes home and he's feeling full of the joys of spring and I'm an absolute dampener on his spirits. I *know* I am. You see he likes to stay up late. We always used to stay up late. Now I get tired by ten, really. And by half past twelve I want to go to bed. I want to go to bed by eleven, but you see Lawrence has hardly been in from the office. Lawrence feels he's somehow failed me and I feel likewise – that I'm not making him happy and yet we still love each other. I don't think it's affected our love. He feels a failure because I'm not the happy bouncing me that I was. And because I'm not happy and bouncing and cheerful I'm not making him happy, bouncing and cheerful: I mean we're still happy in our own way.....

The emotional relationship between mother and father seems to improve during pregnancy to a peak at or shortly after birth, and then to deteriorate. Birth, a joint achievement, unites husband and wife; the baby, a maternal responsibility, divides them. From the euphoria following birth there is an abrupt fall to the tired anxiety and disorganised routine of the early weeks of the baby's life. To remember, through all this, how happy you both really are (or ought to be) is difficult: a drop in marital happiness was described by 73 per cent of the wives. Alison Mountjoy alludes to one reason for this: problems with sex.

Vaginal politics

The passage out of which the baby emerges is the most intimate channel of communication a couple possess. But unhappily the baby leaves physical scars and many women – 72 per cent of this sample – have trouble with stitches and with intercourse afterwards.

I: I suppose this is a silly question since your stitches haven't healed properly yet, but what about sex?
MANDY GREEN: Well it hasn't stopped the desire. Nothing ever stops the desire; I tell you, that's the trouble.
HARRY: We're both going round the bend. But it's worth it, isn't it kid?
MANDY: You speak for yourself!

NICOLA BELL:
I wondered if I'd ever be normal again. When I went for my postnatal, well, we had attempted intercourse before, at about five weeks, and it was very painful; I went for the postnatal and when they inserted that thing into me that hurt me again and the doctor examined me and he said it *shouldn't* hurt me. He said it shouldn't be hurting, is it the stitches? And I said yes I think it is. And he felt round the stitches and it wasn't the stitches. He said does that hurt and I said no; he put his finger up and said is it here? And I said yes. It wasn't at the neck of the womb, that was alright. It was further down and he said you've got a tight vagina, and I'd got to persevere with intercourse to stretch it, and if it hadn't stretched in three weeks to go

back and they'd stretch it for me. It's still a little bit painful. . . .

I: What did he mean when he said you'd got a tight vagina?

NICOLA: I don't know. I don't know if it's got anything to do with the stitching. Has it? Do they stitch you inside? I couldn't really understand that. You know, when we do have intercourse once it's in, it's okay, but it's *getting* it in. At first it was painful the whole time but now once it's in, it's alright.

I: So you don't enjoy sex at the moment?

NICOLA: Oh yes I do *enjoy* it, but I suppose not to the same extent as I did before, because you're always thinking oh dear! You remember I complained when that doctor was stitching me? I shouted. And I think that perhaps because I shouted he didn't do his job properly. I don't feel as though I was stitched up properly. It is bad really when you think about it. I mean it could ruin the whole relationship, couldn't it?

SUE JOHNSON:

Do you know what they did to me at that hospital? They stitched my fanny up so that I'm sort of a virgin – or worse than a virgin.

When I went for my postnatal they told me I was tense – and it was just all my fault. So I went away thinking well I'm *tense* you know. That was really weird. I don't *feel* I'm tense but I am! So I went through *months* – we went to France and all the time it was like every time we made love I'd sort of grit my teeth and it was absolute *agony* – I mean *real physical pain*. And so when we got back here I thought I'd go to my private gynaecologist and she told me that they'd stitched me up so small that I've hardly got any opening at all. She gave me these glass expanders – she gave me a small size to begin with; I couldn't *believe* it, I could only just get it in. It was *tiny* and I could only just get it in.

I haven't been able to have sex properly for *six months*. When I discovered that that was what had happened it really freaked me out, it really did. I really felt just terrible. Because that could have completely ruined my relationship. In any case because of it Martin was having affairs with two of my friends. I discovered that when I got back to London. I think to do something like that to a woman is really *appalling*. I mean probably the only person I could go to bed with is a Chinaman: everyone else is too big! I thought of putting an ad in the paper, 'experienced virgin. . . .'

TWO'S COMPANY...

Life with a young baby is difficult enough without these complications. A new mother may feel everyone is claiming different bits of her body when all she wants to do is sleep. Torn between husband and baby, she may feel she cannot satisfy either. Seventy per cent of the sample mothers felt some conflict of this kind. Tiredness saps self-confidence, and the cliché that twenty-four-hour-a-day baby care has to be experienced to be believed, divides the sexes.

He never shows his feelings

The father becomes jealous of the baby or perhaps the mother learns to resent the way father walks in and starts playing with the baby; she feels left out: she does all the work, he gets all the fun. Part of the communication gap is men's 'trained incapacity to share'.³ Men are brought up not to talk about their feelings, women to look upon such talk as therapeutic. Masculinity means the domination of the mind over the heart, or keeping one's feelings to oneself; femininity means having feelings and letting them out. So especially at a time when life is stressful, the chasm of different concerns and attitudes that separates mother and father may be greater than the common interest that joins them together. Pat and Alex Jenkins' marriage, five months after Wayne's birth, has this pattern.

I: How does he feel about being a father?

PAT JENKINS: I think he's very proud, but he doesn't tell me how he feels. I phoned him up at work one day and his boss answered the phone and he said we hear about your baby all the time because Alex never stops talking about him. So he must talk about us, you know, but to me he doesn't say anything. I suppose to other people he does. But I just wish he'd say it to me more often.

Alex was the one who wanted the baby, he's the one who kept on and on about it, because I wasn't going to start a family so soon. I wanted to wait until I was about 26 or so, because I felt I wasn't ready yet, you know. But in the end I had to, well I wanted him myself, but I thought well I'll have to give in, because he just kept on and on about it. But to want one so much, he doesn't – well he *loves* him, don't get me wrong, he's very *proud* of him, but he just doesn't *show* it enough, you know. He doesn't play with him enough I don't think. You know when he comes in at night, and he's there, he probably wouldn't acknowledge the fact he was there, and I'd say oh Alex, look, he can do this or he can do that, and he'll have a wee look and he'll smile, and he'll say something and then he'll go back to reading his paper or watching the television.

I: And how do you feel about that?

PAT: Well it hurts me, you know. I'm going to talk about it to him, but I just have to pick the right moment, because Alex is funny that way. The other night I kept the baby up and I said when he came in, I said I've kept him up for you, you know, but he never bothered playing with him. So I mightn't have bothered keeping him up, you know. I don't understand. But Alex doesn't show his feelings a lot anyway, you know. Like I know he loves Wayne and I know he's really proud and thinks the world of him, but I don't think he shows it enough.

I didn't know if I loved Alex any more, thinking all these stupid things. He wasn't telling me he loved me, he wasn't even having much to do with me, because he was hardly talking to me, and then when I wanted to bring everything up, he just shouted at me. I just couldn't say anything to him. He'd bite my head off all the time. And then he'd say oh you talk a lot of rubbish when I wanted to talk with him. I know I'm not going out and I can't – when you're at work, you've got something to talk about. It's true. All I wanted to talk about was what Wayne did and to me that is the most important, but to him, he just wasn't interested. He must come in and tell me all he did at work, and I just have to sit and listen and try and be enthusiastic, and I didn't know what he was talking about sometimes, but I pretended to know, and he could do the same for me couldn't he? When I get depressed, when I feel depressed, he just thinks I'm silly: that's all there is to it. One time I was going to walk out, I was taking Wayne with me, and he said you can go, but leave Wayne! He didn't ask me why I was going, or what was wrong, or anything. And then he lifted up Wayne and kept him by his side so that I wouldn't go!

I: What did you feel about that?

PAT: Well I felt hurt, because he wasn't really bothered about what I was feeling, you know.

I: But you didn't go?

PAT: No. I just wanted him to do something, you know. Because every night he was coming home – although I admit he does work very hard, and he's very tired himself – but he's coming in at ten o'clock you know, or nine o'clock, eleven o'clock some nights, and he wasn't even saying hallo to me or anything. And he'd go and sit over there and he'd be working on papers or something. And then in the mornings he always kissed me goodbye, but he wasn't saying goodbye to me really.

Children make a marriage

Children have a symbolic value. They are prized because the family is an ideal – but this does not mean they have an ideal effect on marriage.

I TO BARBARA HOOD: Do you feel that being a mother has any particular advantages or disadvantages?

GEORGE HOOD [walking into room]: Yes, I tell you one disadvantage, I don't get my dinner on time. [Sits down.]

BARBARA TO GEORGE: You're not stopping, are you?

GEORGE: I'm starving, I want me dinner.

BARBARA: Oh I asked you earlier and you said you didn't want any.

I TO BARBARA: Do you want to go and get him some dinner?

GEORGE: No, it's alright, go on, get this over with.

BARBARA: I think the only thing I can give you is egg, ham and chips.

GEORGE: That's nice, isn't it? Isn't it nice, that? What were you going on about this chicken for? Weren't you going to get some chicken? Or was that last night?

BARBARA: Chicken? You had some chicken last night.

GEORGE: I've had some dinner but I still feel hungry.

BARBARA: Well, get some fish and chips then.

GEORGE [still sitting there] to I: Is this for your book, then?

I: Eventually.

GEORGE: How is it going? Is it going alright? Is it taking, are the right things happening?

I: It's very interesting.

GEORGE: Is it? Have you got a family of your own as well?

I: Yes.

GEORGE: So you know it all? What's the idea of this book, then, what are you trying to do?

[Interviewer explains]

GEORGE: Yes, it's a lot of hard work. . . . Is your husband looking after the children?

I: Yes.

GEORGE: It's amazed me actually, the number of people, I wouldn't say they're anti-children, but they say, you know, they can get

through a marriage without children . . . I think it *makes* a marriage. I
don't see how a marriage can *work* without children.
I TO BARBARA: Would you agree with that?
BARBARA: Not really, no. If a couple agree that they don't want
them . . .
I: Will you have a second baby?
BARBARA: If we're still together!
GEORGE: See what I mean? See if there *wasn't* children I think you'd
be a bit more – oh blow it – and do your own thing.
BARBARA: Oh yes?
GEORGE: Yes, you would be, let's face it.
BARBARA: Clear out?
GEORGE: Yes, exactly. You want your way and I want my way and
there's that continual . . .
BARBARA: But we're always like that.
GEORGE: Well, there you are! I want my breakfast in bed and you
want yours in bed. Now who gets their breakfast in bed?

ROLES AND IDENTITIES

*Some marriages weather the advent of a baby better than others. The more
romantic the vision, the worse the prognosis. A 'good' relationship acts as a
shock-absorber, and the changed dynamics are not less resilient but more so. In our
society where the nuclear family is seen as the only proper nursery for children, the
major effect of parenthood is to set husband and wife on different paths: the roles
are divided, the overlap between their daily lives is reduced. Since for most couples
the division is according to the formula female–housewife/male–breadwinner,
there is a tendency to see the consequences in sexist terms. The woman complains
that she only has the milkman to talk to because that is how women behave; the
man comes home and wonders what she's been doing all day because men are all
chauvinists at heart. But Jo Ingram and Steve show up the falsity of this
deduction – not intellectually, but in the way they experience parenthood. Jo is a
further education teacher and Steve looks after the baby.*

A mirror image

I: Has the baby affected your relationship?
JO: Well you say no and I'll say yes or I'll say no and you say yes and

we'll scream at each other. Maybe I ought to go up the shop and get some cigarettes while you answer that question, and then you can go up while I do. I'm not sure that either of us will give an honest answer! [She goes.]

STEVE: I just think of the good times, any time up to six months ago. The past. I think of the good times and forget the bad. I think we're both under a lot of pressure at the moment.

I: Is that just the baby?

STEVE: Oh Christ, I don't know. I think it's a mixture of everything. But I probably blame it – I don't know, I mean I really couldn't give you an honest answer. I mean I could just list a load of things and you'd have to sort it out yourself.

There's a lot of tension at the moment: tension builds up very quickly between us. We sort of step back, take a breather, and then we come at it again. I mean I find that I seem to be resenting a lot of things now, and I don't know whether that's because of Jo and the situation that we're in or whether it's because of my own limits. The thing I resent more than anything else I think is Jo coming home, and I can see it almost like a mirror image of what in fact I'd probably do – coming home, not in a mood so much, but in a *different* mood. Like if you're sitting at home here all day you're orientated between here and the bedroom and the kitchen, you know, and the shops, or whatever: and really you can talk to the grocer, you can talk to the paperman, you can talk to the milkman, you can talk to people who come to the house – that's fine, you can talk to people who come and visit you – but nevertheless it's almost like you're having a conversation with yourself and then somebody rudely bursts in.

For instance like yesterday, Jo's got a habit of coming home and working her arse off until it's time to go to bed. It could be political work, it could be stitching up those curtains, it could be cleaning bottles, it could be emptying the nappy bucket, because it hasn't been done in time, or washing up, and it's like it's pushing *me* into the activity as well . . . because I think to myself I resent that because really I should be doing it, I feel that I should be doing it. And that sort of builds up inside of me and so I can't just bottle it up and I just turn round and say get out of the fucking way . . . I do find I resent Jo coming home like that. But I can also see that that's what *I* used to do; I used to come home and I could feel the change in me as soon as I stepped in the door; it's almost like you're as happy as a pig in shit all day and then I'd come home and there was a clamp. [Compare this with Emma Buckingham's remark, pp. 226–7.]

And then if I meet old work friends, I mean alright they're only working-class blokes if you like – they say when are you going back to work Steve? This sort of thing. I say I *am* working, I'm working fucking harder now than I've ever worked. Their attitude is yeah yeah I know, but when are you coming back to work? And I say I *am* working . . . I don't think they understand. . . .

The home is a private place, so the work of child care is socially invisible, and can be discounted. But it is perfectly real to the person who does it. Although having a first baby permanently alters the emotional interior of a couple's relationship, it is the social division in parental roles that threatens it most. Husband and wife can pretend to be equal: mother and father know they are not.

CHAPTER 10

Into a Routine

It's like when you have a new recipe – a complicated recipe – and you keep looking at the book at first and then you can whip it up in no time.

When I think about it now – you see I don't think a lot at the moment – my life does seem trivial. I mean what is your life for? Now my life isn't my own any more; my life is to be devoted to my children now.

DAILY LIFE

JULIET MORLEY, ex-rebate officer, mother of David, five months: The alarm goes off at ten past seven. We get up after the half past seven news. I made some tea, made Paul a piece of toast, had a piece of toast myself. David woke up about eight o'clock – no, that's wrong, he woke later than that this morning, because I cleaned up last night's dishes and things first. Had my wash. So he must have woken about half past eight, quarter to nine. After that I had my jeans in the machine and I was waiting for them to dry so I was wearing my dressing gown, and I did a bit of sewing while he was in a good mood after breakfast. He usually has a bath, I didn't give him a bath this morning, I gave him an all-over wash instead about ten o'clock. About quarter to eleven he had his nap for about half an hour, then we went down to the village to do a bit of shopping, about half past eleven. [Juliet moved from London to a Somerset village after her son's birth.] And he was hungry by this time. So he had his meal just before twelve. And then I put some more washing in the machine. He sat in his chair and played with rattles and chewed bits of celery. And then I took him round the garden, looked at the branches of the trees, that sort of thing; then I put him back to sleep.

I did some housework – I was doing the kitchen. He had his tea at four o'clock so I probably spent some time playing with him before that – if you play with him afterwards he's sick. He had his tea, changed him, brought him back down again, I had to get Paul's meal on time yesterday because he was going out. At six. So I think I did the preparations, then played with him and put him to sleep just before Paul came in. We had our meal at six. He slept till seven. Then he's very grumpy for an hour: I spent all that hour playing with him. He was tired, he was in between sleep and waking for an hour; for that last hour in the day he doesn't usually play on his own. You see he has part of my attention the whole day really. After that I had a bath and I went to bed early – about nine.

LOIS MANSON, part-time educational research worker, mother of Jane, five months:
At half past two yesterday I was at work observing a large class of unruly children. I went with them into a room to see some slides of battered children for a project called 'personal relationships'. That was a *traumatic* experience, really miserable, I couldn't watch it, it was all so awful and I related everything I saw entirely to Jane. I quickly followed them out of the room after that and went back to what we'd intended to do. I read them something from a book called *The Big Switch* where women take over the world from men. We talked about women's position in the world, and again everything I said was related entirely to Jane and being a mum back at work. And then it was the end of the day, three thirty, and I went into the greenhouse at the school where David [her husband works with her on the same research project] and I are transplanting tomato plants because we're going to grow all the tomatoes for the school and for us: we sell them cheaply to the staff. Then I did a little bit of shopping on the way home. Took back a cucumber and waved it at the proprietor of the shop and got a new one in its place.
  Got home here at four thirty. Mum had been looking after Jane. David took Jane for a little walk round the garden, into the greenhouse, and chatted to her for a bit. Then I fed her, probably about a quarter to five. Then I did a meal for Mum, David and I, and we had our meal. Then David said he was going to sleep for a little while because he wanted to do some work, and he went to sleep in front of the television, and I started to do some work. We played with Jane and she went to sleep very quickly about five thirty, just before the meal. And I did some paperwork in connection with a committee I'm on: I wrote some letters. And I wrote a letter of complaint about

some photos that weren't very good and that took me quite a long while. Then I came in here and it was probably by that time nineish, and I watched – did I watch something on television? I'm not sure. And then I was going to do some knitting. I got the knitting out and started to do it. Then I fell asleep. Oh that's right, I wanted to see the programme on schizophrenia, and I started watching that – that's what I came in to watch and I fell asleep half way through. Woke up and had a chat with David; by that time it was probably ten thirty, eleven. And we woke Jane up because it was late and I was tired and I thought we'd play with her and what have you, because we like to play with her before she goes to sleep in the evening. And so we had a little play with Jane, and I fed her, then I went to bed probably about midnight. And David came to bed and we made love – that's not the most usual thing every night, so I include that. You wanted every detail, didn't you?

This morning I woke up about four o'clock and I fed her and she went back to sleep again, but she woke up again about six plus and David played with her most of the time because he was going to have to get up at seven, so I rationalised and said well you can get up a little bit earlier. I went back to sleep on and off; I was vaguely aware of Jane being there. I fed her again about eight. In the meantime David brought her down here and played with her while he had his breakfast and what have you. And then I came down because he was cooking breakfast and it smelt so nice and I thought I'd cook myself some, and I opened up the post and there was a letter of complaint from a chap I'd written to last night: I'd written a letter to do with my committee work, but I'd left it for ages, and this letter was complaining that I hadn't written, and it was a nasty little letter and it really upset me. So I was going back to bed: for a long while I've been going to have a rest because I've had a busy weekend, my sister-in-law's been down from Liverpool and it really has been a hectic weekend. But I really couldn't lay up there and think about that letter, so I came down again and David was going off to the school, and I got him to post this letter that I wrote last night. I was agitated about that.

I started doing some housework, tidying around. I did some washing. I've been on the phone to someone who wants me to talk at a money management conference and I've been in touch with him to say that I would willingly talk at this conference but what about Jane? Could I take her along, or could they organise it so they could pick me up and bring me back. And I chatted to him and made arrangements and I've made arrangements to take Jane, so that's fine. Then I finished doing my washing; I played with Jane, she went to sleep after I'd fed her about nine; then she woke up again at ten thirty. She usually sleeps till about eleven. But when I fed her this morning she wasn't very hungry at all and I thought well perhaps she's hungry. So I made her a drink, gave her some rosehip syrup, and she didn't want to go to sleep, obviously, so I played with her down here and put the television on because she loves television, and we started watching the telly. She likes the news because of the faces. And I started watching a programme, I don't know whether it was a schools programme, on King Farouk, and Jane was getting frustrated because I *insisted* that she watch this programme with me. And so we watched King Farouk between us, walking around the room and what have you. And then I gave Jane a bath about eleven-thirty and fed her about twelve and put her to sleep. And then I did a bit more work, committee work; I don't do that often but it so happened that I'd got all the stuff out. So I finished off that, sorted through some papers, started writing a letter, and then you arrived.

CHRISTINA LYNCH, ex-traffic warden, mother of Adrian, five months:
I worked all day yesterday, I didn't stop. I did a load of washing, I did all *his* washing by hand, and I put it on the line. And then I did a machine load of washing, then I did dusting and vacuuming. I can't remember in what order. Isn't it stupid, it was only twenty-four hours ago, I can't remember. Yes, I think that was all the afternoon. It doesn't sound much, does it? What was I doing while the machine was going round? Oh having something to eat. Because I had breakfast at half past ten, I didn't eat until four: cheese and biscuits. Keith was coming in late, so I had a meal with him at about eight o'clock. I fed the baby in between times: I think at nine, one and five: he went to bed at six. Keith came in about half past seven. My friend had ordered a bed and he said we'd take it in for her, and it'd just been delivered, so they came round to take it away and he helped them and he said you owe me a pint now.

After our meal I think I did the vacuuming then, I cleaned the bathroom and the toilet. Yes, because Keith went out and then I did the vacuuming: I was still doing it when he came in at eleven o'clock. He said why are you doing it up on the landing? You'll wake the baby. I said that's the idea. I left the landing till last so I'd do it just before his feed so it'd wake him up, but when I opened the door he was still fast asleep.

To me it doesn't sound much, but I was busy all the time. I went to bed about half past twelve, got up at seven. I got up three times in the night and put the dummy back. I thought if it happens a third time I'll get up and feed him and it did but I didn't feed him. I fed him about a quarter to nine. Fed him, washed my hair, I had a couple of biscuits. I fed him and then I dashed down to the shops. I'd run out of everything, and as soon as we came back it was time to feed him again. That was it. That was an untypical day, I did all my work yesterday.

I: So what is a typical day like?

CHRISTINA: I don't really know. I don't seem to do anything. The time just goes. I go out every day shopping: I make myself go out. Because otherwise I'd just sit there and rot.

KIRSTY MILLER, ex-pattern grader, mother of Martin, five months: I get up about half nine, ten o'clock, any time like that. Get him dressed, washed and dressed. Get dressed meself. Give him his breakfast and then a bottle, and then I'm off for the day.

I: To?

KIRSTY: My sister's.

I: Every day?

KIRSTY: Yes.

I: What do you do there?

KIRSTY: Nothing. Hardly anything. Just sort of look after him and that's it. Sometimes we go out shopping.

I: How many children has she got?

KIRSTY: Six. They run everywhere. Well, she's got two at home and four at school. I get there about twelve, after breakfast, after I've sorted everything else out. Done some washing. Just his. His lunch, it all depends what time he has the last feed: round about twelve, one o'clock, something like that. All depends. Usually after one o'clock he'll go to sleep. In the pram, outside in the hallway.

I: And what do you do then?

KIRSTY: Don't know. Anything and everything. Just chatting away. He has his next feed about four. I come home about five. Sit there and have our tea. He might drop off, it all depends. If not, he'll sit in front of the telly, and that's how he'll stay until about eight. And then he'll go to sleep. At eleven he'll wake up and then I'll give him a bottle and he goes for the night.

THE MEANING OF MOTHERHOOD

Five months after the birth life has become ordinary again. The achievement of producing the baby is in the past, and the present must be devoted to growing and guiding the baby towards childhood, adolescence and adulthood. Accounts of daily routines given at this stage will reflect the different dispositions and social circumstances of mothers, but all record a sense of life being focused on the baby. Either activities are organised around the baby's needs or the baby's needs are stage-managed to make other activities possible, but in both cases the baby is dictator. In every family it is the mother who is seen and who sees herself as responsible for satisfying the baby's needs. (Even the Ingrams, who 'reversed roles' (see pp. 232−4), found it difficult to share the reponsibility.) This responsibility is rarely delegated to anyone else, but some of the work load may be. Fathers, as we have seen, 'help' to differing degrees. Baby-sitters can take over for a few hours: by five months, 91 per cent of mothers had left their babies with someone, 93 per cent of these with mothers, mothers-in-law, other close relatives or husbands. By five months, 31 per cent of the sample women had taken on some kind of paid work. Only 2 per cent worked full time, and only eleven of the employed mothers worked outside the home − ten of these doing part-time or occasional work.[1] Most mothers either took their babies with them to work or left them with their husbands or mothers at home. Only two mothers had to find someone else to care for the baby − a neighbour and a friend, and on an occasional basis only. Leaving the baby − whether to go out to work or for a social occasion − is, then, predominantly a family affair. Few women feel able to leave their babies with a stranger − a person employed solely for baby-sitting, who has no other connection with the family. Few women are willing to take employment if this means finding such substitute care for their child − many who envisaged it in pregnancy reject it once they have their babies. (This does not mean they give up the ambition to become 'workers' again; nearly half of those without work said they would like a job, but had been prevented from taking one by the difficulty of finding work compatible with their idea of motherhood.)

For most women, then, the meaning of early motherhood lies in constant contact with the child.

You see now, he's playing by himself: he's quite happy. [Baby playing with newspaper on the floor.] I could be doing something else, but I've got to be in the room. He can see me and make his noises and get a bit of attention. So he's happy. If I went out of the room and left him there he wouldn't be happy. I have to have him with me. (*Juliet Morley*)

It's the restrictions it puts on you – social restrictions really. It's just the feeling that you're always there and you're always on duty. If I could go back to not being a mother I think I would be more independent from my husband, because I would have had the opportunity to be. Now that I've got the baby I can't. I don't *resent* it. I mean I'd go out on my own a bit more and things like that. I don't know why I was like that before. Looking inwards towards the family I suppose. Now that I've got the family, I can look outwards again. (*Jane Tarrant*)

You're on the go from seven in the morning and you're on call more or less all night, every night, whereas you're not when you're working. Your boss isn't going to ring you up at eleven o'clock at night and say come and take a letter. Whereas if the baby cries, you can't say I've finished for the day, tough luck. (*Deirdre James*)

Sometimes I just feel like having a rest from her. I used to have this fantasy of being in St Tropez and just lying there – you know on a private beach in a lounge chair, and you sort of snap your fingers and somebody comes with your lunch. (*Louise Thompson*)

Mothers are caught in a double bind. Because they are with their babies all the time they sometimes resent the loss of freedom. But because the tie with the baby is so close, they are only happy when the baby is with them.

I: What about going out without her?
TANYA KEMP: Oh no. I did once.
I: And what happened?
TANYA: I had a miserable time. I think I spent half of it in tears.
I: How old was she?
TANYA: About four and a half months.
I: Was that the first time you'd gone out without her?
TANYA: Yes.
I: The very first time since you'd had her?
TANYA: Yes.
I: That must have been some occasion!
TANYA: My husband said it's about time we went out, so I said only if you look after her.
I: So you didn't go out with him?
TANYA: No, I went out with a girlfriend and we went to the pictures and I left half way through. I cried all the way to her house in the car. I

wasn't very good company I'm afraid. She's got children of her own.
She understood.

*Babies need their mothers: therefore mothers need their babies. This is the
ideological formula that in modern industrialised society makes child care
women's work. For the happy housewife–wife–mother is the emblem and
foundation of capitalism; without her industry would crumble and the population
would die out. But although women may believe that a mother's place is with her
child before they become mothers (see pp. 59–66) it is only through the experience
of motherhood that the emotional logic becomes binding.*

*Janet Streeter, a dance instructor, planned to work two days a week after she had
her baby. She felt that it would be important for her to go on working – for the
interest and mental stimulation it would provide. Five months after Piers was
born:*

I can't remember what I said when I was pregnant, but I do know
that my ideas have changed somewhat. Whereas before I was *adamant*
about working I really am not all that keen to do it now, as long as I've
got some other interests and I'm not sitting around at home all day
long. I do feel now that it'd be *unfair* – whether to me or Piers I'm not
sure – to not look after him all the time. My ideal before I had him was
that I would work two days a week and leave him one day with the
woman next door, one day with somebody else, but I just don't feel I
could do that now. I think that would bother him. And I think I would
miss looking after him quite honestly. I do enjoy it. And I enjoy *him.*

*Ellen George had not been as adamant about working as Janet Streeter, but
during her pregnancy she felt she might well turn out to be bored by domesticity,
and in that case she said she would not hesitate to go back to her old job as a health
visitor. But motherhood convinced her:*

I used to see a lot of children in the course of my work who were in
care, attended to by different people all the time. And now, seeing
Emma's reaction when she really has been upset and I've come into
the room: it's alright, Mummy's back again – it makes me feel how
important it is: I mean I *knew* academically it was bad for them to
have different people looking after them all the time, but I can *see* it
now.

Do you think babies need their mothers?

PAULINE DIGGORY:
As opposed to what?

I: Other people.

PAULINE: Yes I do. Well, you mean a natural mother or a person acting as a mother? Well, what do you mean by a mother? I don't know. Is it me, or is it – I tend to be in bed sometimes and I listen to her in her cot and I *know* what she's feeling. And I think that may be because I'm her biological mother. I don't know if I'd feel that if I'd just adopted her.

BARBARA HOOD:
I think they need that security, don't they? A feeling of security. Personally I don't think I'd *like* anyone else to look after him. I don't know about you, but you don't think anybody else can do it the same way. They might be able to do it *better*, but it's not the same.

KATE PRINCE:
No. I think it's the other way around. I think the mothers need their babies. Well I know that I don't want to give her to everybody, but it's only for *me* – *she'd* be perfectly alright.

MAUREEN PATERSON:
Yes I think they do. Well I'd *like* to think so really.

The need a child has for its mother is one side of the coin: the other is the maternal instinct. Whereas the feeling that babies need their mothers grows over time, the belief in the maternal instinct diminishes, reflecting the difficulty with which maternal feeling and abilities are developed. While three-fifths of the women believed in the existence of a maternal instinct before they had their babies, less than half did so afterwards. The biggest shock here is the discovery that maternal love is not an instant product. When the baby is first placed in the mother's arms she feels bewildered and detached, and interest, devotion and love all take time to develop. In the same way, knowing how to look after a baby (how to hold it, how to feed it, how to fold a nappy, how to stop the crying) is not a natural, i.e. automatic, consequence of giving birth. These are skills that have to be learnt along with the character and personality of the baby – for the baby is not only the product of its mother's body but also a person in its own right.

So the bond that unites mother and child is not that of instinct. Three processes happen in the early months. In the first place, the mother learns how to take care of her baby, and the baby makes it plain by sleeping better, crying less and eating more, that the mother is satisfying it – this in turn boosts maternal confidence. Secondly, the baby becomes more responsive, smiling and laughing and reward-ing the mother for all her work. And, thirdly, the baby begins to demonstrate a dependence on the mother, which makes the mother feel she is necessary to the baby. (Or, in other words, the formula is realised: mother and baby come to need each other.)

All these processes have begun by five weeks (the stage described in chapter 7); by then babies, still to some extent bundles of unpredictable needs and messes, are beginning *to seem human. What the mother does gradually seems to have more effect and the baby's responses have begun to suggest that he or she is grateful for (though not yet psychologically dependent on) maternal attention. But by five months most babies are much more accommodating. Their demands for food, sleep, stimulation or clean nappies are easier to predict, and daily crying time has fallen from over two hours to less than three-quarters; night sleeping is up from under six to nearly ten hours. All this serves to make babies more acceptably human and mothers begin to feel more human again too. Moreover, babies make it plain that they recognise and like their mothers, which all helps to make a mother feel she is doing a worthwhile job.*

Ties thus developed with the baby fit long-held notions about the nature of motherhood. The idea of such closeness between mother and baby may be cultural (there are societies in which it would be very out-of-place),[2] but, nevertheless, the force of the bond once it is established is immensely strong. It is for this reason that most mothers feel they should not work outside the home. Although they cite unfairness to the child, most mothers seem to take the decision in the light of their own needs – or desires – to be with the child.

MARY ROSEN:
I still feel I don't want to work until they [she plans to have two or more children] are at senior school. But I can see why people go back – they want *freedom* from the baby. I mean they give up work because they want freedom from work but I think it's the reverse working. But I mean I do think it's my job to bring him up. Unless we're in dire financial straits I think it's my job: I should be with him. There's no point in having a baby and giving it to a grandmother or someone else to bring it up.

ALISON MOUNTJOY:
When I was pregnant, I think I thought mothers who wanted to stay at home shouldn't feel pressured to work. But now I think mothers should be *encouraged* to do it – I mean who else is *mad* enough to do it? Far too many people have babies for the wrong reasons. I think anybody who has a baby and goes back to work say six weeks after they've had it just shouldn't really have a baby. I mean what have they had a baby for? I mean I really would like to know what they had a baby for. I mean do *you* know why people have babies if they don't

want to look after them? I don't wish to be dogmatic about it but. . . .

Kate Prince works two days a week as her husband's secretary:
The first thing I say is that I work two days a week and they go,
where? What do you do with the baby? And as soon as I say oh she
comes with us they express a mixture of surprise and approval.

*Lois Manson works two-and-a-half days a week. Her mother has the baby one
day a week, a neighbour another day, and she takes the baby to work with her for
half a day. She is still breastfeeding Jane and returns home at lunchtime to feed
the baby.*

I think really it is the *ideal* arrangement: whose law is it, the law that
says the more time you've got to do things in the more you find to do?
That applies to me. I spend my whole time whizzing around doing
housework and my time is absolutely filled and I really don't know
how. But it is. And I *hate* the thought that if I had those other two and
a half days at home I would just continue in that sort of existence. But
I don't think I'd be as bored and frustrated as I thought I would. But I
think I would be a little bit bored and frustrated. That sounds very
confused, but I change to fit circumstances. Work has become so
secondary to everything else. I still enjoy it, I mean I don't enjoy
having to get up in the morning and the routine and what have you.
And I also don't really like the idea of Jane having to go to somebody
else on a Wednesday – I think I might even still try to come home at
lunchtime even if I'm not breastfeeding. That's something that never
would have occurred to me before – that I'd want to do that; but in
fact I think I would. But I very rarely work in the evenings or at
weekends now, and I make sure that my work on the project is kept
down to a minimum; I get there at the last minute and I leave as soon
as possible. I *know* I'm not doing my best from that point of view. But I
do what I can.

See pp. 60–2 and 62–3 for Kate's and Lois's attitudes to work before *they
had their babies.*

LOSING YOUR L-PLATES

How do you feel you're coping with the baby generally?
Very good. Excellent. I feel I'm a very good mother. *(Nina Brady)*

Fine. I've got quite a good routine. *(Deirdre James)*

I think I'm coping *marvellously. (Sophy Fisher)*

Very well. There's nothing I feel anxious about. I feel more confident about me looking after her than anybody else. *(Angela King)*

Well I think I'm getting on alright. I do all me washing early, get that out of the way, and then I bath him every day before his breakfast. Get that done and he'll probably go off to sleep for a little while and I can get all me work done. *(Janette Watson)*

Well, I felt very confident actually a few weeks ago and then I started him on solid food and I thought my God am I giving him the right thing? Does he need protein in his food or is he getting protein in his milk? My confidence was completely shaken. So I realised that I'm only confident in the present, you know, and that my confidence is easily shaken the next day when he does something different, because they change so much.

But on the whole I suppose I'm fairly confident. I just feel as though I've been looking after him for years now. Strange. And I feel I know him very well, I know his habits. A friend left her baby here the other day and I found lots of times when I was doing something I didn't know what the baby would like, and I felt very disconcerted. Like when I was putting him in his cot for his afternoon sleep I didn't know whether he would normally have a little cry and then go to sleep, or whether . . . because he did cry as soon as I put him in the cot. And I didn't know whether to pick him up or not when of course with *him*, I know. *(Rosalind Kimber)*

Well I'm giving him so much time that I'm coping quite well with *him*. With everything else – no chance. But with *him*: I've got him just there. Or he's got me just there! *(Sarah Moore)*

Okay. I feel confident: it's not that hard. It used to be when I was with her she was crying and she was horrible: it was like an ordeal. Now she's not crying, now it's okay. *(Louise Thompson)*

I feel now I'm coping with him. At first I didn't. I didn't think I was. You know, I felt I was doing what I was supposed to be doing, if you know what I mean, but I couldn't relax and enjoy it, do you know what I mean? Because I kept thinking what's going to happen next. But you see now, as I say, he's in a routine now. *(Lily Mitchell)*

As mother and child grow together, love deepens and maternal anxiety lessens. Three-fifths of mothers were less anxious about their babies at five months than at five weeks; more than a third expressed stronger positive feelings towards them.

But a deepening of the relationship, a change in the quality of the bond, cannot of course necessarily be summed up as more love; it must be spelt out as an alteration in its nature.

What sort of relationship do you feel you have with the baby now?

I definitely feel much more maternal now than I did. I just felt like nothing when she was first born. I feel *protective* and like that she really *depends* on me. *(Angela King)*

I think she knows me more. It's quite an ego-trip! *(Louise Thompson)*

She knows me. Well, I know sometimes that I'm the only one who is any good. No one else will do: I am the one that matters. Which is great for me, it makes me feel good. *(Clare Dawson)*

Well she's got a bit *better* hasn't she? I think she knows her Mum. I mean she does stop crying when I pick her up. I think at the beginning you forget: every time she cried in the night or woke up in the morning too early I used to think oh my goodness me it's going to stop tomorrow or it's going to stop at the end of the week – she's going to sort of *go away* or something. But now I've got used to it. *(Pauline Diggory)*

I had no feelings at first. My mother used to say the instinct will come later on. This motherly instinct – it never came to me! It's here now, yes. I'm getting fonder and fonder of him every day. I don't know why. Is that natural? This is my work, dear, now. This is my job. I've accepted now that there is no more going back to work for me – this *is* my work, and I've got used to it and I'm into a routine now, if you know what I mean. He's very good you know. He's the perfect child. *(Nina Brady)* [Compare this with Nina's earlier refusal to accept staying at home – in pregnancy (p. 64–65) and five weeks after the birth (p. 156).]

I think I've got a better relationship with him now because at the beginning I was terrified of him. I didn't know what to do with him – I didn't know how to hold him, how to change him or anything. But I think I've got more used to him now, so we're sort of more friendly.

Last night his aunt, she was picking him up, and she said you don't want your Mum, do you, you love me, don't you, and I know it's really a joke, but when I go over and take him he sort of turns round and puts his arms out and I feel all pleased with meself. *(Vera Abbatt)*

I think it's better now because I don't worry about every movement and gurgle and spot. I think it's just getting used to her. I think it's just so frightening at the beginning because every time you pick up a magazine you read about cot death or an accident or something and you think how can this child possibly still be alive a year from today? *(José Bryce)*

The baby changes as well as the mother. As sleeping, eating and excreting habits become more established, a personality is seen to unfold. The baby comes to terms with life outside the womb, and the mother comes to terms with the baby, being able to see past the babyness to the person within. Detecting the baby's emerging personality is a great game (who is he or she like?) and serves to put mother and baby on an equal footing as people, cementing the mutuality of the relationship.

What kind of person is your baby?

SOPHY FISHER, about Tiffany:
She's more *interesting* than I thought a baby would be. I find all her little developments fascinating. She understands jokes now: if you sort of rub noses with her she laughs and likes it. Her grabbing for things has become so much more accurate; she sees it and wants it and gets it. We've got her one of those bouncers that you put on the door frame and she *adores* that; she'll play in it for ages. And she can actually pull herself up now into a sitting position.

It's like watching a chrysalis: it's like watching a butterfly coming out. Because she's getting so much more interested in the outside world and so much more responsive to it. She's turning into a person in her own right. She has things that *she* likes to do – times when she likes to play or stand up or sleep or whatever. I think that will determine our relationship as much as I will – I mean I can't try and make her what *I* want her to be. I just enjoy her, I think she's fantastic. She seems to think I'm quite fantastic too; we have a great mutual admiration society!

LOIS MANSON, about Jane:
I think of her being much older than she is. I think of her having a very definite personality. I sometimes think gosh she's only four and a half months – she's only a little baby. And yet when I am with her on my own, I talk to her and I think about her: I think of her being a much older person – not someone with a specific age, but just someone in her own right more, with her own feelings, thoughts, mind. I don't think I thought that before. When you asked me before I tried to tell you how I felt about her personality, but the feeling wasn't nearly as strong as it is now.

JANET STREETER, about Piers:
He's got *terrific* character. I'm sure he's going to be an absolute little devil. He's stubborn as a mule. And he's got such a *look* about him. And there are times when I know damn well he's taking absolutely no notice *on purpose*. I mean you come into the room and say something to him and he'll look at you and then he'll look away. And then after ages he'll laugh – but I'm sure he knows perfectly well what's going on. He just has, I think, a great deal of character.

JULIET MORLEY, about David:
I think he's got my husband's personality. He's very gregarious – he doesn't like being on his own. I don't think he's going to be a particularly *timid* child. He doesn't seem to be at all *nervous*.

PAULINE DIGGORY, about Hannah:
She's like a little animal now – a little cat! She's got a very *naughty* personality, and she's always *thinking*.

CARY WIMBORNE, about Miranda:
I look on her as a real character. I don't look on her as a baby. I look on her more as another person to talk to.

IT'S THE IMAGE, REALLY

Motherhood is like a new recipe – or like a new job; it takes some time to get used to it. Having a baby turns a woman into a biological mother, but she only becomes a mother in the social sense when she begins to care for the child, when she is seen by other people to be a mother – and when she thinks of herself as a mother. Taking on this occupational identity does have parallels with other jobs – doctor, teacher, greengrocer. But it is crucially different in one way, for mothers are what women are supposed to be.

GILLIAN HARTLEY:
You're stereotyped. You go up the High Road with your pram and there it is – everything you've been taught to hate since you were eighteen. There it is! Last time I went up the High Road with the pram some stupid lady was doing consumer research and she said I'm doing a survey of housewives. And I said wait a minute, I'm not a housewife. Which is a stupid thing to say, I know – I mean what does it matter if she thought I was a housewife? But it makes me angry.

Two-thirds of mothers felt that people (neighbours, friends, shopkeepers, strangers) treated them as mothers:

Do people treat you as a mother?	
Yes	69%
No	31%

PAULINE DIGGORY:

I just don't feel I look a mother. Do you know what I mean? I'm worried about being able to get it together – the mother and the woman thing. We was walking through the park the other day and I was holding her and she was getting tired and she was falling asleep on me, and there was my sister and her boyfriend and Jeff, and I thought well here I am, everyone's looking at me, I've got a child in my arms, I'm a *real* mother. Whereas last year I'd been walking along here without one and people were looking at me completely differently. You know, as you pass by somebody what clicks in your mind is either it's a girl walking along or it's a woman walking along with a baby in her arms. It's the image, really.

I don't *feel* like a mother, I feel like a *friend* really. This is what put me off getting a papoose because I thought I want to be a woman again now and if you had a papoose you couldn't be. You just couldn't be: the image is not the same. And I strove to get back into what I was before. I'm not so paranoid about it now – the butcher said oh you've got your figure back quick. And remarks like that. I thought that's something. I was a bit pleased with that.

You asked me whether I think mothers are discriminated against. I do think they are really. I was walking along with my pram through the park to the clinic – I'm conscious of it, that I am walking with the pram, half the time I'm sure everyone thinks I'm the au pair, especially in *this* area – but, apart from that, everyone was a baby themselves and everyone assumes that you've got to have babies to keep the world going. And yet there's an unusual attitude towards a mother these days – there's this attitude that everyone's got to have babies to perpetuate the world, and yet there's this other attitude that you're a bit odd.

Maybe I'm not maternal enough. This is another fallacy that I think exists. Some people are maternal and some people aren't. I think that's a load of old rubbish. There are ways of loving a baby without – I mean I know I'm not terribly good at the physical things, I know I'm impatient when she takes ages on the breast, but I feel that's not as important as just intelligent understanding.

KATE PRINCE:
I quite like the idea of being able to cope so well *and* being a mother. The other day I got into a taxi, I'd been at the office and I had to get back, Mark was minding Gillian, and this taxi driver started to chat me up and everything. I was joking and all that, then he got a bit sort of fruity, and I started to play it down, and then I thought well I'd say about my husband and the baby – and he *visibly* got more miserable about it. And I was very very *pleased* because I thought oh gosh somebody's chatting me up and there's me a mum and a housewife and all that! And I was saying that to Mum and she said oh that's stupid, ridiculous to think like that: why shouldn't they? But without realising it I'd got into this thing about nobody's interested in me and my life's finished – which is *silly*. It made me think, gosh I can *still* be chatted up even though I've got this baby.

And another thing which is quite interesting. When I first came out of hospital I had that terrible depression – I was really miserable, I thought that's it, my life's over now, I've got her till I'm about ninety. And I was talking to a friend of mine and saying how sad I felt and she said oh don't be silly, look at Lady Antonia Fraser, she knocks kids out *and* novels, and all the rest of it *and* she's having an affair with so-and-so. And I thought I don't know how she does it, it's just *amazing*. I shall *never* be like that – able to do things *and* have children. And that's all gone now. I was thinking the other day how I thought it was impossible *ever* to get back to normal again. It's the role thing, isn't it? Because it just seems to me so natural. Why does anybody *ever* make a big deal about it? I don't mean about the *physical* effort involved – because that is a big deal, but the whole thing around motherhood. It shouldn't be like that. It should be just played down. It's just something you *do* isn't it? It's like getting a sofa or going to Waitrose.

LOUISE THOMPSON:
I was walking down the King's Road on Saturday and I was wearing this kind of shiny panée velvet halter thing with no bra on, and I was pushing the pram. And these three Scotsmen were outside a pub and one of them – because my breasts are so big, and Polly was just wearing pants and everyone thinks she's a boy anyway – this Scotsman said well the little lad certainly isn't bottlefed!

And sometimes this social attitude to women as mothers negates a woman's identity: she is no one, her life is finished.

ANNE BLOOMFIELD:
I like her but I don't like looking after her. I don't like the fact that she has to rely on me for everything. I mean you don't *exist* when you have a baby, do you?

ALISON MOUNTJOY:
One sometimes forgets that one is actually a *person* other than her mother.

TAMSIN ATTWOOD:
They seem to think that's it, you know: that's the end of my life. My Mum goes on about the price of vegetables and that: women of the world and that. I'm one of them now. I've made the grade now.

I: If you had to fill in a form and put your occupation now, what would you put?
SASHA MORRIS: I don't know. What would you class me as? I don't know what I am. I know I'm a mother but I don't think of myself as a mother. I don't think I'm maternal. I've reached this conclusion myself – that I'm not filled with maternal love and wanting to have loads of babies.

I do like having the baby, I should hate to give the wrong impression. I love the baby but I'm not totally occupied with her, and I don't regard this as the thing I want to do most in life, and that I have now *finished*: I think I'm far too young to give up the ghost.

I'm just not cut out for it. It's only now that I'm beginning to appreciate her. She is a remarkably good baby – what I'd have been like with a crying baby I don't know. I find myself impatient with her, wanting to *kill* her sometimes, and she's a *good* baby. I'm too *impatient* with children and I expect them to do everything that I think they should do. At the moment, if I was told I couldn't have any more children I wouldn't be upset.

So if we ask how satisfied women are with their jobs as mothers, the answer has to be a mixed one. By five months, they have all fallen in love with their babies and the idea of being without them has become abhorrent. The smile from the cot in the morning, the classic noises of post-feed contentment, the clear healthy skin in the clean clothes that become almost daily too small as the scales in the baby clinic weigh out a measure of maternal care: these are the addictive pleasures of motherhood. 'She's healthy, she's growing, I fed her, she's all my creation.' A mother's labour is not alienated in this sense: her product, the baby, is her possession. And for a long while it is impossible to realise that the baby will grow up and cease to be the mother's possession. But the conditions *of a mother's labour can be as alienating as those of any factory worker. The work of child care*

can be monotonous; the pace of the job too fast; the effect of having constantly to interrupt other tasks may be experienced as incredibly frustrating. In addition, the mother is never free of her work as the factory worker is: she may feel she has no time to herself, she is tied down by the baby, all her interests and activities have been changed by the baby's incessant demands. And while the factory is other people's workplace too, the home is not. On her own a mother may feel lonely and isolated from adult company.

A mother's working conditions	
Monotony*	40%
Pace	66%
Social isolation*	36%
Being tied down	80%
Having no time to self	67%
Changed interests	55%

*These figures are probably an underestimate. The questions were asked at five weeks and not again at five months, and at five weeks many mothers said they thought as the baby got older they would find motherhood more monotonous and lonely.

PASSING THE TIME

Lily Mitchell, an ex-civil-servant, describes many of these aspects of her life with five-month-old William:

This is what I'm trying to get over to him at the moment. That there's seven days doing the same thing, you know. And you're not complaining, but life seems a little bit, you know, sort of stale and drab. I really feel like going out, like one Saturday at nine in the morning and not coming back till nine at night. I really feel like doing it. For one day only, just to see how *he* puts those twelve hours in.

I find you're tied hand and foot every minute of the day. I find I do less now than what I used to do when I was working. I don't do half of what I'd like to do at all. You know, people say you're at home all day, but I don't *start* the things – if it is something I really want to get stuck into I don't start it. And then after I find out I would have got it done I think I should have started it – do you know what I mean? But I find then if William was to wake up I'd be annoyed at him waking even though he was due to wake. I started sewing the other day and once I start sewing I really do get into it, and I want to carry on. When he cried for his feed I thought oh: and I was getting on so well, you know. And it's not his fault that he woke up, so I think is it worth getting involved? By the time the evening comes you haven't done anything all day. You seem to get through your day without doing anything, and you keep thinking of all the things you've still got to do or that you'd like to do. You get tired but you don't know what you're doing to *make* you feel tired, you know.

I have to go out every day because I get too annoyed to stay in. I think well, where can I go today? I mean there's a few people that I can go to, you know. I can usually go somewhere once a week. I think the one thing you miss is adult companionship you know, because you small talk to people, the neighbours, you say good morning, how are you, nice day, but you don't really *talk* to anyone.

Sometimes I think you wonder, why try and make somewhere to go every day – because that's really what I'm doing. Some days you don't mind if it's a nice day – you think oh it's lovely to get out, but then if it's not a very nice day you're just really drifting from one feed time to the next: passing the time. I just get a bit fed up with things, you know. There's nothing I want to do and nowhere that I want to go and there's nobody I want to see. It's not a nice way to think; it's not a nice way to feel in fact.

I: Do you like looking after the baby?

LILY: I do. I do and I don't. When I say I don't, it would be unfair, but you know what I mean. I think it's difficult adjusting to being at home. I'm having to adjust really. And there's times when I miss a little of my own independence. I really do miss it now, I think. You know, I've never really put it into words for anybody before, but there's times when I feel if you went out for an afternoon twice a week, just you, you'd be much better the other times; you'd give anything just for somebody to take him for two hours, just to think for two hours you can do your own thing. Go to the shops and try on a dress or something like that.

But it's society – it's the way it's been going on for years. I don't think it's suddenly going to change over night. This is a mother's twenty-four-hour job. I mean men can be half an hour late or an hour late, but I can't be with him. I have to have him with me and he has to be fed at particular times all the time. I tell Kenneth if he comes in late and he wakes him up, he's your baby, if you wake him coming in, he's yours, you know. I don't like being hard like this but it annoys me, because I've had him all day. Having the baby falls into the background as everybody used to tell me, because having the baby is only a twelve-hour, eighteen-hour deal. I think it's bringing him up every day and in the end that becomes more of a test.

CHAPTER 11

Lessons Learnt

*I've joined women all over the world. I feel I'm no longer an individual like
I used to be, because my idea of what I was was a woman going out to work
— I feel that's all gone now.*

*I even feel like warning people — before they become pregnant; saying, well,
you know, I expected it to be all joy and roses straight away.*

*Looking back on the process of becoming a mother, women come to understand the
visions they had — of motherhood as a bed of roses, of birth as agony or ecstasy, of
pregnancy as a flowering or a burden. After the event these images are brought
sharply into focus by the contrast medium of reality, which exposes the outline of
what was, too often, a romantic dream.*

*More than a third of the women said they found becoming a mother a difficult
experience. Eight out of ten said it had been different from what they had
expected. The same proportion thought the pictures of pregnancy, birth and
motherhood conveyed in antenatal literature, women's magazines and the media in*
general were too romantic, painting an
over-optimistic portrait of happy
mothers and fathers, quiet contented
babies and neat and shining homes that
bore little resemblance to the chaos, dis-
ruption and confusion of first-time
motherhood.

Becoming a mother	
Was difficult	36%
Was different from expected	84%
Is too romanticised	84%

FAIRY STORIES

NINA BRADY, ex-shop assistant:
What's romantic about changing that nappy down there? What's

romantic about it? I think people should be told about the hard life it is to be a mother. It's not easy to be a mother. I don't think it is, I think it's very difficult. It takes all your energy out of you. The responsibility and the work: because you are kept going. If that child cries at three o'clock you have got to get up and feed it if it continues to cry, haven't you? Isn't that a responsibility? Well you can't dial nine nine nine and tell them to come, the baby's crying: you've got to do it. I think they should be *warned* more: because when you go to those classes, they tell you about your baby and they make it sound so nice, like the adverts on television, they make everything sound so nice. But it's not. When your baby is born in hospital it took me a long time to get to want to see it at all. I'm telling you the truth; it took me about four or five days before I wanted to look at that child; I didn't want to know.

ANGELA KING, ex-cashier:
Everything is so *straightforward* in those books you get at the clinic. It's all the water breaks, and then you get this and then you get that. Maybe seven out of ten get it like that but most people don't. I mean when you read those books, you get a picture in your mind that it's going to *be* like that – you're going to get the first stage and how long the first stage is: but I think a lot of the time, well most of the time, it doesn't run like that. I think you're better off buying a book like that Gordon Bourne book [*Pregnancy*, Pan Books, 1975]; I mean I know it can frighten you to death, but it describes every aspect of labour, everything to do with childbirth. I mean I know it can be frightening, especially to mothers that are nervous, but I think you're better off knowing about it before than going and having a really rough time and not expecting it. You're better off going in frightened because then nine times out of ten it's better than you expected.

Then those books go on about the feeding, and that's all wrong as well, because no baby – well I should think maybe there's a few – but no baby is straightforward at feeding. You know they say get into a routine, and one, it gives you a routine for the day: washing at ten and a cup of coffee at eleven, I mean it's *ridiculous*. I don't know how you could *ever* do it. Because she was never on a routine really. Maybe she'd have a bottle after three hours and then another one after four hours and you never get them into a four-hourly routine properly – well I didn't, maybe a few do.

RACHEL SHARPE, ex-copywriter:
I suppose it's quite a difficult thing to convey to people who don't

have the experience, but I think it *is* far too romantic the way they portray it. Especially those *sickly* booklets they give you in the hospital: they're *disgraceful*, they really are [*You and Your Baby* Part I and Part II, British Medical Association 'Family Doctor' publication]. You know, everybody looking sort of starry-eyed. I think they should do something to correct that image: that the only time you spend with the baby is whenever he needs to be fed, and that's at ten and two and six and on and on like that. Just things like that. And also I think you're under the impression too that a newborn sleeps twenty hours a day which I didn't find was true.

SHARON WARRINGTON, ex-audiotypist:
Yes, they only give you little bits. If the baby suffers from wind pat its back, you know, not that you have to sit up all night giving him his bottle. They don't tell you that. Sleepless nights. And half of them – midwives, nurses – they say what are you complaining for? Childbirth doesn't *hurt*! They've never had a child, they don't know. And that really irritates me, especially the bitch I had. She was a Miss. I said I'm in pain: she just looked at me as if I was stupid, you know. Oh she was horrible, I'll never forget her. Like a major in the army.

JOSÉ BRYCE, ex-manicurist:
I think they don't say much, in anything I've read, about how you get depressed. They just sort of say this is perfectly natural and you might feel a bit weepy for a couple of days when you're in hospital and that's about all that anyone seems to say. If you knew how long it was going on, you'd feel alright. But it was just the fact that day after day after day I felt the same. That was the worst thing. Every morning that sort of dread: another day. And then I used to say now tomorrow I'm really going to make the effort, I can't do it now, tomorrow will be better. And I did make myself go out just to stop crying really. I mean I just used to walk around the streets pushing her just so I wouldn't cry.

GILLIAN HARTLEY, illustrator:
No, I don't think it's too romantic. I mean it's not the whole picture, obviously, but it *is* romantic and sentimental to be a mother in many respects. The feeling you have for the child is a very romantic one. With all the realism, you do love the child and that's a very romantic thing – just the way romantic novels do not present a very *accurate* picture of love, but they present a *portion* of it. I think they might do

well to tell you more about the realities and then let you find out about the nice things which will come.

DEIRDRE JAMES, ex-jewellery assembler:
You don't see someone on the telly changing a dirty gooey nappy, do you? Or when you pick him up and he's sick all down your back? You get all the nice things, gooey and sweet, and not the other side of it.

HELEN FOWLER, ex-nursing auxiliary:
I think they play on the fact that everyone has as much time as they want and so everything's lovely because you have as much time as you want for your child. And you can rest all through pregnancy and there's never any problems. It sort of goes on like that. Even the pictures that they show have lovely fields and a couple walking along sort of thing, completely sentimental. But I think it's probably better to have an idealistic image, because if it said oh terrible, terrible, probably no one would have children, you know.

PAULINE DIGGORY, ex-market researcher:
I don't think there's enough said about the pain of childbirth myself – I still remember it. I make sure I remember it myself because I've heard this tale, oh it's a terrible pain but you forget it so quickly, I thought I'm not going to forget it quickly, no way.

KIRSTY MILLER, ex-pattern grader:
They don't tell you when they induce you and all those sorts of things, you know: you don't expect it. They don't give enough *detail*.

ELLEN GEORGE, ex-health visitor:
They treat you like a person with the lowest possible intelligence I think. I think they should tell you more of the sheer hard facts of the whole business – of the whole process from start to finish. They tell you bits that they choose to tell you, but they leave out quite a lot. They don't tell you about the aftermath, and they don't tell you enough about breastfeeding.

SASHA MORRIS, ex-air hostess:
You always see mothers and babies looking terribly happy. They look collected and together. But it's not the case at all. The photographs of me and the baby in the beginning, I always looked haggard and the baby looked marvellous. I was the haggard one.

FELICITY CHAMBERS, ex-receptionist:
It's a bit like a fairy story: they always bring out the good points. They

never bring out the other points.

HILARY JACKSON, ex-catering manager:
I think they should tell you just what hard work it is *basically*. You can't just lay around all day cuddling them; things like that. It's basically hard work.

Would you say becoming a mother has been pretty much as you expected it to be?

PAT JENKINS, ex-shop assistant:
It's very hard work. Well I knew it was hard work, because I've looked after a lot of kids, you know. But I mean you could always hand them over. It's different with your own. If you're tired there's no one you can give him to. You know he's your own and you've got to put up with it. That's not right, put up with it, but you know what I mean: you can't hand him over when you feel oh I've had enough.

ALISON MOUNTJOY, ex-fashion designer:
It's been harder work, I mean just *totally* different. No, it hasn't been *totally* different, because I've got the sort of love for her that I expected and I hoped I would have, so I mean from that point of view it's as I expected. And that's about all. The pregnancy was nothing like I expected, I expected it to be much more idyllic – I didn't expect to get depressed and fed up. And the piles. I thought I'd float through it on a silver cloud, or a cloud with a silver lining: is that what I mean?

ROSALIND KIMBER, ex-social worker:
The pregnancy was worse in that I thought women who were sick were neurotic and I was so sick the whole nine months. The birth wasn't nearly as bad as I expected because I was really dreading it, but it wasn't nearly as bad, and actually *having* a baby I couldn't really imagine.

SARAH MOORE, ex-civil servant:
There haven't been any nasty shocks. It's been much more rewarding than I thought it was going to be, and much more pleasurable. Everybody knows that when you're at home looking after a baby you tend to get very bored. I think maybe I had a very jaundiced view of it, and I didn't take into account the pleasure that a baby can give.

MARY ROSEN, ex-exhibition organiser:
There haven't been any surprises, but I think no one realises how

much there is to do really. I mean it's not a toy, it's not like a doll. It's something you've got to keep alive and everything else.

RACHEL SHARPE:
I think the biggest shock first was the amount of time that it required to look after a newborn baby. I just never dreamed that I'd be spending every waking minute and every *sleeping* minute just about looking after him, doing one thing or another for him. I mean the first day home was especially bad. I found I spent most of the day weeping; I found that really difficult, and I think at first there was that really *overwhelming* sense of responsibility caused by the fact that they're so *completely* helpless.

PAULINE DIGGORY:
They do assume, you see, because these hospitals are male-dominated, they do assume that the minute you have a baby you know what to do. I don't believe in the maternal instinct. I wish there was a book that tells you that it's *common* that some of them are sick or that half of them don't wind, and don't be frightened of it. I mean I feel like saying to some mothers, if I was writing for them, maybe they're not as frightened as I was? – don't be frightened of the baby as long as it's eating and sleeping, that's a good rule of thumb. You seem *incompetent* you see if you moan to outsiders: this is why mothers do talk to each other, because they can let the barrier down. But people, they do tend to expect – *I* expected – that once you have a baby you know it all. I *suspected* that you didn't, but everyone behaved as though they knew it all once they'd had one, and nobody *said* it. And then I thought well I'm just as intelligent as most mothers, why aren't I managing? Maybe I'm not maternal enough. This is another fallacy I think that exists. Those books, it's all don't worry, everything's fine. That annoys me, they don't allow for the unusual, which is always happening as far as I can tell. Like that she brings up so much milk, that she didn't take to the breast: I thought that was uncommon until I realised that half the ward were having the same trouble. All those sorts of things. It annoys me because you go through all those worries to find out that you needn't have gone through it at all. I get angry with that.

NINA BRADY:
Having a baby is supposed to be a great experience – I didn't find it no great experience, dear. It was very cruel. I had that injection and

before that I think I would have died. I think I really would have been one of those mothers that died in birth.

JOSÉ BRYCE:
I think it's more dramatic, the whole thing: having her; yes, I just think the whole thing has been more, it's changed everything *more* than I thought. I thought I would carry on as normal but with a baby. But I just feel differently about lots of things, not just her.

Has it been an easy or difficult experience, becoming a mother?

Well, difficult in the way that it's changed my whole life, I would say completely. (*Polly Field, ex-telecommunications supervisor*) Difficult at first until you get into a routine and then it's alright. (*Kirsty Miller, ex-pattern grader*)
I suppose it's been difficult really. Well I suppose it is a difficult thing trying to bring up a baby: making sure they're eating enough, all sorts of things like that, keeping them warm. . . . (*Janette Watson, ex-machinist*)
It has been a hard experience, darling, but I like it now; I'm very relaxed now: I've got everything organised. I've got him into a nice routine: everything's lovely; it's worth it now. (*Nina Brady, ex-shop assistant*)
It's been easy for *me* because I've got other people with me. [She and her husband live with her parents and her younger brother and sister.] He's not the type of baby – you leave him in a chair or you leave him on the floor and you've got to be there talking to him all the time. He won't be left on his own for long – five minutes and that's it, he starts. So you can imagine, doing the housework and having to look after him as well, it'd be very difficult, I think. (*Grace Bower, switchboard operator*)
It's alright in the hospital. You've got a nice rosy picture, you know. The nurses are there and you don't have to do anything: there's no washing to do, your meals are cooked for you, you're looked after. But once you come home you've got to cook and look after your husband and do all the washing. I think it's different then, isn't it? (*Pat Jenkins, ex-shop assistant*)
It's been difficult. It's been hateful. Not just the whole business of the nine months carrying and waiting, you know: all the check ups you have to have. Alright, the birth was difficult, but the birth is the

least of it. And then of course it should have been better after that, but she was so difficult and she had the colic and it was one thing after another. So up until now I really haven't had any of the so-called joys of motherhood. (*Mandy Green, ex-hairdresser*)

Oh it's a very difficult experience. When I say it doesn't *live up to* one's expectations, it's not the *same* as one's expectations, because it's such a totally *new* experience. I mean there can be *nothing* that anybody has to experience that can be as new and as different. When people say once they had their first baby they felt life was never the same again and never will be, it's *true*: it *can't* be the same again. (*Alison Mountjoy, ex-fashion designer*)

JOINING THE CLUB

Life is changed because motherhood is a new job and often the only job for a period of years: a baby transforms a private relationship between man and woman into 'family life' with all its traps and trappings; economically a woman with a baby is dependent in a way that a woman without a baby is not. But the job of mother has other, more pervasive consequences. Women's views about themselves, their ideas about themselves as people also change. Again, this process is a gradual one, beginning in pregnancy before motherhood has even happened. By five weeks there may be a firm sense of maternal identity but this is unlikely (see pp. 155-6). For some women the association between their sense of personal identity and the cultural image of mothers remains weak. Others simply take longer to settle down to the idea that they are mothers; one in three of the sample women had distinctly stronger notions of themselves as mothers five months after the birth than they did earlier.[1]

CHRISTINA LYNCH:
I suppose I do feel differently. Even if he's not with me. I feel as though I am a mother, you know, I'm *equal* to everyone else. I feel a bit more cocky. I surprised myself by going to this Pippa Dee party. Normally, I would never go on my own. But I feel more confident. Yes, I think that's another thing about being a mother: I feel more *self*-confident in that respect: I feel as if I could go up to anyone and talk to them.

VERA ABBATT:
It's great, terrific! I wish I'd done it before, I think I *needed* some

responsibility. I was a bit of a nut case at one time, it's quietened me down a bit! I'm not quite as daft as I used to be. I used to class myself in a completely different class from my mother, I could never see myself as my mother is, whereas now I can.

ANGELA KING:
It's made me feel more fulfilled. It's given me something in life; I feel that I've *achieved* something now. Whereas before, I mean work and everything, maybe it was the jobs I had, but I always felt like I was in a rut and was never *achieving* anything. But I feel as though I've done something *useful*; and if I can turn her into a nice person and put her into the world I'll feel that I've really achieved something.

EMMA BUCKINGHAM:
Apart from feeling awfully proud, you feel terribly *important*. I think I feel much securer having her. In many ways life's more relaxed. Well, you really feel *proud* of your baby: it's something you've done together. I'm more contented.

JANE TARRANT:
I suppose you've got a slight mystique about you once you've had a baby, which I think people had for me before I had one. And to people who *have* got babies you've joined the club so to speak – excuse the pun!

DEIRDRE JAMES:
I feel older; you're more responsible: you've got someone to be responsible *for*. I suppose when you work, you just pop out for a drink lunchtime, yet I wouldn't *think* of doing something like that now. *It's really like living in a different world.*

You have to experience it. I was trying to explain it to my friend. She was saying that she doesn't think she's the mothering type. But I think she is because she's so good with children. I said it's just such a special bond between the mother and the baby. . . .

And the bond of love that grows between mother and baby reaches outwards to the world:

JOSÉ BRYCE:
I didn't think I could feel so *passionately* about something. I'd always assumed that if I had a baby I'd love it, but I never thought I would actually feel like I do about it. If someone said cut your arm off otherwise something would happen to her you'd do it. It's a different

sort of love from, say, you feel for your parents or your husband. I didn't realise I could feel so *deeply* about something. I look at her sometimes and think – I don't know how to describe it really. But how can people get over something like if their child dies or something? I don't know how anyone can get over a thing like that.

I'm more *emotional* now. Like I can watch the news now and if I see anything to do with children or babies, whereas before I'd think how awful, how sad; now I feel a real *twist*. . . .

SANDY WRIGHT:
The miracle of it: I look at her and I think you're *mine*, you're nobody else's, or you're *ours*, rather. We produced her and it's a wonderful feeling. I don't think you can understand it until you've actually had one, no matter how much someone tells you. And how that also affects other things; when you hear something awful's happened to a child you think, oh God, that could be you. Before when I heard about baby battering and so on I would discuss it and feel terrible about it, but it didn't affect *me*. Now when I hear about I have a *pain* almost.

It's definitely fulfilled something in me. If I hadn't had a child I would always have wanted one or wondered how it would have been. It gives a bit more meaning to life, I suppose. I think it's made me perhaps a bit more *sensitive* towards people. I'm sometimes impatient with people but I'm not so much now.

GILLIAN HARTLEY:
I think when you're a parent you're conscious of so many good things. I think what struck me particularly since the baby's been born is – I really have wondered how men can kill each other: I've wondered how there could be wars. I can't understand how people can kill each other.

The baby is the pebble in the pool and the proverbial ripples are an unexpected bonus of motherhood.[2] For having a child of one's own is, despite all the sleepless nights, the sacrifice of self, the end to freedom, the most rewarding af all human experiences.

I don't think one can describe what it's like to be a mother. I mean to me it's a very rewarding and wonderful feeling, and Leslie finds this as well, being a father. We love going for walks with the baby; we just feel incredibly fulfilled, and we don't worry about money, or houses, or holidays or anything. We feel incredibly happy with the baby. (*Rosalind Kimber*)

I: If you were going to describe to somebody who didn't have any children what it's like to be a mum, what would you say?

JOSEPHINE LLOYD: It is something that you can't describe until you have a child of your own. And I've never been one for children before, but it is an absolutely *fantastic* feeling when you've got a child of your own. I don't think that you can even *begin* to describe it to somebody. But I did write a letter to a friend, she'd just had her baby, and I was writing to her saying oh it's fantastic, and even now when he laughs it brings the tears to my eyes.

A few weeks ago I was just feeding her and I suddenly was sort of overwhelmed with love for her and I thought this is good, this is great, this is what life is all about. It's so rewarding, the feeling of her dependence on you and the way she's growing and the way you're bringing her up, the way she responds to you. I've always wanted to be a mother: I wanted a family and I wanted to be a mother to fulfil my life. (*Clare Dawson*)

Living through the babyhood of one's own child is reliving one's own babyhood: through the actions and emotions of oneself as a mother the experience of being mothered is reawakened. So bridging the generation gap is another unanticipated consequence of first-time motherhood.

ROSALIND KIMBER:
I feel closer to my mother: I identify with her much more now. I feel I understand an awful lot more about her, and I feel much more sympathy for her now. Sometimes I look at the baby and I think my goodness my mother must have thought that about not just me, but all my brothers and sisters. And then I will make an effort to telephone her and that sort of thing. How much she must miss not having us at home, and how hurt she must be if we don't telephone her. Because I mean it's very easy to just forget and not bother. I find I bother much more now: I write to her and send her photographs of the baby.

LILY MITCHELL:
I think it's the closest I've ever felt to her, if you know what I mean. Because now you can sort of half-understand, really, some of her feelings. Because I used to say why do you worry about John [her brother] even though he's 24? I said why do you worry about him? But mothers worry about their children until they die because they're still their children no matter what age they are. And this is what we're

like now with William. You know what I mean: you're still going to worry about him, even after he's got married. And I think it's made me see that a little bit more now.

VERA ABBATT:

The last time I saw her I didn't feel it was my mother, she was more like a friend. I can see all the things that used to rile me with her now, I can see why she did them all now, whereas I could never see it before. I could never understand why she had to tell me to do this and why she had to tell me to do that. But sometimes I sit here and think what I would do if he did something like that: didn't go to school, stayed out all night at a party, fell off a train.

JULIET MORLEY:

I certainly understand far better than I used to things that happened when we were children. I can certainly remember as a child thinking my mother wasn't very easy to please and was always being *cross* – this sort of thing. Well now I can understand it. Four children and a large house and going out to work.

LOUISE THOMPSON:

I think she must have been a good mother – she was never angry, she was always loving and we were close, and I feel the same way to Polly: that's why I assume she was like that.

PAT JENKINS:

I think it's because I've experienced the same as my Mum, you know, and when we're talking we know what we're talking about, because she knows that I've gone through it as well. I've always been close to my Mum anyway. But it's nice; because we can talk about it more I tell her what I went through and things like that. Mum went through a terrible time with us, having us. I don't know – I said I don't know how she did it!

DEIRDRE JAMES:

She treats me as though I'm a more responsible person. She'll talk to me about things of the world really: on the news and that, whereas she didn't before.

She'll phone up and ask how he is and I'll say he's dribbling and she'll say oh yes, teething. Whereas it used to be I went to the pictures the other night, nothing of great interest: I think the baby is something to talk about.

HELEN FOWLER:
It's like joining a club type of thing: she lets me in on little secrets: we talk about things we didn't talk about before.

But what sort of club is this? Mothers and daughters share the secret society of those who are guardians of future generations: they are united in their protectiveness, in that special sort of anxious devotion that is the birthright of children in our culture. Yet in becoming a mother, a woman acquires a new kind of citizenship; or is deprived of one. When she is childless and out at work she can pretend (or believe) that everything in the garden is lovely. When she is 'just a housewife', the vision of equality fades a little and motherhood, deeply rewarding as it is, becomes an imperfect occupation.

WOMEN OF THE WORLD

Some women noted in fairly unexplicit ways the specific place of mothers in our culture (by complaining that they had to ask their husbands for money, or that their unmarried female friends no longer invited them out, for example). But nearly half the sample said that becoming a mother had definitely changed their attitudes to the position of women.

Since you became a mother, have your views about the position of women changed at all?

SARAH MOORE:
Yes, definitely. I've never been anti-women's lib, ever, and I still think they tend to preach to the converted, that they're not getting at the real sort of poor downtrodden housewife and mother: they preach to the middle class who've got the education and the money to get out. But, my God, I've got so much more sympathy with them now!

My views have changed, become more radical. I do think that women are – oppressed is a very emotive word, isn't it? But they are to a certain extent. I mean I *do* work twelve hours a day; I've *never* worked twelve hours a day: I never thought I would. And I'm buggered if I like it! I mean I *do* it because the work's got to be done, and I try to do the housework so I haven't got any to do at weekends. I realise that my twelve hours isn't nearly as hard as other women; I've got a washing machine, I've got carpets which are a darn sight easier to clean than scrubbing floors and polishing them. I realise that the work I put in is far less than my mother did or hundreds of other women do, but nevertheless you *are* working. I mean I don't think *anybody* should have to work twelve hours a day.

My views are changing towards society as well. I mean I knew that society was definitely anti-children: I knew that before he was born. But there are so many things now that you can't do because you've got a child. Shopping for example. I mean I don't like shopping – I don't mean food shopping, that's *got* to be done – but window shopping, that never used to appeal to me, I didn't go very often; but now I know I *can't* go, even if I want to, because I've got a kid.

I do think you're thought of as a second-class citizen. You're described as a housewife. Oh well, you've got plenty of time on your hands, you can sit down and knit all day. I mean I *work*!!! I don't think you should be paid, but I think that national insurance contributions, we should get those, so that then you can claim benefit when you're sick. I went down with gastric flu, that really brought it home to me. I felt so ill. Dick, it happened, couldn't take a day off from work that day: he had a lot on. And I was sort of running to the loo, being sick – oh God, you haven't got time to be ill when you've got' kids, and this is what *really* brought it home to me. I mean I thought if you go out to work you take a day off and you don't even lose your *pay* if you take a day off, if you're sick. You can't take a day off when you've got kids.

It's taken Jonathan for me, and for me to be at *home* for me to realise this. It's strange, isn't it, because before when I was working, I wouldn't say I was a liberated woman by any means, but I was certainly holding my own at work and running a home. And so I should have then been in favour of women's lib. Let's be honest, once you've got the education behind you, you're not discriminated against as much as other women, are you? And you don't *experience* it: it's all very chatty, you go down to the pub at lunchtime with the fellows from work and what's this women's lib all about? My God.

JO INGRAM:
It's been a consciousness-raising experience for me; it's shown me tremendously that I'm just one of millions.

I just feel I understand the difficulties women have. I was thinking the other day about how I'd never totally accepted what some people said – that even if women are working their main interest is still going to be the children and the housework and all the rest of it – and I never *really* took that too seriously, although I sort of half-accepted it: I never really knew what it *meant*. But now I think it's probably true for the majority of women. I mean the thing that's most likely to turn them on is something to do with kids, that's my personal experience; that's what worries *me* far more than my job conditions – is what sort of chance he's getting, nursery facilities and so on.

LOIS MANSON:
I suppose I feel a little bit more strongly on issues to do with women working and childminding facilities for women than I did before, because I didn't identify with those as *problems* particularly before and I do much more so now. I've never been a *militant* or *ardent* women's liberationist and that's possibly because my relationship with David has always been such that I've never felt that there was anything particularly lacking in *my* life, and perhaps I looked at it from a very selfish point of view. I do feel that women on the whole are treated as second-class citizens. I get very annoyed with people who don't hold doors open when I've got the pram and I want to go into shops and things. Little things. I suppose my attitudes have been more reinforced than changed. I've become more aware of difficulties.

JULIET MORLEY:
I miss having an independent life, that's the thing. I don't miss the work I was doing particularly, it's having an independent life: something outside the home, something that's mine as opposed to something I share with Paul. Well I don't *have* an independent life at the moment, really.

But things like women not getting to the top in their careers just don't seem as important at the moment as they used to be. Things to do with the position of women in that sense don't seem so important. I think things could be made a lot easier for *mothers*. Even in the sense of providing access to buildings; I've certainly thought about people in wheelchairs a lot more since I've had a pram to push. Shopping could be made a lot easier and when new buildings are designed people ought to think about prams and wheelchairs a great deal more. I never realised, I thought these bloody people with prams: I wish they'd get out of the way!

HELEN FOWLER:
I feel much more sympathetic to people with children now than I did before, I think.

I: People?

HELEN: Oh women. I think on the whole men get the easy side of it.

LOUISE THOMPSON:

I think I've become a feminist. I really get annoyed at men's roles –
like in school [she is a law student] lots of men are married there and
you never see their kids, they have this total freedom. To Oliver she's
like a little toy, he can play with her.

CAROLINE SAUNDERS:

I tend to favour female politicians more than I did before and I
respect them more; I think because I tend to think of women being
stronger now, able to cope more. Because I'm sure if I was left in a
position now where I had to cope I probably would.

PAULINE DIGGORY:

This business about pills and depression, it puts women down, you
know: Victorian women coped, didn't they? I'm annoyed at women
not having the strength, because I'm beginning to think women are
superior to men now. I used to think they were equal, but now I'm
beginning to think they're superior.

I: Why?

PAULINE: Well, they can have a baby for a start!

GILLIAN HARTLEY:

Having experienced childbirth, the potentialities of being a woman
are so much greater. Women are so lucky to have been the ones able to
give birth, to have a child: that's marvellous.

KATE PRINCE:

Well my views have become stronger. I think it's far more important
that you're doing this kind of thing: I would *love* to do a lot of myth
shattering. I've grown to resent tremendously all this silly nonsense. I
mean it's fine when people think oh I'm unhappy, I wonder why I am,
and then get out of it, but what's worse is when people put on this
cloak of motherhood. Men are brought up to think they're the
breadwinners: they think well I'm not going to have the baby, and so
they think really hard about choosing a career. And I've been
blaming *other* people for my career and my type of life beforehand, but
really it's silly because I probably had at the back of my mind, oh well
I'm going to have a baby one day so it doesn't *matter* what I do,
whereas I *should* have said, well I'm going to concentrate and I'm

going to do medicine or something – not because my husband might leave me or because he might die, but just because I've got to do it in the same way *he's* got to do it.

SOPHY FISHER:
The disadvantages are the same as with being a housewife. I don't like being categorised, because people then generalise about categories. I say I don't think of myself as a mother, of course I do, but not in the social category sense. I must have had about eight million things through the post saying wouldn't I like to do my shopping at home with Janet Frazer or somebody else's catalogue. No I *wouldn't*. And because I've had a baby, I'm no more likely to do my shopping through Janet Frazer's catalogue than I ever was.

JOSEPHINE LLOYD:
I think probably more and more I've realised how women do get taken for granted. For example, when Howard and I go out shopping and he wants a drink on the way home, we sit in the pub and he might meet a couple of friends and sometimes I get the feeling that they're not interested in me: I'm just his wife and I've got a baby, and I'm not a person. I think that women definitely get taken for granted.

We don't get a lot of money anyway, but it does annoy me, because before, when I was working, I always had my own money. Howard gets the money on Monday, he gets about £28 social security [he is unemployed] and he gives me about £13 and keeps the rest. And he forgets that the money that he's given me isn't for me: they always seem to say that money is for you and it isn't. I never have even £1 for myself for make-up or anything: I haven't had any new clothes, nothing, whereas the money that he's got is for him. I mean I know friends of mine, their husbands give them housekeeping money and money for clothes but I've never had that. He says if there's some money left, he says oh spend it on yourself: but I've never had enough housekeeping to do that. If I did spend it on myself, he'd wonder why there wasn't any food in the house, so I can't win. I think I do miss that independence, you know, relying on him, even though he is not supporting us. I went to the social security and said look, we've had so many arguments over money, he's been borrowing and borrowing, he goes into the pub for some cigarettes and then when he's got the money on Monday he'll repay it, and I don't have anything, and I've drawn out all my savings to spend on food. So I asked if I can have half, just for the food, but they didn't want to know: they said no, we can't do that. So I have to rely on him giving me the money.

Power lies where money is. The birth of a first child divides the sexes, making mother economically dependent on father – and even if she goes out to work and he stays at home the weight of tax laws, national insurance and social security rulings goes against her.³ The conventional arrangement of father's job plus mother's domesticity works when communication between the partners is good, when husbands are generous (and when mothers are happy at home). But if there are cracks in the marital foundation, division adds to division. Emotional dependence matches economic dependence: bringing up a child in our culture is socially isolated work. Most first-time mothers have few friends in the community. The stereotype of middle-class mothers' coffee mornings is at odds with even middle-class reality: how to break down the isolation of each housewife locked behind her own front door is the problem. For working-class mothers, the range of contacts is even narrower. One or two childhood friends, a married sister with children, mothers or other relatives – these may be the only available confidantes. People, strangers, peer into the pram as it is wheeled down the street and make noises at the baby, but this breach in social manners is not the beginning of a beautiful friendship. There are simply few escapes from the burden of loneliness. The world shrinks to the size of the home: mother, father and baby. However much the baby was 'wanted', the resulting reduction in life's opportunities and options may not be.

Deborah Smyth was married at eighteen and she was nineteen when Dominic was born. She used to work as a checker in a factory; her husband works in a greengrocer's:

My friend was getting married last Saturday. And she saw the baby – it was the first time she'd seen him, and she said oh I want to start a family. And I said to her: don't start a family yet.

I: Why did you say that?

DEBORAH: I don't know. [long pause] We did it quickly. I like him – I like having him at home, you know. And I like looking after him and everything else. I don't know why I said that.

Sometimes I think about before we got married and that, you know: I think about going to work every morning. I never want to do it again, you know: I just *think* about it.

Janette Watson, an ex-factory machinist, was also married at eighteen and a mother a year later:

Well, I always think of what I'm missing. You know, before I was married I used to go out with friends: I don't do it any more. They all go out in crowds. I miss that really, because I don't get out much. I miss that a lot, I suppose.

They're all going abroad for their holidays – that's what I miss, I think: I've never been abroad. Mind you, when I started going out with Dan I always wanted to be with him more than with them. So I suppose you can't have everything.

I think sometimes I've thought I should have waited for a little while to get married and have a baby. But we both wanted to get married. I think of what I'm missing – going abroad and everything. But I like it: I like being married now. I mean I'll still be young when he grows up. I hope.

CHAPTER 12

Mothers and Medical People

It's your first experience, and you feel as if you're the only one in the world having a baby. I think they should make you feel as if you're a little bit important. [A patient]

Who knows what is important? Well, if a doctor doesn't know what's important, what is so important about doctors? [A doctor[1]]

It has become improper in the modern world to have a baby without consulting medical experts. Even women who want to go against the tide and have babies at home seek doctors or midwives to attend them. Throughout most of history and in most cultures childbirth has not had, does not have, this medical aspect: those who manage childbirth are experienced women in the community. But in many places today having a first baby brings a woman into a direct encounter with medicine, probably the first or the most thorough she has had in her life. Pregnancy involves a series of visits to hospital or general practitioners, birth is a hospital affair, and the advisers on postnatal health and baby care are also experts. Child-rearing, like childbirth, has become a scientific field in the twentieth century. How people bring up their children has ceased to be simply one facet of social behaviour and has become instead a technical exercise. Certain practices are regarded by medical experts as correct, and it is the role of midwives, doctors and health visitors to spread the word among mothers. Moral virtues have become technical necessities: breastfeeding is scientifically superior to bottlefeeding, and not just a maternal duty; later, rather than earlier, toilet training is advised on grounds of what is known about the child's psychological development; and the innate moral superiority of cleanliness is overriden by the rational superiority of paediatric science.

These encounters with health professionals are a central theme in the transition to motherhood. How mothers feel about their health care has become an

274

inseparable part of having and rearing a baby. Everybody knows that reproduction is a medical business, but not everybody feels the same way about it. The satisfactions and dissatisfactions mothers exhibit towards hospital doctors, GPs, midwives and health visitors, depend on the attitudes they have towards them. While some are happy to place themselves and their babies in medical hands, others suspect that useful advice can be given without medical training; some may argue that experts are only experts by virtue of their own belief in a false image.

DOCTOR KNOWS BEST?

LOIS MANSON, research worker:
I haven't got a high regard for any doctor particularly. When I was at university I used to do film extra work in the holidays and I got into it through a medic friend because loads of medical students from the London hospitals do this film extra work. And I was *amazed*, because I used to think that doctors saw the body as a sort of diagram of veins and muscles and what have you, but they were the most pornographic bunch of people you'd ever come across. And they were incredibly immature as well. It's a real eye-opener, isn't it? I'm afraid I've had no respect for doctors; I know it's a vast generalisation – I shouldn't say that – but it really did lower them in my esteem.

Added to that was the fact that when I was at school there were so many good people who *couldn't* get into medical school because their fathers weren't doctors and they weren't related. And the fools that *did* get in – when you've got friends and you know that that one is just as good as the next one and he gets in because he happens to be the son of a doctor, you sort of put that together with other things. And there's this *annoying* attitude that people have towards doctors: terrific *reverence* and not questioning what they say. It really annoys me intensely. And they play on it and they talk to you in this way as though you're not to know anything about it, because they are a very special elite. It makes me very cross, and it makes me very intolerant, which is a shame. I know some very very good doctors, and it's an awful thing to tarnish them all with the same brush.
I: So how do you feel about your medical care so far?
LOIS: I would say that it's difficult to expect a lot more. You know, I come home and I complain to David every time and he says really I

can't *expect* very much more, because of the time factor and what have you. It annoys me intensely that I've not seen the same doctor twice. I mean, they're very efficient and what have you, but I really do feel as if I've travelled quite a long way to be dealt with in a matter of minutes and that they're very loath to sit and chat with you or answer any questions or give you an opportunity to ask questions. I know I'm a bit over-sensitive about this sort of thing, and I'm sure I'm a *pain* as far as that is concerned, but I *do* think they could be nicer. I'm sure that *they* think I'm a pain!

So generally I suppose my opinion of the medical profession is sort of reflected in what happens when I go to the hospital. So *ideally* no, I'm not in the least bit satisfied, but I suppose it's relatively efficient, and I don't have to wait around for hours. I think it's a shame, particularly in that aspect of medicine, because it's such an emotional thing, isn't it? And you would think, I suppose, that doctors who go into antenatal work and who work at that hospital are interested in not *just* the physical side. Perhaps it's too much to expect. Are you interested to find out, I mean I don't know whether it's any part of your work, but it would be interesting to find out about the backgrounds of the various doctors, you know, how many of them are married and have children.

LOUISE THOMPSON, law student:
I personally don't like to have that much attention from doctors. The less, the better. Being on a conveyor belt is just fine. The faster the better.

It's like a mystique. That's what I think is so funny. Like going to law school, which is a profession, you realise that you just learn the right language and then it becomes very mystical, and that's how I think the medical profession is as well: if you just use the right words, people believe you. I mean if they talked very simply, people wouldn't go to doctors. The less I have to do with medicine and doctors the better.

SOPHY FISHER, television producer:
I have a basic belief in doctors and experts. I suppose if they advised me that it [induction] would be best for the baby and me then I would accept it – the advice and the reasons given. I sort of trust them to know what's best really. If they say that's good, then that's fine by me. If you can't trust them – if you *don't* trust them, who *can* you trust?

NINA BRADY, shop assistant:
I would be happy to have whatever the doctors say, because doctors, the hospital, you can't beat them; whatever they say I would do. I trust them that much. They're bound to know. I would leave it to the doctors, for surely they would do what is best for you, wouldn't they?

Doctor knows best: safe deliveries only happen in hospital. Ninety one per cent of the sample women did not even consider the alternative of a home birth (although 21 per cent said afterwards that they would think about it for their next baby).

It didn't cross my mind. I was expecting to go into hospital. In hospital they've got everything. (*Deirdre James*)

I like to know that I'm in a place where I'm being looked after. They've got everything there. You couldn't have your first one at home, could you? I don't think *I* could. I just want to know there's a doctor there or a nurse there: they know what they're doing. (*Veronica Pratt*)

Being the first one and my advanced age [30] I thought the best thing would be to go into hospital. Because I'm not one who wants to know what's going on, anyway. If anything goes wrong, they've got all the equipment there. I like to think they're well equipped to cope with anything that might go wrong. (*Hilary Jackson*)

I thought okay, first baby, the best thing to do is to have it in hospital, because it's far more of an unknown quantity. It's the done thing these days to have your first baby in hospital, because you think oh God if anything *did* happen, perhaps it would be better. So I decided to fight down my initial dislike of hospitals for the sake of the *baby*. But now I keep saying to Luke I wish I'd decided to have it at home. It just turns me off. It's this concern with medicine that seems to override everything else – the natural process. (*Alison Mountjoy*)

Defending childbirth as a natural process is not easy. Being critical of its medicalisation, of the control doctors believe they should properly exercise over it, places the patient in an attitude of confrontation: battles produce stress and anxiety. It is easier for the patient to act passively. As Alison Mountjoy puts it:

Who do you believe? That's part of the trouble of having a baby, that somehow each book and each medical person, they all say something a bit different. I mean you're not taking an A-level in having a baby, are you? I mean it's the sort of thing you want a certain amount of knowledge for, but you don't want contradictions, do you? Because you start to think well, which is it? Am I doing the right thing? Am I doing the wrong thing? Who do I believe?

I don't really *want* to lose confidence in them, because then I might start panicking. I'm lucky I've got all this confidence – I don't normally have confidence in doctors. I think it's important to *believe* in the hospital because it's so easy to become sceptical . . . (*Jane Tarrant*)

I felt it important that I felt positive about the hospital, and I know I tend to be rather critical, probably, coming from a doctor's family. I felt that this was a disadvantage, that I *wasn't* a bit more gullible and innocent and everything, because I would be critical and I'd probably lose out in the end. It's in my own interest to try and believe in them. (*Ellen George*)

·*Not believing that doctors always know best means thinking sometimes that their treatment might be wrong. It means suspecting that doctors do not tell the whole truth, and nothing but the truth: it means believing that behind what the doctor says and does lies a primary need to keep the patient in her place, a place where she knows less about her body than the doctor does, where the inside of a medical dictionary is as foreign to her as her own inside must be.*

A first pregnancy is a time for acquiring knowledge. The sample women were asked if they understood a list of twenty-one medical terms; scores were higher five months after the birth than seven months before it. For example, whereas 39 per cent knew what 'uterus' meant the first time, 69 per cent did after they had had their babies. Information of this kind is picked up haphazardly through the cubicle curtains in the hospital clinic, from discussions with one's best friend, by being sensitised to television programmes about having a baby and by reading antenatal advice literature (all but two of the women mentioned reading at least one book or pamphlet on birth). But it is also provided more systematically in antenatal classes. Two-thirds of the women went to one or more of the hospital's four 'parentcraft' classes (an 'introductory talk', talks on labour and feeding, and a tour of the hospital), and nearly half attended local authority antenatal classes (these usually combine relaxation/breathing exercises with talks on aspects of baby care). Five women also paid to join classes in psychoprophylaxis run by the National Childbirth Trust. Most were glad to have gone to these classes, although only a minority found the breathing exercises a help in controlling labour pain.

But knowledge is a double-edged sword. The medical ideal is a patient who knows enough but not too much.

RACHEL SHARPE:
When I was in labour this fellow came along with this apparatus and although I was dopey, I said what are you doing? Oh he said, I'm just

going to put up a drip in your arm. So I asked him what kind of drip it was and he sort of looked at me and said, oh it's a glucose drip, and I told him I didn't think I really needed one because I'd just eaten a meal before I'd come. And he asked why I thought I knew, why I thought I knew what was best for me in this situation? So I just told him that I'd done a lot of reading and everything. Anyway, he talked me into having this drip, because he said you don't know how long – it's good that you've had enough nourishment to sustain you up until now, he said, but you don't know how much longer you're going to be in labour. And if it gets much later we can't put it in. *That's* certainly not true – but anyway, he said are you going to let me put it in now? And I said yes, you can. And then I saw that he wasn't going to give me a local anaesthetic. So I said I'd like one. And he said what makes you think you need one? Why should you know what's best for you? So I just said that I'd had a drip set up before and I thought it was quite painful. I was so fed up arguing that I just said firmly I'd like to have a local anaesthetic, please. So he went off and he came back and he waved this little bottle in front of my face and said you've got what you wanted! Actually it was a good thing that I did have one because it took him five times before he found the place where he could get it in.

The fellow I didn't like, he put the monitor on, and while he was doing it, when he was putting that monitor on, the pain was absolutely *excruciating*. And I screamed and he said to me – well at first he didn't say anything, he just sort of looked up at me, and then when I hollered again he said to me why are you screaming? Well I said it's very painful. Can you not be a bit gentler? Oh he said I'm doing the best I can.

I mean doctors don't have any sort of human relations grounding, do they? When you think of it, to be a doctor all you need is a good memory. They don't say that you have to be exceptionally sympathetic: I mean you're *supposed* to be but as long as you give the *impression* of being that and as long as your memory's good enough to retain all that you're supposed to know, then that's all there is to it, really.

THANK YOU, DOCTOR?

Satisfaction with medical care reflects these attitudes of criticism or deference. It also mirrors the extent to which women want to know what is happening to them, and whether or not they feel that their questions are adequately answered.

Thirty per cent of the sample women had 'shared care' – they went to their own GPs for most of their antenatal care. In the GP's surgery the depersonalising features of hospital treatment are much less likely; reflecting this, 88 per cent of the women who had shared care would go to their GPs for a future pregnancy. So far as hospital care is concerned, there is, as the figures in the table show, a tendency for women to become less happy as the pregnancy advances and medical encounters multiply. But through most of the medical experiences of first-time motherhood, satisfaction with midwife care is higher, suggesting a bias towards the female management of birth even (or especially?) within the high technology of the modern hospital system.

How do you feel about your care from hospital doctors and midwives?		
Time	Satisfied with doctor care	Satisfied with midwife care
Early pregnancy	80%	82%
Late pregnancy	63%	63%
Birth	60%	80%
After the birth	59%	74%

The three most common complaints about hospital treatment are:
(1) feeling depersonalised, like items on a conveyor belt or assembly line;
(2) not being able to ask questions or not having questions answered satisfactorily;
(3) seeing too many doctors.
Women who had all their antenatal care at the hospital saw an average of nine different doctors. The average length of these antenatal consultations* is 3.9 minutes. Nearly half of all questions asked by mothers in one series of antenatal encounters* were requests for information about the progress of the pregnancy, about the physiology of pregnancy and birth in general, or about related medical procedures. Twelve per cent of all statements made by mothers concerned pain and discomfort, which was discounted by the doctor as clinically unimportant.[2]

A typical antenatal consultation goes like this:
DOCTOR [entering cubicle]: Hello.
PATIENT: Hello.
DOCTOR [reading notes]: Mrs Watkins?
PATIENT: Yes.
DOCTOR: Well, how are you?
PATIENT: Fine, thank you.
DOCTOR: Can I feel your tummy? [He undoes the buttons on her dressing gown and does so] Any complaints?
PATIENT: No.
DOCTOR [filling in notes]: Have you felt the baby move yet?

* *As observed by A.O. in 1974–5.*

PATIENT: Yes.
DOCTOR: How long have you felt it?
PATIENT: Two weeks.
DOCTOR [feeling patient's ankles]: All the tests we did last time were okay.
PATIENT: Good.
DOCTOR: Okay [leaves cubicle].

Being computerised

CHRISTINA LYNCH:
It's like a cattle market, a production line. You queue up and in you go and out you go. They just say are you alright? And most people say yes I'm alright unless they've had something drastically wrong. The doctor has a quick feel around and he says right we'll see you in four weeks' time. And that's it, in and out in a couple of minutes. Well, I suppose they must know what they're doing: if there was anything wrong they would have said so. I haven't had any *bad* treatment; they're all very kind. But I suppose they get so many people, when they say their bit at the end it's all automatic, like a parrot, no tone in the voice. They just say it off pat: they don't have time to get *involved* with people. There's no *personal* touch at all. You're just a body to them. A body with a name.

PAULINE DIGGORY:
It was very efficient, but there was an awful lot going on; people coming in and going out, and it was so funny, because these cubicles that you go in to be examined in are just in an open room with curtains, so everyone can hear what's going on next door: there was this funny doctor next door with this woman; he was shouting out, saying can I have a nurse please? Is there any nurses on this ward? Like something out of a film. Like that film 'Hospital' when that doctor died. Some other doctor shouted well you can blame Barbara Castle for that.
You seem to see somebody different every time. I'd rather have continuity. They probably don't remember you, but you remember them, don't you? Because you do feel a bit production-linish. They walk along the cubicles and say: have you been done yet?

HILARY JACKSON:
You just go in and out type of thing. It's all rushed through: you're all

prepared for the doctor, blood pressure taken quickly, so you're all ready for the doctors when they come.

TAMSIN ATTWOOD:
It's like a butcher's shop, you're laid out on slabs.

LOIS MANSON:
I was having to peer round them during an ultrasound scan to see what was going on, and they weren't the *least* bit interested in me and they were talking about *my* baby. And I wanted to say to them look, it's mine: that's *my womb* you've got up there.

ELIZABETH FARRELL:
When the patient is lying down they're at a disadvantage. Their personality I would say is *deprived* of them almost, in that horizontal position.

MARGARET SAMSON:
I felt as though I was a kind of computer. I felt as though I was just being computerised. I felt it was terribly impersonal. I came out thinking it was a great big computer line churning people out.

GRACE BOWER:
I wanted special treatment and I didn't get it. I think I was a bit upset about that. Maybe because the baby's so special to me. I thought it must be special to everyone else.

Questions unasked and unanswered

SHARON WARRINGTON:
Any questions I've asked him is about the size of the baby, and this doctor, he kept asking how tall I was. I said why? He said: just answer that, you answer me. I said no: you answer *me*. So he said, well he said, all we want to know is how tall you are. So I said if I tell you how tall I am will you tell me why you want to know? And he said yes. And I said I'm five foot one. And he hummed and harred and hummed and harred and I said right: you tell me now why you want to know. And he said well we won't be able to tell you till your next visit, he said, we'll give you an internal examination. You won't be able to tell me what?

I: Did you ask him any questions?
NANCY CARTER: [Pause] Um, I said I was worried about being

pregnant so soon after the appendicitis. And he said it just showed
what a healthy person I was.

I: What did you feel about that?

NANCY: Well, it wasn't really answering my question.

I: It didn't reassure you?

NANCY: Not really, no.

BARBARA HOOD:

I went in one day and the doctor said my blood pressure was up and I
had some protein in my water. I'm still not sure what that is, protein
in the water. Do you know what it is? They asked me to do another
specimen then, midstream. They don't tell you anything. Then they
asked me to do a twenty-four-hour urine collection. Anyway it cleared
up: when I went back the next time, they said it was alright.

I don't know whether these doctors *should* say these things. Either
they tell you *nothing* or they tell you some diabolical thing to frighten
the life out of you. Because this doctor said it leads to some kind of
disease or something, some Latin word . . . it can lead to that which
means that the baby will stop growing and could be susceptible to fits.
It frightened the life out of me.

They don't realise you go down to these places and you're a little bit
nervous, and it's all a bit above your head type of thing, and you can't
really talk as freely as you would like, and all the questions seem to
come an hour after you've left, you know, the questions you wanted to
ask, and I don't think they really appreciate this.

ELLEN GEORGE:

She tried to pump some kind of tranquillisers into me and I refused
them. She said here, take this: this'll make you feel better. And I
resisted it and she practically *physically* forced it into me. And I
thought well I'm just not bloody taking this. I didn't want to take it
because she wouldn't tell me what it was. I thought well that's just the
giddy limit. She wouldn't tell me what it was and I just didn't want to
take something when I didn't know what it was. I suppose I just want
to be told more about what's happening, about what they're doing.

JULIET MORLEY:

If they give you your notes to take somewhere they give them to you in
a big sealed brown envelope stapled up, and if you want to read them
you have to get them down from the rack in the cubicle and you get
caught.

I: Have you done that?

JULIET: Yes. There's nothing in them. The staff nurse came in and said oh you mustn't read those, and she got very cross. She said you're much better off if you don't know anything; nurses and midwives are the worst patients. And she told me about a case at Hillingdon hospital where a chap who had his arm and his leg in plaster read his notes and they'd written POP off – plaster of paris off – and he thought it meant that he was going to die!

PAULINE DIGGORY:
They gave me this thing you stick up and also some cream and of course I didn't use it, I forgot. And he wrote on my form – I'm always reading my form, they don't like you reading your form, and he'd written 'she says she forgets to take it' exclamation mark. They leave your notes lying about in that cubicle thing. The nurses tell you off. One doctor did find me, he said do you find it interesting? I said well it's my form, I'm not going to look at someone else's.

JOSÉ BRYCE:
He's a bloody whizz kid, he is, he came breezing in and he said: right, we'll see you next week. I said well I hope not, she's due before next week. And he said oh really? So I know he didn't even look at my notes enough to know when she was due, and then I said well what about the X-rays? And he said what X-rays? And I said look, I've had four X-rays and one ultrasound test supposedly to see whether I'm going to have a caesarean or not. Don't you worry about that, my dear, we'll worry about that. Like I'm a real idiot, and he couldn't possibly discuss me with me. And he breezed off.

MICHELLE CRAIG:
Er, I don't know how to put this really. After sexual intercourse I had some bleeding, three times, only a few little drops, and I didn't tell the hospital because I didn't know how to put it to them. It worried me first off, as soon as I saw it I just cried. I don't know if I'd be able to tell them. You see I've also got a sore down there and a discharge and you know I wash there lots of times a day. You think I should tell the hospital? I could never speak to my own doctor about it. You see I feel like this, but I can talk to you about it and I can talk to my sister about it.

ANNE BLOOMFIELD:
I've been getting really bad stomach pains like I'm coming on. I said

that to the doctor; I said I had bad stomach pains. He said it's usual.
But I mean they're getting worse. He said you do get this. It might be
usual but . . .

They don't tell you *why* you get the pain, but then they don't tell you
anything unless you ask them and when you ask them they answer
you as if you're silly. I ask which way the baby's lying and how much
it weighs now. Just natural questions. Well it's about *this* big, and it
weighs about a pound, and it lies *this* way. They make you feel silly, so
I don't ask now. They just answer you as though they don't really
want you to ask them.

Nameless faces

DEBORAH SMYTH:
You seem to get a different doctor every time you go. They don't really
examine you, they just look at your stomach and say you're alright
and that's it. That's all I've ever had. They could, you know, talk to
you. Because if you start to talk to them about something they say well
ask the girl at the desk. They treat you as another pregnant body
really. The nurses are always nice, they come and take your blood
pressure, they always talk to you as though you're somebody and not
just a patient. The first time I went I had a nice doctor: he was very
nice. But since then they've all been – just in, look at your stomach,
you're alright, see you in two weeks' time which you don't, because
you don't see the same doctor.

JOSEPHINE LLOYD:
I really think I would have preferred to have seen the same doctor
every time and I think that would be better from their point of view,
because if the same doctor followed it through, they'd know. I'm not
saying that they've got time, that they should go into the social side of
it, but if they know a bit more about your state of mind, perhaps it
would help them. I don't know anything about it from the medical
side. I just feel that if the same doctor saw you every time you'd feel a
bit more important and you'd feel you could say hallo, you know, and
he'd say, are you feeling any better from last time, or anything of this
kind.

JANE TARRANT:
The first doctor I met was really very nice actually. And since then
I've seen a chap who sometimes wears shorts. In the hot weather he

came in in shorts: he's almost boorish in that he walks in, he doesn't even say hallo. I say good morning and he just – yes, you're alright, off you go. Well I don't expect them to spend a long time. I realise that they *are* very pushed, but it is a pity that you don't seem able to have a relationship with the doctor at all.

BARBARA HOOD:
The doctor I saw when I was first in labour, he was very nice. When he came in he came over and introduced himself. I thought he was nice. He introduced himself the first time which is very unusual. On the Sunday afternoon two doctors came in and they didn't introduce themselves and I didn't know who they were. I think that's not polite. They know who *you* are, don't they?

I: How did you feel about your medical care during the birth?
GRACE BOWER: I suppose to them it's just a job. They come in and walk out and go to the other one. It's just a job: come three o'clock they had to change; some had to go and others had to come back. And then at nine o'clock they had to change again. No one seemed to care; they said well I'm off duty, it doesn't matter what happens to *her*: wait till someone else comes.

Three-quarters of the women had never seen the person who delivered their baby before. This is an innovation in the management of childbirth, for the traditional custom is for there to be some special relationship between the woman having the baby and her birth attendant. The baby is not helped into the world by a total stranger who walks in out of the blue, and then walks out never to be seen again. Of all the features of hospital birth today, this is perhaps one of the hardest to tolerate.

ALISON MOUNTJOY:
Isn't it funny that you do feel this sort of emotional tie with the person who delivers you? It's strange. That was one of the things that I do remember saying at the hospital, at the clinics: that it would be really nice to know who was going to deliver you because it would be one less thing to be scared about; if you knew who it was you'd get to know them. So it really was a bonus to find that the person I did feel at ease with was in fact going to deliver her.

JANE TARRANT:
They had to call a doctor in the end because I was too small and I had an assisted delivery. Anyway this doctor I knew, he was the nice one

I'd seen in the clinic, he came in and said oh hallo Jane, which I thought was awfully nice; it made me feel, do you know what I mean?

ELIZABETH FARRELL:

If you've got a husband who isn't there – I mean I would have liked my mother to have been there if my husband wasn't there. Really *you* were the substitute for my mother being there [A.O. attended the birth]; that sounds funny, but I mean it was *horrific* that the midwife and the pupil midwife who were there I'd never seen in my life before and I've never seen them again since. And yet they were *the* people in about the most vital and powerful experience in my life so far.

JO INGRAM:

I went up to this nurse and said can I see the doctor who'll deliver the baby? And she said well we don't know who it'll be, because it depends on when you come in. I said you've got no idea at all? She said not really. So I can't ask the doctor, I can't ask anybody the things I'm worried about? She said oh you shouldn't be worried . . .

GILLIAN HARTLEY:

I'm going to ask if I can meet the doctor who'll deliver the baby. You can't just have this figure appearing from nowhere. They'll probably say no, and that'll upset me tremendously. If I could just see him for five minutes just to say I want to know your face when you come in. It's very important. You want a personal relationship with the person who delivers your baby.

In the event, Gillian's baby was delivered by a midwife as were 43 per cent of the sample babies, but her midwife was a familiar face: she had run the antenatal classes Gillian had attended.

When I saw that that midwife was there I thought that was marvellous. I thought I *know* her, I can ask her things; I don't have to feel she's a stranger, and I thought that made a great deal of difference.

LABOUR NEGOTIATIONS

From the medical point of view however, who delivers the baby is less important than how it is done. Medical technology has now developed to the point where two key areas of maternal expertise can be challenged: the dating of the pregnancy, and the physical sensation of giving birth. Doctors now have the means to control both these.

The technique of ultrasonic scanning measures the size of the baby and its growth in the uterus, and claims to be able to date within a few days the time of conception and thus the expected time of delivery. Sixty-six per cent of the sample women were given ultrasound in pregnancy. The medical rationale for this varied: a short interval between coming off the pill and pregnancy (so that regular periods had not yet been re-established); a discrepancy between size and dates; a suspected complication – like placental failure or too much amniotic fluid. Whatever the reason, having ultrasound and working out what ultrasound means figure prominently in antenatal care at this hospital. In one series of antenatal clinic encounters (referred to earlier, pp. 280–1), 6 per cent of the questions mothers asked doctors in the clinic concerned the 'proper' expected delivery date. Mothers regard this as a matter for, at best, the person whose body is growing the baby, and, at worst, for negotiation between mother and doctor. They do not agree that a machine can so automatically arbitrate a time for birth.

Clare Dawson's last period began on 20 February 1975, which gave an expected delivery date of 27 November.

When I went to the hospital the first time they said I was fourteen weeks by dates and eleven weeks by size, so I was confused; I didn't know whether to take fourteen weeks or eleven weeks. I saw the sister after I saw the doctor and she said the doctor wants you to have an ultrasound, and she phoned the ultrasound place and she said this patient's got to have an ultrasound because she's fourteen weeks by her dates and eleven weeks by size. I thought I don't know where I am. I said to her what date am I supposed to take? I've got to give in my notice at work and I have to let them know this week when I'm leaving. She said take the fourteen weeks, but I don't know what she meant really – fourteen weeks by dates, eleven weeks by size. I was a bit confused.

Later on in the pregnancy:

I had three ultrasounds and they finally decided that it's due on the 27th *December*. The first time she said she only did a rough one but she said if you come the next time then you'll know definitely. So I went again and they said I was definitely a month out. But I think it's due earlier than that: I feel so huge.

The doctor and the nurse had an argument about it after the third ultrasound. She said you are twenty-two weeks pregnant, and then I said well the ultrasound has just told me that I am eighteen-and-a-half weeks, and so she said well the doctor has written down that you are twenty-two. I said well I don't know, sort it out amongst yourselves, and so she called the staff nurse or somebody and she called in a group of them and they had little discussions and they called the doctor out. And he said if I've written she's twenty-two weeks, she's twenty-two weeks. So she said well ultrasound said that she is only eighteen-and-a-half. So then he turned round and said the policy in this hospital is to take the ultrasound date, and if that is what ultrasound says, that's what the date is. So she said well why didn't you write that down? He said ours is not to reason why. He said you just put it where you want to: you know as well as I do to take the ultrasound date. So she put it in the folder and presumably the sister was going to decide which date they were going to take. She said don't worry about it, that's for us to sort out. And when I went back the next time they had decided to go for the ultrasound date – the 27th December.

Mary was born on 1 December, a full-term baby.

As far as I'm concerned it's stupid to be that far out. Really. And at six pounds ten ounces she wasn't a particularly small baby – she wasn't five pounds or something like that. She was so convinced, this woman in ultrasound. So it makes me wonder really what the value of it is.

Women are routinely asked in the antenatal clinic for the date of their last period. But they are not asked if they have any idea of the date of conception – nor are they asked to date the pregnancy from the time when symptoms first appear.

JANET STREETER:

I'm sure I'm twelve weeks because my bust started to hurt early in the month – earlier than it would on a twenty-eight-day cycle. I'm sure I'm right. If only they went by one's symptoms a bit more, I'm sure they could do without some of these tests. I don't know why they do these endless ultrasounds. Ultrasound make it a week later: I think, quite honestly, if there's any excuse to do any of these tests they do them.

Her period date gave an expected birth date of 10 December. Ultrasound provided the 17th. The baby, weighing 7lbs 1oz, was born on 2 December, in line with her statement that he was conceived early in the month.

RACHEL SHARPE:

I've had six ultrasounds and had I known from the beginning that they were not almost spot on I would never have consented to them. I think the first thing is, it's just something new. And although they say it doesn't do anything to the baby I think the *less* things that are done to the unborn baby the better. And there's no point in having it if it doesn't give you an accurate date. I think they should tell you at the very beginning that it isn't accurate, the only thing you get is the emphasis that it doesn't hurt the baby and it doesn't hurt you, it's just like getting an X-ray. Bla, bla, bla. I mean they don't account for things like some babies have bigger heads. And I was just thinking that my head is a bit bigger than average and so is Francis's, so there's a very good chance that this baby would have a bigger than average head. So when they tell me the end of November I think a baby with a big head might be a week later or something.

Her last period began on 12 February, but she said she thought conception had occurred mid-March. Julian was eventually born, weighing 9lbs 6ozs, on 10 December, which gives a conception date of 19 March.

More complex than the problem of dating pregnancy is the emotive topic of pain in childbirth. While it is not a woman's destiny to suffer as she reproduces, most mothers certainly feel some pain – 70 per cent feel moderate, severe or intolerable pain according to one estimate.[3] Drugs for reducing the pain of labour have been available for a long time, but it is only the advent of epidural analgesia that promises the fulfilment of a dream: mothers giving birth totally conscious but feeling no pain at all. The birth accounts in chapter 5 clearly show that this dream can turn into a nightmare. Too much pain relief may relieve nothing but the doctor's unease in the face of pain. Childbirth is not experienced if the feeling of giving birth is missing.

GILLIAN HARTLEY:

I'd like to have nothing – no drugs for the birth. I don't like the idea of epidurals – I know at that hospital they do them every day and they're very safe, but I don't like the idea of needles in my spine, and I don't like the idea of not feeling anything but pressure and you can't push. It's almost a spartan feeling – that your body is doing something that is natural to it: presumably if your pelvis is wide enough and everything else is alright then labour should go alright. You're denying yourself the response of your body if you start tampering with its mechanisms, and the experience is something that is unique: you're denying yourself the total experience if you have an epidural ... I think if you can go through labour without it, it seems to me it must be more rewarding to do it nature's way. Pain is a natural thing.

If it gets painful I'd like the assurance that I could scream and that no one would really get upset about it. They get so upset if you make the slightest noise. Screaming doesn't necessarily mean you want anything: it's just a way of reacting. If the baby's in an uncomfortable position or it kicks me hard and it hurts, I make a noise. Max says what's the matter, what's the matter, and I say it hurts!

After the birth:
I started to scream when they stitched me and they can't bear you screaming. I think they should have let me scream if I'd wanted to, because it really was very painful. It's terrible because it did hurt and it wouldn't have hurt if I'd screamed a little. It would have made me feel better. I felt that during the labour itself too.

Perhaps we have lost touch with pain, with the pain of childbirth, in the same way as we have lost touch with death and dying? The beginnings and the ends of life are horrible and marvellous, too much to bear: so we hospitalise and anaesthetise them out of sight: out of sight, out of mind.

Not all women see pain productively, of course. Before the baby is born they may say there is no reason why women should be martyrs: suffering ennobles no one. Ninety-eight per cent of the sample women had some kind of pain relief; less than half were satisfied with the pain relief they had. While 29 per cent intended to have an epidural, 79 per cent actually had one. The gap is explained in part by pressure from hospital staff to succumb to the temptation (or promise) of painless childbirth. Seventy-two per cent said they were given a 'sales talk' for epidurals.

SOPHY FISHER:
They talked me into the epidural. A doctor came round the day before and said will you have one? And I said well I had intended to have a go without. And he said well it makes things easier for us if you do because we'll probably have to use forceps [her baby was in a breech position] and we would recommend it unless you are very very set against it. So in the face of that it seemed foolish to argue. I took him to mean that I would be less likely to *hinder* them if I had an epidural: that I would be more *passive* really.

SUE JOHNSON:
When I went to the hospital last time I said to the doctor are there any exercises I can do to help with the birth? He said oh you don't want to bother with all that. I said why not? And he said well all our women have epidurals. I said I don't want an epidural and he said why ever not? You don't want to bother with all that exercise rubbish.

GRACE BOWER:
I just went into hospital to see what was wrong and they said to me
how long have you been in labour? And I said I haven't, I haven't got
any pains. She said you have, you know. Oh, have I? I said all I know
is this morning when I woke up I kept going to the toilet. It was just
like you were constipated. They said do you want an epidural, as *soon*
as I got in. And I said to them I can't feel any pain: what's the point in
having it? And she said oh you soon will do, you soon will feel pain. I
said well wait and see, wait and see. And about eight I said alright.
I: So did you feel pain then?
GRACE: No, I just felt that I was constipated. Pressure, not pain. I just
gave into them. It didn't work, I'm glad to say. Everyone else in the
ward who had it had to have a forceps delivery. I wasn't *going* to have
it. Right up until the last minute I said no, no. Then I think one of the
girls really persuaded me – she made me feel so guilty for not having
it. She kept saying oh it's going to be much better for you and all the
way round it's going to be much better. So I said alright.

*Antenatal educators have a hard time. On the one hand it is their self-appointed
duty to dispel anxiety – and being afraid of the pain must be the oldest and greatest
anxiety there is. Yet, perversely, they are there to promote techniques for relieving
and controlling pain: breathing exercises, relaxation, pethidine, nitrous oxide,
epidurals. Here a registrar at the research hospital is addressing pregnant women
and their husbands at an antenatal class on labour, and what he has to say
demonstrates very well the tension between the two formulae: childbirth hurts so
you must have drugs to relieve it; and childbirth doesn't hurt very much so don't be
afraid of it.*

The best method we know of pain relief at the present time is an
epidural. Except for a few very fortunate labourers, labour is painful.
There is no doubt about it, that labour is painful. And only a few go
through labour without experiencing any pain at all. And therefore
we have to provide analgesia or pain relief to mothers who are
labouring. Either to *support* what they've been taught in psychoprophylaxis – I don't want to *knock* psychoprophylaxis – I think that
psychoprophylaxis has a value in that it helps you relax and helps you
to anticipate what's to come and *may* reduce your awareness of the
pain, but you may still require some support. And I personally prefer
to see a patient not experiencing pain and enjoying their labour,
enjoying the final outcome; rather than to have someone who is in
pain, is distressed, is *un-co-operative* and *renders the job of the nursing and*

medical staff far more difficult, and makes it far more difficult for the doctors and the nurses to spot the problems, to monitor them properly and to assist their labour with syntocinon to expedite delivery. Now are there any questions on epidurals? I think we'll deal with those first.

PATIENT: I'm not worried about the medical side – how safe it is – but don't you get *any* feedback in the way of regret that they haven't experienced it – that it does completely cut out sensation – you have to be told when to push?

DOCTOR: A very small proportion *do* regret it, but if you then allow them to have a painful labour without any analgesia they change their minds. Yes, there can be regrets that you've disturbed nature's natural process, but until you experience the pain of labour it's difficult to know what it's like, or what it can be like. It's very difficult when you're having your first baby. Are you all having your first baby? Yes. Well, I personally like to see a relaxed happy patient who maybe isn't *experiencing* her labour fully, by not having the pain, or the *feeling*, but who is happy and relaxed.

GRACE BOWER:

They all seemed to be for injections at that class, but they never said you could do it without injections. Because I hate injections of any sort, especially that one in the spine, oh I couldn't have that one, that one I'd never have. I said to my husband, I'd rather die than have an injection in my back: it'd kill me. It seemed to me from what they said that you had to have one of the three – the gas, the one in the back or the other one. My husband said to me do you *have* to have one of them? I said I don't know. They didn't mention you *not* having them. I'd rather not have them if I could. They could have explained that you can give birth without these injections: it's not *so* painful, or maybe it is: I don't really know.

One girl, she said she wanted to have the epidural and she said could she have it right until the baby's more or less born and then *not* have it, to stop: not to have it any more. And she said oh it's no good that way, you can't take the pain away from someone and then at the last minute give it back to them. And I thought oh is it going to be that painful then? [It wasn't, see p. 292.]

ANGELA KING:

Not knowing what the pain's going to be like, you don't know. I feel completely confused. You know, they're talking about the pain and this and that and you start to think well will it be *really* painful? I'd like not to have it really. The anaesthetist, he said he'd done 600 and he'd never heard of one that went wrong. Because you hear all these stories about them missing and people being paralysed and all that. But you know, they were really *selling* it. I suppose it is his job to sell it.

The last two girls from the relaxation classes who've had their babies, they didn't have anything. They said the breathing exercises really helped. That could be psychological, I suppose, because the obstetrician at the hospital talk, he said it doesn't *really* help. Another thing I asked them about the cost, and they said it cost £30,000 a year or £60,000, I can't remember now, whereas pethidine or gas and air would only cost in the sum of hundreds. So why, I mean the NHS is in a terrible state anyway, so *why* do they do it, waste all that; well, I know it's not wasted, in some cases it would be vital or really necessary, but why push people into having it?

Of those who had epidurals, 46 per cent were unhappy about having had them. This unhappiness is often a product of reflection; asked five months later women's answers may be different from the minute, or the day, after the birth. (This may of course be one reason why dissatisfaction with epidurals is news to many obstetricians, who measure satisfaction with birth immediately afterwards only.)

DEBORAH SMYTH, seven weeks later:
They said do you want an epidural? I was getting the pains every two minutes and I said yes, I'll have an epidural. That was horrible, I think that was more painful than actually having the baby.
I: Why did you decide to have an epidural?
DEBORAH: Because it was so painful at the time, and they said do you want one and I said yes, you know, not really thinking about it. I said yes because I was getting this pain. I had it and then the pain came back in half an hour. They put some more stuff in it and after a little while the pain came back again. They made out that it was quite a good thing, you know. They told me, they said as soon as the pain comes back we'll put some more in you and the pain'll go away and it didn't. They explained it to me and I said yes – I didn't even know what it was; they said it's an injection into your back and it makes your legs numb and from your waist down numb. Then I had to have a drip, she didn't say that until I actually went into the delivery room, you know. Next time I won't have it. I'll have the next one at home and I'll try and have nothing.

CHRISTINA LYNCH, five months later:
I think I wouldn't have it again because I think I missed out. I couldn't feel the contractions for a start, and I felt so awkward: like a lump of lead, and having that blooming drip in my arm, I can still feel the pain of the drip; and having to be humped around every twenty-five minutes, foetal heart beat, blood pressure, and not being able to help myself because I was numb from the waist downwards. And having a lot of trouble afterwards. I thought it was lovely at the time, but I think I would like to experience – it sounds idiotic – but I think I would like to experience more pain; I don't know why.

MICHELLE CRAIG, five months later:
I had the epidural and I couldn't feel it properly. I mean you don't know what's happening at the other end. Sometimes I wish, I'd prefer not to have had it. My sister told me that when she was in there was a woman in her ward, she was blind or deaf or something, and she wanted to feel the pain to know that it was hers.

If I think about it I might like to have gone without the epidural just to know what it's like, because I mean you're missing out, aren't you?

SANDY WRIGHT, five months later:
I still wish I hadn't had an epidural, I feel silly, when people discuss their births, you know when someone's just had a baby, and I feel I can't really say anything about that because I didn't really experience it properly. If I had another baby I think I would – I wasn't *ever* going to have an epidural anyway: it's easy when you're not in the throes of labour pains.

I just have the same feeling really, that I wish I hadn't had an epidural, I think maybe they do it for their own convenience, because it's easier to deal with a patient who's not feeling great pain. I don't think I felt probably the same sense of elation or whatever, because although I had pushed her out myself I hadn't really felt it. I think that might have affected me somehow.

To have the experience but miss the meaning can be a lasting reproach. For birth is not just any experience: the creation of life is one of life's most indelible moments. And first birth stands out because it sets a precedent for future births, because it marks the passage to an era, the era of parenthood, and because through it a woman first encounters the challenge of loving an infant of her own. The baby's birth and the baby's status as a person are theoretically separate questions, but in a mother's mind they may become interlocked, so that a bad experience of one leads into a bad experience of the other. For this reason as well, every *aspect of childbirth management is potentially important. Less than half the mothers said they enjoyed the experience of having a baby in hospital. More than a third felt that feelings about the management of the birth in some way overflowed into their relationship with the baby:*

I think you have more of a *bond* if you have experienced a bit of pain; you feel as though you've really done something. I mean when they held her up I just sort of looked at her – maybe it was a state of shock or something, but I just couldn't believe it because I hadn't felt anything. Obviously the maternal instinct's grown since then, but I think possibly it would have been there from the very beginning if I had experienced pain, some sensation of actually having her. (*Cary Wimborne*)

SEXUAL POLITICS

Invasions of privacy

One of the doctor's tasks in treating women who are having babies is to examine them vaginally. This is done for a variety of reasons: for instance, in pregnancy to make sure the baby is in the right place or that the cervix is closed; during labour to monitor the opening of the cervix; at the postnatal examination to check that any lacerations have healed. Though a technical exercise, both doctor and patient have their own views on the vaginal examination.

The doctor didn't seem to remember me, but you remember them don't you? I mean they see so many women that it's all just fannies to them, isn't it? (*Anne Bloomfield*)

What I'm interested in is the doctor's reaction. They see all these women – how on earth he ever makes love to his girl-friend I don't know. Do you know what I mean? It interests me so much. His professional mind, all these women, must affect his emotional side when he sees his girl-friend, if you know what I mean. (*Pauline Diggory*)

Lois Gould in her novel Necessary Objects *describes the vaginal examination of women's army recruits:*

All those rubbery arms lost at sea. Disappearing inside dark underwater caves, many of them never before explored. If you squint, all those doctors look like amputees, or Peeping Toms imprisoned in the stocks. But I could tell a lot of the girls were really scared; they would gasp, and some of them actually screamed. . . . And the doctors had to work fast, which hurts more. I figured out that if they did it slowly, I mean if they were careful, or gentle, then maybe some of the girls would have misunderstood. Ahem, this isn't for fun, young lady, it hurts me as much as it does you . . . Smiles could be interpreted as indicating the doctor likes to . . . imagine getting paid to do *that*. Wow – like being a movie critic. . . .

There was a girl lying on the next table who asked the doctor if this was what intercourse felt like. He made some noise that was authorized instead of a laugh. 'Not' he said in this gruff voice 'exactly'.[4]

The problem of the vaginal examination is that the doctor's hand or speculum are exceptions to a general rule – that what penetrates a woman's vagina she or her lover choose to put there. This is a problem both for the patient and for the doctor. It is thus in both their interests to define the vaginal examination as non-sexual.[5]

I hadn't the faintest idea what happened. People had said they examine you and take tests and this and that but they never actually said what happens. . . . (*Grace Bower*)

And then he gave me the internal and he was fiddling about there for about twenty minutes and of course at the time, it was the first time a doctor's really examined me like that, I went bright red and I was looking up at the ceiling and I didn't know whether to pull the towel over my face and close my eyes – I just didn't know what to do. And he went out and got another doctor in. I said to the nurse is he treating me like a guinea pig? She just laughed and then an Indian doctor came in. He was quite nice, he said good morning, which the other one didn't say: I was noting all these things. After the first doctor examined me, he wouldn't sort of look at my face. Then the second doctor examined me and I felt embarrassed first of all, but as soon as he started he didn't make me feel embarrassed, he was talking to me at the same time. . . . (*Michelle Craig*)

A nurse came in and she said she'd come and hold my hand. She took my blood pressure and went out, and then the doctor came in and he was just writing a few notes down in his book, and she came in and said do you need my assistance? And he said yes, I was just going to call you. He said will you hold her hand? Perhaps they hold everybody's hand? (*Deborah Smyth*)

Apprehension about internal examinations was very commonly mentioned by women in their accounts of medical care. Most simply find it very difficult to regard the doctor's intrusion as a clinical exercise. It seems much more like rape – or enforced adultery.

I don't like doctors mucking about with me. My husband doesn't like it either. He says to me every time I come back from the hospital, or when I've to go, what are they going to do to you? Why have they got to do that to you? They've done it once. And all things like that. (*Michelle Craig*)

DEBORAH SMYTH: Patrick wanted to stay for the birth, but you turned a bit green at the end, didn't you?
PATRICK: Only because of the afterbirth.
DEBORAH: The cord broke.
PATRICK: Something happened and they couldn't get it out. There were these two women fiddling around, trying to get it out, and a doctor, and he puts his hand inside Debbie and that hurt, it hurt *me*: I come out in a sweat, I felt sick. They sent me out every time they examined her, it upset her.
DEBORAH: Yes it did. He said if the doctors can see you, I can.

She said he only won't be allowed to be there during the internal examination. So I said why won't he be allowed to be there during the internal examination? It's absolutely disgusting. It must be because they're frightened of the blokes being jealous; I can't think of any other reason. Not jealous, but feeling a bit funny about the doctor sticking his . . . when I asked her *why* he couldn't be there during the internal she said because the doctors don't like them to be there. (*Jo Ingram*)

Alison Mountjoy had sixteen vaginal examinations during her pregnancy; because she had once had an abortion, the doctor in charge of her care thought she might have an 'incompetent cervix' as a result (which could cause premature labour):

It's awful, because half of you wants to get used to internals, because it makes it less uncomfortable, but you get so used to flinching or taking yourself away from that part of your body that when you don't want to take yourself away you've got to consciously bring yourself back: say it's not going to hurt, and it is your husband, it's not a doctor.

I said to this doctor the other day I'll *never* get used to this, and he said let's face it, do you really *want* to get used to it? And he really understood. But some doctors, they've said well you don't mind if your husband puts his hand up you? I mean you try to explain to them that it is actually totally different. You say well your husband doesn't put plastic gloves on. Why *should* one have to get used to all these things? That's what annoys me about it. Like having internals every five minutes, why should one have to get used to it? It's not a very nice thing to have to get used to.

Mandy Green has a particular reason for disliking internals:
When I was younger I had to have an internal, when I was about eight. There were some boys that sort of waylaid us, a girlfriend and myself. It wasn't actually that that upset me, but the doctor who examined me afterwards. And although I didn't realise it at the time, when I look back it was probably something to do with that. Because, you know, you get your face covered up, and your mother and he are going pss-pss-pss and it's all very ugh. As I say, it wasn't the boys, because I didn't know very much about sex when I was seven... That seemed perfectly normal, what the boys did, it didn't bother me. It was the examination afterwards – the secrecy and how nasty it was, although I didn't appear in court. The climax was being examined by the doctor, and that was terrible. I mean, I knew it was terrible, it wasn't what the boys had done, but it was the terrible thing of having to be examined by a police doctor. So I think that could have something to do with me not liking to have internals. I've certainly tried to avoid them like the plague.

Vera Abbatt had 'phobia of vaginal examinations' written on her medical notes:
It used to terrify me, the idea of having a baby, to be quite honest with you. Lying on your back with people peering at you. I felt that way when I went to the hospital and I could see there were other people around in the same position, but it didn't help much: I still felt it was disgusting, to be quite honest. But I phoned my mother up and she said not to worry about it – you're not the only one they see all day, sort of thing. I think it *is* embarrassing. I don't think I could ever get used to it.

He was quite nice at first, then, when he found out he was going to have a bit of a problem with me, he sort of got a bit nasty; I think he was a bit browned off, I think he'd probably had a bad morning and I didn't help matters much. He said he didn't know how I got bloody pregnant in the first place, which I thought coming from a doctor was a bit of a cheek. I didn't think it was at all ethical. That didn't help matters; that made me worse actually. I thought if you're going to be rude, I can be just as rude back. I refused to submit to anything he wanted to do then: I was so disgusted with it all. And that was when he said oh get dressed and pranced out.

The doctor who did it, he picked up this stainless steel thing they listen to the heart with, and I thought that was what he was going to do the examination with. I thought where the hell is he going to put that? It looked so huge. Of course now I know what it's for – but this one, he was standing over me with this steel instrument in his hand asking me how are you sort of thing.

After the baby was born I thought about it a lot. I kept thinking *why* was I like that? When they came in to examine my stitches, to me that was as bad as any internal. To me it's the hospital, to me it's just any hospital and doctors in general. I'm alright, as I say, with my husband. To me, it's not me, it's the idea of the hospital.

Funnily enough they wanted to give me an internal at my postnatal. Then I was right back to square one, I couldn't. I was alright at first when he said we'll give you an internal: you had some problems during your pregnancy? I said yes, but I'm alright now. I really thought I was, because I had managed with this epidural. And as soon as they tried it I just froze, I couldn't relax. And he said oh I think you've still got the problem. I felt such a twit. So he didn't do one. He said it wasn't really necessary. He only wanted to do it for routine.

It's just doctors, the atmosphere of the hospital: as soon as I go in, I just go cold.

To Hilary Jackson, it is an allergy:
I'd never had an internal before because I'd never been to a family planning clinic, you see. I was probably tense and a bit embarrassed. It was just the thought of that light shining down. I thought you've got a better view than I have!

I feel it's *barbaric*, it really is, you know. I think the trouble is that they don't think of you as individuals, they don't think that anyone's got any feelings. You know, they don't think one's a modest person, that you *still* feel embarrassed after everything that's gone on.

They did an internal every week towards the end – I don't know why. I think the word went round that I was allergic to them, and so every week someone would come in and have this session. And some people were very gentle, and some people were like a bull in a china shop. This Dr Stancomb eventually broke the water and he was fine. But the one before that was like a great big rugby player, a huge great rugby player. When I go back if I see that rugby player coming in with his great big fists, I shall be out of that bed in five seconds flat. . . . Some of them are gentle and some of them are diabolical. Dr Thompson is good and so is Andrews and one of the coloured sisters did it and she was very very good. But I think it's when they suddenly *surge* in, I mean I don't think they *ever* think what they're doing. To them it's just like feeling your tummy, or like listening to your chest, it's just another part of the examination. But to the person lying there that is the part that you want someone to be the most gentle with you. And when you come out of it you feel really rotten. You know, you feel *indignant* and everything else. And I get down to the car and I start crying. My husband says what are you crying for? What's he done? And I just say, oh nothing. They don't think of what they're doing, they just don't. I don't think *any* woman *ever* gets used to that, I really don't. The amazing thing is they ask you if you're allergic to plaster or something *stupid* like that. But they don't ask you if you're allergic to *that*. I said to him, this doctor, I was allergic to them, internals, so he said I think we all are aren't we? So I said well how the hell can *you* be? I don't suppose you've ever had one. He just laughed.

Styles vary; so does the sex of the doctor, although most obstetricians are male.[6]

NINA BRADY:
The doctor in the family planning, she was a lady doctor: she was *so* nice, so nice. I can't explain it to you. She was an elderly woman and it was my sister told me to go on a Wednesday if you could and she said you'll get this lady doctor. Isn't she nice? She said I presume you're a Catholic and if it's going to cause problems between you and your husband, she said, why don't you talk about it? And all this. Before her, I think I'd be pregnant now and having another baby, if it weren't for that lady doctor. I'd never have been able to stand that, when they put the coil in. She was so nice, and she was so understanding. It didn't hurt, and all the other eternals [*sic*] I had, they all hurted. That's why I had the epidural so quick when I was having the baby: I couldn't bear to have an eternal. It didn't hurt, it really didn't hurt. She was so nice. She fitted it straight away, and it didn't hurt. And when I went in she said now you'll come back here in six weeks' time for a check-up. But instead I went to my own doctor; she said I could go there if I liked as well. So I went there and he was going to

examine me, and he couldn't examine me: my nerves, oh! I was up on the table, and I had to get down again. He said I'm sorry, but you'll have to go to the hospital to be examined. And I went and no problems. That lady doctor: no problems. I think it's because she's experienced, she knows her job, I think. I couldn't tell you how good that woman is. (*See pp. 44–5 for Nina's first experience of an internal examination.*)

JANETTE WATSON:

He was the only gentle one there. It never felt sore when he felt your tummy, the only one with gentle hands: he was so gentle, it was unbelievable, I didn't feel a thing. He was ever so nice. I was glad when I saw him. Oh I was so pleased.

When I went to the clinic and had those internals, the last one I had at thirty-six weeks, I couldn't relax for, it hurt so much. I had to have X-rays. I couldn't relax. He was really rough, this doctor. He didn't say much, he kept saying can you relax? One of the midwives was holding my hand. Oh I thought he was rough. But when I had my waters broke, I didn't feel a thing. Dr Thompson, do you know him, he was so nice, everyone liked him. He was so sweet. My friend used to be embarrassed with him, because he used to smile a lot and he always looked so shy. He was so nice.

ALISON MOUNTJOY:

My consultant came down; he didn't even say hallo. The nurse brought him in, he said well, what am I here for? She had to remind him I was lying there and you know that blue towel they give you? Well I had it over my feet because I'd been waiting for so long *I* was alright, but my feet were freezing, your feet do get cold. So he looked at me and he said you look a bit *naked*. So he picked up this towel and threw it at my tits which seemed to offend him. He was terribly, terribly brusque. And I was being quite a good girl, drawing my legs up to be examined and all the rest of it. Anyway, he put his plastic gloves on and *jammed* his hand in and *really* hurt. It was pretty painful. And when his hands came out they were absolutely *covered* in blood. Oh you might bleed for a bit – don't worry about it. And I was lying there absolutely shattered; I was in a terrible state.

Inflicting discomfort is one way the doctor has of desexualising the vaginal examination. Another is to joke about it.

When you have internals they have a metal thing that they put inside, and I don't know what the nurse thought of him, but he undid the bag, and it was a tiny little thing, and he said, what are you supposed to do with this, look down somebody's ear? (*Mandy Green*)

It was quite funny actually, because I had an internal, then I had a cervical smear test, and it hurt, and the doctor had a sense of humour, and he said just look on me as a male chauvinist pig, and was laughing, so it was quite funny. (*Nancy Carter*)

After the birth come the stitches. In sewing up the perineum, the doctor restores the husband's territory to him – or not, as the case may be.

DOCTOR [stitching] TO SARAH MOORE: We've got to make sure it works again, me dear, or your husband'll be back complaining.
DOCTOR TO RESEARCHER: Come and look at this! There you are [points to the stitches], you're the expert, does that look as though it'll work again?

Of course not everybody has trouble with their stitches. But 72 per cent of the sample women did, and in discussing their preferences for male or female doctors, this is one of the reasons why women are preferred. It is felt that a male doctor is unlikely to understand how a woman feels about vaginal examinations, episiotomies and stitches, and that he will not attach the same degree of importance to that part of her anatomy as she does.

How do you feel about male and female doctors and midwives?

I think I would have certainly felt better if I'd had a qualified doctor to stitch. Since then I've met another young doctor on a social occasion, and she told me that she was only ever shown how to do an episiotomy when she was a student and she had to think back to her school sewing lessons when she was setting about the next one. I think they should train the midwives to do it. I think *any* woman would be better at it than a man. They just don't understand. I mean if you think how they would feel if anyone did the equivalent to them . . . ! (*Juliet Morley*)

The midwife can do the actual cut but she can't stitch. So it's the junior doctor who stitches, and if it's a junior doctor who's not done it often before and makes a hell of a mess, the midwife looks on and sympathises and thinks how she could do it better. I don't see how some of these doctors can understand how you feel anyway. (*Sandy Wright*)

I think there are certain problems that you can only appreciate if you've had them, like period pains and things like that. And I just don't see how all the teaching in the world can help you advise someone about that.

The young married doctors tend to be a bit more helpful. Like this gynaecologist in the family planning clinic, he was terrific, his wife had just had a baby you see, and as it happened she had fractured her coccyx as well, you see, so he was almost *glad* that I'd done mine: it was something he knew all about! (*Rachel Sharpe*)

The student nurses are very gentle – that's what I like. Better than the doctors, they just dig in. They've got gentle, soft hands. They put themselves in the patient's place because they're women. The doctors, they just prod you, you're just another woman having a baby. (*Christina Lynch*)

I think I react differently to a woman. I don't know, I suppose you feel more relaxed with a woman, it's less embarrassing. (*Lily Mitchell*)

I am slightly embarrassed with a woman. The first time she walked in I thought Christ, a woman! (*Grace Bower*)

Some women like it better if they have a man than a woman. I'm just embarrassed all round. (*Nina Brady*)

On the whole I'd prefer a male doctor. I think it's what most people say, don't they? Simply because among the male and female doctors I've come across, the male doctors tend to be a bit older and more experienced. (*Catherine Andrews*)

I prefer male doctors. I don't like female doctors – I don't like women particularly. They make me nervous. You can get some that are so bitchy and when you get a bitchy woman, you really get a bitchy woman. You get bad male doctors but they can never be as bad as a woman.

There was a woman on the radio yesterday who said she thought men should be excluded from gynaecology and midwifery: I don't see why men should be excluded from it. I think that saying men can't *feel* as much – I mean you can say equally that a woman doesn't feel as much because she hasn't experienced it. (*Cary Wimborne*)

DEBORAH SMYTH:
Female doctors are much nicer: male doctors, they're flippant, they just brush you off, say a few words and that's it.
I: So if you'd had a male midwife. . . ?
DEBORAH: I don't suppose I'd have felt much different. [Pause] No, I

think I would have done, because a load of men – doctors, students, came in afterwards, didn't they?

PATRICK: I didn't see why they should be laughing and joking. It wasn't really a time for laughing and joking, was it?

DEBORAH: They were laughing and joking amongst themselves as they walked in. It didn't seem right, did it? How are you feeling, love? Bloody cheek. No, I wouldn't like a male midwife. Women know, don't they, if they've had children of their own.

JO INGRAM:
I mean I really am a complete chauvinist about that. I really do think that men should fucking keep out of birth. I think it's none of their fucking business. I really am quite angry about it. I just don't think they're very sympathetic; they just don't care enough about it. If it was a different society, I mean if it was the kind of society that I'm hopefully working for, and we eventually get a breed of men who are fairly non-chauvinist and cared about people and were more *human* then it'd be okay. But in the present situation. . . .

I: So are there any changes you would like to see in the way women are treated in childbirth?

JO: Yes, they should eliminate the men!

I think if they *want* to, there's no reason why men shouldn't be midwives. A lot of men are very sympathetic, very easy to talk to, very easy to put your trust in and if they are those sorts of men, they might just as well be midwives as those sorts of women. I don't like sexual distinctions. I believe in people, not categories. (*Sophy Fisher*)

Not if it's just some sort of odd bloke who fancies looking up people's fannies. I think it's possibly better if women who've had babies deliver your baby, because they know what it's all about. But if it's a choice between an unsympathetic woman who's never had a baby and a man who, okay, has never had a baby either, but his wife's had a hard time having a baby and he's a midwife, then okay I'll have a man, who cares? (*Kate Prince*)

Attitude to sex of doctor		Attitude to sex of midwife	
Preference:		Preference:	
Female doctor	23%	Female midwife	27%
Male doctor	21%	Male midwife	4%
Don't mind	55%	Don't mind	70%

YOU CAN'T ASK A BOOK A QUESTION

Experience breeds sympathy: that is the message. Throughout the process of becoming a mother, the people who are valued are those whose expertise is of the personal and practical kind. The contradictions are not between the expert and the non-expert, but between one kind of expert and another: theory should be grounded in practice, not practice in theory.

HEALTH VISITOR: Does she not settle if the wind's not brought up?
EMMA BUCKINGHAM with DINAH, aged five months, screaming: She can't *eat* till she's got her wind up.
HV: Oh, really? People don't seem to worry so much about wind these days. Hugh Jolly at Charing Cross is dead against winding. He doesn't think it's necessary at all.
EMMA: Well would you like to take this little thing? She's blue in the face!
HV: She's okay, is she?
EMMA: Yes. She's just got wind!
[Later] If health visitors had children they might be a good deal better!

ELIZABETH FARRELL:
The health visitor is a bit of a dilettante sort of person, isn't she? A bit of a buffer, really. You go with your problems to get reassurance. She hasn't been able to help this friend of mine over feeding. That's one thing I do think: you've got to have been through having children yourself to understand what it means and entails.

In hospitals the only real help I got with breastfeeding was from two nursing auxiliaries – women who both had a couple of children each and they'd talk about their children, and they were just ideally suited to the job. One of them sat down and really showed me what to do: she was terribly good. The best people are the least qualified people I think.

CLARE DAWSON:
The nursing auxiliaries I thought were very very good. Most of them were very helpful and there was one nurse particularly, a state enrolled nurse, who was absolutely super, and had about eight

children herself and would sort of say to you on the quiet, well don't tell so and so I've told you this, but I wouldn't do that, I'd do so and so. For instance, the baby milk. You didn't – the nursery nurse said you don't need to warm it up as long as you give it at room temperature that's all you need to do. And Mary, she was getting tummy ache, she'd started her colic by then, and this nurse with eight children said to me why don't you warm it up? She said your baby's got a new tummy and milk's going into it and everything's new to her; you know, give her a chance and have it a bit warm. So I did, which actually did the trick. And it was tips like that which she gave me and she was really super. Sort of a mother figure.

MARY ROSEN:
One doctor at the clinic has a ten month old and said she sees clinic work in a completely different light now.

JANE TARRANT:
I think it makes a difference, I feel that about the health visitor. There's one there, she's very sweet, but she's not even married. I know it sounds wrong to say it, but it *must* be different. I think that the health visitor who's had her own child she was *so* much more sympathetic. She could see that I was really worried about the baby's weight gain. And also practical experience of day to day things. You can read anything in a book but then I feel they're just trotting advice out of a book. They haven't *actually* had to deal with a baby themselves.

Practice may not make perfect, but at least it improves on theories. Motherhood means listening to the baby and not the experts; or, babies are interpreters and revisers of what the experts say. If any single phrase can sum up the message of becoming a mother it is this: the value of experience.

There are three particular ways in which the women whose accounts make up this book come to see this as the catch-phrase, the key to their passage through child-bearing to the social role of mother. In the first place, no one can tell you what it (pregnancy, birth, motherhood) will be like. Or, to put it another way, they can tell you, but the words have no meaning, are even not remembered, because becoming a mother is like entering a foreign country. Travelling there is like nothing you have ever done before. There is thus no common language to describe it in – Chinese or Swahili or Serbo-Croat only make sense, after all, to those who already know from experience what concepts are referred to by the words. 'A baby of one's own', 'the movements of the child in the womb', 'the contractions of labour', 'being a housewife' – such terms have an infinite resonance after the event, but little before.

Secondly, communication of these experiences is hindered by the gap between mother and expert. For the best teacher is not the one who has read books and attended lectures, but the one who has been taught by experience. While the mother has gone through, or will go through, the experience, whether or not the expert has is deemed to be irrelevant to the giving of professional advice. The obstetrician who writes a book about pregnancy does not indicate how close is his or her personal involvement in parenthood. The health visitor who calls at the home is there as a health visitor, although she may be a mother as well. But in fact experience does alter the way people (experts and others) behave: this is part of the scientific method, that theories should be tested empirically, not just once under artificial conditions, but constantly in the real world of heat and cold and light and dark – of contrasts and instabilities and unpredicted, unforeseeable moments.

It is from *their own experience in this world that most people (who are not scientists) develop their theories, build up their generalisations, become confident about asserting particular things to be generally true. The impact of experience on people is the third way in which first-time mothers learn to place a value on experience. They discover that it is not just a case of having the baby and carrying on as if nothing had happened: something* has *happened, a historical event. Attitudes are altered – to doctors, to husbands, to mothers, to television programmes, to politics, to the past, to the future. Producing a baby is re-producing, looking differently at one's body, one's identity, one's way of living in the society of which one is a part. And in becoming a mother a woman takes her place among all women, conscious in a new way of the divisions between men and women, more sharply aware both of the ties of human kinship and of the special solidarity of sisterhood. Motherhood is a handicap but also a strength; a trial and an error; an achievement and a prize.*

Endnote – Being Researched

Well, quite honestly, I said I hope this research is worth it. I said to my Mum I've got this lady coming to see me this morning. She said, what about? I said I hope it's not a load of old rubbish. Because there's been so much research on such rubbishy things I feel money's been wasted. So she said, oh it probably is. . . . Well, it's a bit indulgent isn't it, really, just talking about yourself all the time?

The accounts of motherhood given in this book were obtained from sixty-six women in 233 interviews, which yielded a total of 545 hours 26 minutes of tape-recorded material. The point of the interviews was to gather material for a sociological research project, and it was for this purpose that interviewer and interviewee came together: to construct a conversation that would provide a series of full, vivid and comparable first-hand accounts of the process of becoming a mother.

But how does it feel to interview – and, more important, to be interviewed? Textbooks of sociological methods describe the research interview in mechanical terms as simply an instrument for the production of sociological data. For example:

> Regarded as an information-gathering tool, the interview is designed to minimise the local, concrete, immediate circumstances of the particular encounter – including the respective personalities of the participants – and to emphasise only those aspects that can be kept general enough and demonstrable enough to be counted. As an encounter between these two particular people the typical interview has no meaning; it is conceived in a framework of other, comparable meetings between other couples . . .[1]

Or:

> The interview is not simply a conversation. It is, rather, a pseudo conversation. In order to be successful, it must have all the warmth and personality exchange of a conversation, with the clarity and guidelines of scientific searching. Consequently, the interviewer cannot merely lose himself* in being friendly. He must introduce

* *It seems not to have occurred to many writers of such textbooks that interviewers are often female.*

himself as though beginning a conversation, but from the beginning the additional element of respect, of professional competence, should be maintained. . . . He is a professional researcher in this situation, and he must demand and obtain respect for the task he is trying to perform.[2]

Every interview is the practice that challenges this theory, for the important questions are: does the theory work? Should it be made to work? Is this the best way to get inside other people's experiences, to make available to others the private meanings of being human? These questions do not seem to have been asked by sociologists yet, perhaps because most of those who have discussed methodology have been men, and they have found it easier than many women would to believe that people can (or should be made to) behave like statistics.

Another question also follows from these problems about assuming people to be merely research instruments. For once you start to study people it is at least a possibility that they become so influenced by the fact of being studied that their behaviour or attitudes are changed, and the whole point of doing the research is lost. This *question has been a caveat of sociological method ever since the famous experiments carried out at the Hawthorne Works of the Western Electric Company in Chicago between 1927 and 1932. The Hawthorne experiments attempted to prove a relationship between work conditions and work output, but succeeded only in showing the beneficial effect of the research process in raising workers' interest and morale.*

For, contrary to what the textbooks say, researching and being researched are parts of human *interaction; it may be wishful thinking (or unnecessary pessimism) to think that they can be governed entirely by 'scientific' principles. One feature of these 545 hours 26 minutes of tape-recorded human conversations is the tendency of the interviewed to ask questions back. In all, the tapes include 878 such questions. For example:*

Does ultrasound hurt the baby?
Can you refuse induction?
Who will deliver my baby?
Does the epidural ever paralyse you?
Is it right that the baby doesn't come out of the same hole you pass water out of?
How will I know when I'm in labour?
What is the pain of birth like?
Is breastfeeding sexual?
How long should you wait for sex after the birth?
Can my baby see yet?

Do disposable nappies go down the lavatory?
Does shaking the child harm it?
How do you cook an egg for a baby?
Do you have periods when you're breastfeeding?
What's the difference between the coil and the cap?
How do you clean the baby's nails?
What causes cot death?

Three-quarters of these 878 questions were requests for information. These could be analysed and interpreted in various ways; but perhaps what is most striking is the importance of wanting to know more about medical *practices and about the way in which maternity care is* organised *(who does what, when, how and why) in the clinic and hospital setting. Whatever is provided in the way of formal antenatal education is clearly not meeting these needs adequately; or perhaps there is a level of information that can only be given and received in a more* personal *context.*

Those who were interviewed also appealed directly for advice ('Should I sue the hospital for stitching me up too tightly?'); they asked for information about the research, about the way others had reacted to pregnancy, birth and the daily work of motherhood; they inquired about the researcher herself – her own experiences of reproduction and motherhood ('Are you married?' 'How old are your children?' 'Did you breastfeed?') These questions in particular must be taken as a sign that interviewing is a two-way process.

Questions interviewees asked (total 878)	
Information requests	76%
Personal questions	15%
Questions about the research	6%
Advice questions	4%

Interviewees' requests for information (total 664)	
Medical procedures	31%
Organisational procedures	19%
Physiology of reproduction	15%
Babycare/development/ feeding	21%
Other	15%

Bearing in mind both the shared nature of question-asking in the interviews, and the general sociological caveat that researchers affect what they study, all the women interviewed for this book were asked the following question at the end of their final interview: 'Do you feel that being involved in this research – my coming to see you – has affected your experience of becoming a mother in any way?' Their answers are general comments on the experience of being interviewed, on the value of being researched, on the mechanical theories of the sociological method textbooks, and, of course, incidentally but therefore significantly, on interviewers' own contributions to the interview both as interviewers and as people engaged in conversations with other people.

Has the research affected your experience of becoming a mother?

No	27%
Yes:	73%
thought about it more	30%*
found it reassuring	25%*
a relief to talk	30%*
changed attitudes/ behaviour	7%*

*Percentages do not add up to 100 per cent because some women gave more than one answer.

Becoming aware

JOSÉ BRYCE:

I've enjoyed it. I remember when you went the first time, I thought she must have thought, my God, that woman went on talking and how boring to have to listen – you know, not just to answer your questions, but to go onto other things; when you asked a question, I wouldn't say yes, so-and-so and so-and-so, that's how I feel about that, I'd go on: like a conversation after each question. I thought maybe she only wanted to be here for an hour or something. And she was here for *hours*.

ELIZABETH FARRELL:

First of all, I enjoy talking. I think perhaps not quite so much *now* [baby crying]. I'll probably enjoy this afterwards, in retrospect, but it's difficult, because you're not so free. But before the baby, I really enjoyed talking. And I told you how I felt about you being at the birth: that was quite important.

Just as a person to talk to – yes, I've enjoyed it. Robert said, why don't you want to interview him? So I said well if you're doing a massive research project you've got to draw the line somewhere. It's a research project on *women's* attitudes to childbirth. Of course he might say that I was a hysterical mother or something like that. Spoilt my child unbearably.

How much is what you would like to find or what you think anyway going to influence your selecting material from the tape-recordings? If somebody else listened to your recordings and wrote a book about it, they would interpret it completely differently, wouldn't they?

SOPHY FISHER:

I don't think it's affected the *experience*. I think it's possibly affected my *evaluation* of it: the fact that you make me articulate my responses, or rake about in my memory, or try to rationalise and explain; it makes me more aware of it as an outside experience. You see, questions you've asked me I might not ask myself. I don't think you *change* what I think, but you make me *look* at it. I *believe* in it: it's part of my job anyway, to say this is what's happening to this person, and therefore they use this format of words to convey it. It works backwards in a play because you've got the format of words and you've got to find the emotion underneath. This sort of works the other way – the emotion underneath is there and your questions cause me to find the words. I've tried to be *accurate* in what I've told you.

KATE PRINCE:

You come so rarely that it's not as if we're all in a goldfish bowl being observed with a camera. I think it's very good, actually, because it's put one's thoughts together. And it's interesting to hear you say what I said before, which I'd forgotten about: that's *very* interesting. But it is in a way a monologue. I rabbit on. I suppose you feel everyone's doing you a favour, but really it's a huge ego trip.

CLARE DAWSON:

It's made me think about things that I've never thought about before. For instance, when you said to me does it matter to you if you don't see the same doctor? And I began to think: I wonder if it does? At the time I said no. And then I thought about it more. And I suppose it made me *assess* more what happened. I think I've found it helpful, actually. To talk about it: it's been good to talk about it. . . . I think it would be interesting to see what other people thought or felt. I can't see what *can* come out of it, in a way, because everybody's so different. I can't see how you can compare . . .

Feeling normal

PAULINE DIGGORY:

It's been very, I've really *enjoyed* it. Yes, it has helped me because I probably would have been even more worried. I mean, I think you know a lot. I mean there you are with all these different mothers and I mean all I've got to say is, do you think Hannah's a bit sick, and you say, oh no, I've seen about so many . . . Now that just helps, just to say you've seen a few.

I: But of course I'm not a doctor.

PAULINE: Oh I know. But I mean a doctor's not interested in a baby being sick anyway.

Us against them

I: Do you think that my being at the birth made any difference to the way you felt?

STEVE INGRAM: I don't know. It was their general attitude, I think they treated Jo better. That doctor . . .

JO: Oh yes, I'm sure that doctor was behaving differently. It was much, much better. It was really nice you being there, I think. It was just really good. It made it more of a social event, not something I was on my own doing with a couple of nurses and Steve. More a social thing than a private family affair, which was nice. It made it an awful lot better I'm sure, the fact that you were there: another friendly face.

STEVE: Yes, it did for me.

JO: Not just familiar, friendly: somebody who you felt was on your side.

STEVE: Yes. It was good that you were there, because I don't know how the fuck I would have coped if you hadn't been there.

ELIZABETH FARRELL:

I know I felt so pleased you were there, because I'd expected Robert not to stay. And it made me feel much more secure that you were there. I felt they wouldn't try to pull any fast ones or anything like that if you were there. And so it had a good effect on me. But I forgot you were there, because I couldn't see you.

SARAH MOORE:

You were a fantastic help. It was so nice to see a familiar face in a sea of unknown faces. It was great to see you. I think what I remember most of all was when you and Dick – when it was only us three in the room. I remember that. And I was relying just solely on you two, and not on the professional guidance, the professionalism of anyone else.

A case of change?

LOIS MANSON:

It's the Hawthorne effect question isn't it? [Lois is a sociology graduate.] I don't think it's affected me, save that sometimes there are things you've asked me which I've thought about later. For instance when you asked me about Jane's personality, I think perhaps immediately you'd gone I thought more about that particular question than I would have done otherwise. But I don't think it's affected my *behaviour.* Except do you remember when you asked me if I went to the upstairs clinic or the downstairs clinic? [A complex divison: the 'special' clinic (upstairs) was for medically problematic, but also socially special, patients (i.e. doctors' wives).] And I immediately asked a doctor. I'm sorry if I got you into any hot water. But I suppose that was obviously an effect, wasn't it? And there might be people I suppose that hadn't thought about looking at the hospital in any kind of critical light who might perhaps start thinking, well perhaps there *is* something to criticise.

CHRISTINA LYNCH:
I think it's made me more critical. I suppose it's really someone who I can air my criticisms to, who is not just – I mean, I've said it all to my friends and parents . . . I feel that you would take more notice of me because you are who you are and this is all going in a little book . . . But I know I shall be just another statistic!

Talking it out

ANGELA KING:
I mean I talk a lot I suppose. It puts a lot of things clearer in your mind. Questions that you ask me that I've never thought about: it does help in a way. To think about it, and to talk about it. It's a sort of relief sometimes to talk about things, especially nasty things, because it puts it all into perspective. Nobody else has really got the time, have they? I spoke to Tony's cousin that had a baby two or three weeks ago, and she was full of it: you could tell that she really wanted to talk about it. I think most women do, after a birth; although it might be boring to some people they really want to tell you everything that's happened. And I think it's a relief to them in a way because it's really an emotional thing, and I think your nerves are at their highest pitch and when it's all over it's a kind of relief to talk about it. It makes you *feel* better. Because most people have a bit of a – well I wouldn't say *nasty* – time, but it's a *shock* I think, and it's never what you expected it to be. Like her, she said I would never have dreamed that the pains were that bad, she said, people had told me that the pains were bad, but she said, I couldn't describe them. Yes: it's a shock, and it really helps for people to talk about it and there's not always somebody there *to* talk about it, is there, because a lot of husbands find it a big bore, don't they? And it changes you emotionally, whereas it doesn't really affect them at all.

SANDY WRIGHT:
I don't suppose people like to say yes, do they? I think it's *useful*: it helps to get things off your mind. I *needed* to talk to people those first weeks – I really needed *desperately* to talk to somebody about it: somebody who'd been through the experience. Yes I think it *is* therapeutic. I think it helps to get it out of your system.

GILLIAN HARTLEY:
I think it's improved it if anything. I thought it was marvellous. I really enjoyed being part of the project. I think it's made me more positive about it, because if this kind of research is being done about pregnancy and motherhood, it certainly means that things will probably get better in the future. At least *you'd* have to believe that, or you wouldn't be doing the project in the first place. I think it probably has made me more positive about the experience altogether.

Those lovely long discussions about the baby, and the whole process. Getting things out into the open – questions that I'd had that I felt I really didn't want to bother other people with – those kind of questions. Maybe in a sense middle-class mothers, educated middle-class mothers, suffer in not really having outlets to talk about their feelings. No, I think that's being very biased. Maybe everybody needs a chance to talk about their feelings about pregnancy, and there really isn't anybody who asks them the kind of questions that you do, that you have, rather, in the survey, which acts positively psychologically. You really have asked personal questions about myself that nobody else has – sexual, personal, physical – bringing to the surface things that should have been brought to the surface and not let lie. And there's really no outlet for pregnant and postnatal mothers to talk about these things if they're not going, say to a psychiatrist, who isn't often interested in those things anyway. I think that's one way health care could be improved. If there could be ways for social workers or what have you to talk about it. Or perhaps it's something that women's groups ought to be doing something about – in the same way as rape counselling: it belongs on that level. Your feelings about the experience: getting things out.

I: Right, that's all.
DAWN O'HARA: Thank you very much. I really mean it.
I: Do you feel that being involved in this research . . . has affected your experience?
DAWN: It has, because I regard you as a friend, you know what I

mean? Somebody to speak to. I mean I don't look on you as a doctor, you know, that kind of way? Or a health visitor. I feel I can talk more freely to you.

NINA BRADY:
If I'd known you were coming, I would have made a cake; I was looking forward to your coming, dear. I was wondering about you the other day, and I thought maybe I'd missed you . . . Oh it has helped to talk, it has, it does help you. Turn that thing off, now!

Notes and References

Preface

1 A. Oakley, *The Sociology of Housework,* London: Martin Robertson, 1974; *Housewife,* London: Allen Lane, 1974.
2 See A. Oakley, *Housewife,* 1974, chapter 4, 'The Situation of Women Today'.
3 Perhaps this is partly to do with having worked in the hospital as an observer. Simply knowing all the rituals and routines, the faces and the places, promotes a feeling of confidence. As another researcher–patient put it 'I was able to thread my way safely through a difficult place' (N. Stoller Shaw, *Forced Labour,* New York: Pergamon, 1974, p. 153).
4 C. Wright Mills put this point better than anyone else (*The Sociological Imagination,* New York: Oxford University Press, 1959, esp. p. 226).
5 Those readers who are worried about the ethics of using statistics in small sample research should read J. Galtung, *Theory and Methods of Social Research,* London: Allen and Unwin, 1967.
6 A project of this kind that included fathers would be a different kind of project altogether – a valuable contribution to our knowledge of the way parenthood works, but in a different way from a study of mothers only.

Chapter 1

1 P. H. Chavasse, *Advice to a Wife on the Management of Her Own Health,* London: Cassell, 1911, p. 9.
2 S. Firestone, *The Dialectic of Sex,* London: Paladin, 1972, pp. 189–90.
3 Or at least attempting to do so if there is time. See C. S. Ford, *A Comparative Study of Human Reproduction,* New Haven, Conn.: Yale University Press, 1945; M. Mead and N. Newton, 'Cultural Patterning of Perinatal Behaviour', in S. A. Richardson and A. F. Guttmacher (eds), *Childbearing – Its Social and Psychological Aspects,* Baltimore: Williams and Wilkins, 1967; A. Oakley, 'Cross-Cultural Practice', in T. Chard and M. Richards (eds), *Benefits and Hazards of the New Obstetrics,* London: Heinemann Medical, 1977; Joint Study Group of the International Federation of Gynaecology and Obstetrics and the International Confederation of Midwives, *Maternity Care in the World,* International Federation of Gynaecology and Obstetrics and International Confederation of Midwives, 1976.
4 T. Ferguson and J. C. Logan, 'Mothers Employed Out of the Home', *Glasgow Medical Journal,* June 1953, vol.34, pp. 221–44, p. 239.
5 J. Bernard, *Women, Wives, Mothers,* Chicago: Aldine, 1975, pp. 219–20.
6 A. Rich, *Of Woman Born,* London: Virago, 1977, p. 42.
7 D. Breen, *The Birth of a First Child,* London: Tavistock, 1975.
8 L. Minturn, W. W. Lambert and Associates, *Mothers of Six Cultures,* New York: Wiley, 1964.
9 G. W. Brown and T. Harris, *Social Origins of Depression,* London: Tavistock, 1978.

320   BECOMING A MOTHER

10 A. Rossi, 'Maternalism, Sexuality and the New Feminism', in J. Zubin and J. Money (eds), *Contemporary Sexual Behavior: Critical Issues in the 1970s*, Baltimore: Johns Hopkins, 1973.

11 R. M. Titmuss, *Problems of Social Policy*, London: HMSO, 1950, p. 412.

12 J. Busfield, 'Ideologies and Reproduction', in M. P. M. Richards (ed.), *The Integration of a Child into a Social World*, Cambridge University Press, 1974, p. 13.

13 The US figure includes illegitimate births. The British figure excludes these and takes women married once only, so the actual figure must be higher than 42%. Of a sample of 1544 married and unmarried women interviewed for an infant feeding survey in 1975–6, 46% gave birth to first babies. Office of Population Censuses and Surveys, *Infant Feeding 1975: Attitudes and Practice in England and Wales*, London: HMSO, 1978, p. 7.

14 E. Alberman, 'Facts and Figures', in Chard and Richards (eds), *op. cit.*; Central Statistical Office, *Annual Abstract of Statistics*, London: HMSO, 1971, Table 34.

15 I. Chalmers and M. Richards, 'Intervention and Causal Inference in Obstetric Practice', in Chard and Richards (eds), *op. cit.*

16 M. Versluysen, 'Medical Professionalism and Maternity Hospitals in Eighteenth Century London: a Sociological Interpretation', paper given at Society for the Social History of Medicine, Colloquium 'Society and Medicine in Britain', London, 1977.

17 See A. Oakley, 'Wisewoman and Medicine Man: Changes in the Management of Childbirth', in J. Mitchell and A. Oakley (eds), *The Rights and Wrongs of Women*, Harmondsworth: Penguin, 1976.

18 Joint Committee of the Royal College of Obstetricians and Gynaecologists and the Population Investigation Committee, *Maternity In Great Britain*, Oxford University Press, 1948, p. 48; Joint Study Group of the International Federation of Gynaecology and Obstetrics and the International Confederation of Midwives, *op. cit.*, p. 550.

19 Office of Population Censuses and Surveys, *op. cit.*, p. 168.

20 Figures from Joint Study Group of the International Federation of Gynaecology and Obstetrics and the International Confederation of Midwives, *op. cit.*

21 Chalmers and Richards, *op. cit.*, pp. 39–40.

22 See the DHSS report, *Prevention and Health: Reducing the Risk*, London: HMSO, 1977.

23 See the following sources for arguments about the disadvantages of modern obstetric practice: Chard and Richards (eds), *op. cit.*; P. Dunn, 'Obstetric Delivery Today', *The Lancet*, 10 April 1976, pp. 790–3; D. Haire, *The Cultural Warping of Childbirth*, International Childbirth Education Association, 1972; N. Newton and M. Newton, 'Childbirth in Cross-Cultural Perspective', in J. G. Howells (ed.), *Modern Perspectives in Psycho-Obstetrics*, London: Oliver and Boyd, 1972; M. Richards, 'Innovation in Medical Practice: Obstetricians and the Induction of Labour in Britain', *Social Science and Medicine*, 1975, vol. 9, pp. 595–602; M. Richards, 'A Place of Safety? An Examination of the Risks of Hospital Delivery', in J. Davis and S. Kitzinger (eds), *The Place of Birth*, London: Oxford University Press, 1978; M. H. Shearer, 'Reducing the Drawbacks of Electronic Fetal Monitoring in Labor', in H. Hirsch (ed.), *The Family*, Basel: S. Karger, 1975; P. C. Shervington, 'Diet in Pregnancy: Hygiene; Radiation Effects; and Prophylaxis of Virus Infections', in D. F. Hawkins (ed.), *Obstetric Therapeutics*, London: Baillière Tindall, 1974 (for a discussion of ultrasound); D. Stewart and L. Stewart, *Safe Alternatives in Childbirth*, Chapel Hill: Napsac Inc., 1977.

24 Shearer, *op. cit.*, pp. 458–9.

25 M. G. Kerr 'Problems and Perspectives in Reproductive Medicine', University of Edinburgh Inaugural Lecture, 25 November 1975, pp. 3–5.

26 M. H. Klaus *et al.*, 'Maternal Attachment: Importance of the First Postpartum Days', *New England Journal of Medicine*, 1972, vol. 286, p. 460; J. H. Kennell *et al.*,

'Evidence for a Sensitive Period in the Human Mother', in *Parent-Infant Interaction*, CIBA Foundation symposium, 33, 1975.

27 Select Committee on Violence in the Family, *Violence to Children, vol. I Report*, London: HMSO, 1977, xxxviii.

28 H. Graham, 'Images of Pregnancy in Antenatal Literature' in R. Dingwall, C. Heath, M. Reid and M. Stacey (eds), *Health Care and Health Knowledge*, London: Croom Helm, 1977, p. 29.

29 F. Leboyer, *Birth Without Violence*, New York: Knopf, 1975.

30 A. Rich 'The Theft of Childbirth', *New York Times*, 2 October 1975.

31 N. Newton, 'Interrelationships between Sexual Responsiveness, Birth and Breast-feeding', in Zubin and Money (eds), *op. cit.*

32 L. Gillie and O. Gillie, *The Sunday Times*, 13 October and 20 October 1975; *Horizon*, 'A Time to be Born', BBC television, 27 January 1975.

33 See, for example, contributions to *Spare Rib* over the last few years, which illustrate developments in feminist views of childbirth.

34 Chalmers and Richards, *op. cit.*, p. 48.

Chapter 2

1 Dr H. Flack in 'You and Your Baby', Part I, Family Doctor Publication, British Medical Association, p. 4.

2 It is a complicated question to answer. See A. Cartwright *How Many Children?* (London: Routledge, 1976), and J. Busfield and M. Paddon, *Thinking About Children* (Cambridge University Press, 1977), for two of many studies of 'family' intentions.

3 These figures seem fairly representative of larger samples. G. Bourne (*Pregnancy*, Pan Books, 1975, p. 532) has a table showing that 65% of women in their early twenties conceive by six months (68%, this sample).

Chapter 3

1 J. B. McKinlay, 'The Sick Role – Illness and Pregnancy', *Social Science and Medicine*, 1972, vol. 6, pp. 561–72.

Chapter 4

1 Taken from a set of observations of antenatal encounters collected by A. O. in 1974–5.

2 M. Rutter, in *Maternal Deprivation Reassessed* (Harmondsworth: Penguin Books, 1972), provides a good dispassionate account of the evidence for and against this.

3 Bourne, *op. cit.*, p. 356.

4 This talk was tape-recorded by A. O. as part of the hospital observations carried out in 1974–5.

Chapter 5

1 See Ford, *op. cit.*

Chapter 6

1 D. Llewellyn-Jones, *Everywoman*, London: Faber and Faber, 1971, p. 214.
2 N. E. Williamson reviews the literature on sex preferences in 'Sex Preferences, Sex Control, and the Status of Women' in *SIGNS: Journal of Women in Culture and Society*, Summer 1976, vol. 1, pp. 847–62.
3 The day varies according to the book: Llewellyn-Jones, *op. cit.*, gives the third day; G. Bourne, *op. cit.*, says between day three and day six; H. Brant and M. Brant in *Pregnancy, Childbirth and Contraception* (Corgi Books, 1975), say the fourth or fifth day.
4 I. Yalom, D. T. Lunde, R. H. Moos, D. A. Hamburg, '"Postpartum Blues" Syndrome', *Archives of General Psychiatry*, January 1968, vol. 18, pp. 16–27.
5 Very little research has in fact been done on the relationship between institutional confinement and postnatal depression. B. A. Cone, in a study of Cardiff women, reports a significant difference between the incidence of depression in hospital-delivered women (64% of whom were depressed) and in those delivered at home (19% of these were depressed). B. A. Cone, 'Pueperal Depression' in N. Morris (ed.), *Psychosomatic Medicine in Obstetrics and Gynaecology*, Basel: Karger, 1972. On responses to childbirth in a different culture – the Yequana Indians – see J. Liedloff, *The Continuum Concept*, London: Duckworth, 1975.

Chapter 7

1 Much of the research on postnatal depression is influenced by the idea that it represents some kind of failure in 'proper' feminine development. Very little account, unfortunately, has been taken of social aspects of motherhood as work. See A. Oakley, 'A Case of Maternity: Paradigms of Women as Maternity Cases' *SIGNS: Journal of Women in Culture and Society* (forthcoming).
2 The women who had drug treatment were not of course necessarily suffering from a 'worse' depression than those who had no drugs. Some people are more prone to go to doctors when they feel unwell than others; some GPs are more sympathetic to patients with postnatal depression than others.
3 Again, the paediatric literature has been full of assumptions that crying and not sleeping are in some way the mother's fault. More recent research contradicts this notion. See, for example, M. Richards and J. Bernal, 'Why Some Babies Don't Sleep', *New Society*, 28 February 1974.
4 But the babycare advice books do not reflect this fact, making a rigid distinction between 'normal' and 'abnormal' mothers. See, for example, H. Jolly, *Commonsense about Babies and Children*, Times Newspapers Ltd, 1973, p. 156.
5 This is still a novel idea to many researchers of mother–baby interaction. But on the whole the notion of babies as people with, to some extent, ready-made personalities is gaining ground. See R. Schaffer, *Mothering*, Fontana/Open Books, 1977.

Chapter 8

1 K. Whitehorn, foreword to M. Gunther, *Infant Feeding*, Harmondsworth: Penguin, 1971, p. 11.
2 Department of Health and Social Security, *Present Day Practice in Infant Feeding*, London: HMSO, 1974. This is the report of a Working Party of the Panel of Child Nutrition, Committee on Medical Aspects of Food Policy. It recommends breastfeeding for at least two weeks, preferably four to six months, and no solid food before four months. These recommendations were adopted by the DHSS as 'official policy'.

The report also suggested a national survey of infant feeding, which was subsequently carried out: Office of Population Censuses and Surveys, *op. cit.*

3 The OPCS survey (*op. cit.*) found that more mothers who went to antenatal classes wanted to breastfeed than non-attenders (p. 39). But a large part of the explanation is that mothers from the higher social classes both want to breastfeed and go to antenatal classes. Excluding this effect, it is of course possible that mothers attend antenatal classes to learn about breastfeeding – i.e., the intention precedes the class attendance.

4 These figures compare with 51%, 27% (four weeks) and 13% (four months) in the OPCS survey. However, breastfeeding is higher in London and the South East than in other regions; the proportion breastfeeding at least once in London and the South East was 72%.

5 Newton, *op. cit.*

6 See, for example, the work of Sheila Kitzinger.

7 The OPCS *Infant Feeding* survey (*op. cit.*, p. 100) reported the same finding.

8 In the OPCS survey the most popular time for starting solids was between two and three months (*op. cit.*, p. 100).

9 See M. Hewitt, *Wives and Mothers in Victorian Industry*, London: Rockcliff, 1958.

Chapter 9

1 Husbands' participation in both baby care and housework was assessed from the women's answers to a series of questions about particular tasks. Of course there are problems in assuming that women give a reasonable picture of men's domesticity – a poor relationship between husband and wife may mean, for instance, that she says he does less than he actually does. But it seems that focusing on actual behaviour rather than attitudes minimises this problem. See M. Rutter and G. W. Brown, 'The Reliability and Validity of Measures of Family Life and Relationships in Families Containing Psychiatric Patients', *Social Psychiatry*, 1966, vol. 1, pp. 38–53.

2 See P. Mainardi, 'The Politics of Housework' in R. Morgan (ed.), *Sisterhood is Powerful*, New York: Vintage, 1970.

3 A phrase used by M. Komarovsky in her classic study, *Blue Collar Marriage*, New York: Vintage, 1967.

Chapter 10

1 In the OPCS national feeding survey (*op. cit.*) 10% of mothers of four-month-old babies worked – 3% full time. Half of those working part-time worked at home (p. 22).

2 See A. Oakley, *Sex, Gender and Society*, London: Maurice Temple Smith, 1972, Chapter 5, 'Sex and Social Role'.

Chapter 11

1 The extent to which women think of themselves as mothers was not measured with any complicated psychological test, but simply by asking 'Are you aware of being a mother?', 'Do you think of yourself as a mother?' and 'How do you feel about being a mother?' This may produce limited answers but at least it has the merit of reflecting women's own conscious self-conceptions.

2 If motherhood develops feelings of sympathy and empathy in this way (characteris-

tics universally attributed to women in our culture) then perhaps it is giving birth rather than being female that gives rise to this (so-called) sex difference?
3 See A. Coote and T. Gill, *Women's Rights: A Practical Guide*, Harmondsworth: Penguin Books, 1974; also J. R. Chapman and M. Gates (eds), *Women Into Wives: The Legal and Economic Impact of Marriage*, Beverly Hills: Sage Publications, 1977.

Chapter 12

1 M. Rosen 'The Objective Tangent', *The Lancet*, 24 and 31 December 1977, p. 1341.
2 These and other findings are reported in H. Graham and A. Oakley, 'Competing Ideologies of Reproduction: Medical and Maternal Perspectives on Pregnancy and Childbirth' (forthcoming).
3 This figure applies to first labours. J. and J. Lennane, *Hard Labour*, London: Gollancz, 1977, p. 95.
4 Lois Gould, *Necessary Objects*, London: Cassell, 1974, pp. 229–30.
5 J. Emerson discusses this in 'Behaviour in Private Places: Sustaining Definitions of Reality in Gynaecological Examinations', in H. P. Dreitzel (ed.), *Recent Sociology No. 2*, New York: Macmillan, 1970.
6 In England and Wales in 1977 74·6% of hospital obstetricians were male. The percentage is considerably higher in the top ranks of the medical hierarchy. *Hospital Medical Staff – England and Wales. National Tables, 30 September 1977*, Department of Health and Social Security Statistics and Research Division, February 1978.

Endnote

1 N. K. Denzin, *Sociological Methods: A Source Book*, London: Butterworths, 1970, p. 196.
2 W. J. Goode and P. K. Hatt, *Methods in Social Research*, New York: McGraw-Hill, 1952, p. 191.

APPENDIX

List of Characters

These 60 women all speak in this book. Six other women were interviewed once, but left the sample (through miscarriage, moves, etc). The details given refer to the women when they were first interviewed. Many changed their jobs and/or their housing situations during the project, and some who were single later got married.

VERA ABBATT, 28, canteen worker, married 8 months. Lives in 2 furnished rooms.

CATHERINE ANDREWS, 25, receptionist, married 2 years. Lives in own flat.

TAMSIN ATTWOOD, 20, kiosk attendant, cohabiting 6 months. Lives in 1 furnished room.

NICOLA BELL, 24, contract supervisor, married 4 years. Lives in own house.

ANNE BLOOMFIELD, 23, barmaid, cohabiting 8 months. Lives in furnished flat.

GRACE BOWER, 24, switchboard operator, married 7 months. Lives with her family (parents, younger brother and sister) in their own house.

NINA BRADY, 28, shop assistant, married 8 months. Lives in 2 furnished rooms.

JOSÉ BRYCE, 29, manicurist, married 4 years. Lives in unfurnished flat.

EMMA BUCKINGHAM, 23, audiometrician, married 1 year. Lives in own house.

NANCY CARTER, 26, clerk, married 3 years. Lives in own house.

FELICITY CHAMBERS, 20, receptionist, married 2 years. Lives in unfurnished flat.

JEAN CLARK, 24, conference organiser, married 1 year. Lives in own flat.

MICHELLE CRAIG, 18, florist's assistant, married 3 weeks. Lives in 1 furnished room.

CLARE DAWSON, 29, laboratory assistant, married 6 years. Lives in own house.

PAULINE DIGGORY, 25, market researcher, married 2 years. Lives in own flat.

KAY EDWARDS, 24, cashier, married 2 years. Lives in own flat.

ELIZABETH FARRELL, 28, publisher's assistant, married 5 years. Lives in furnished flat.

POLLY FIELD, 27, telecommunications supervisor, married 6 years. Lives in unfurnished flat.

SOPHY FISHER, 29, TV producer, married 2 years. Lives in own house.

HELEN FOWLER, 22, nursing auxiliary, cohabiting 2 years. Lives in unfurnished flat.

ELLEN GEORGE, 29, health visitor, married 2 years. Lives in own flat.

MANDY GREEN, 30, hairdresser, married 3 years. Lives in own house.

GILLIAN HARTLEY, 26, illustrator, married 3 years. Lives in own flat.

JUNE HATCHARD, 29, teacher, married 3 years. Lives in 3 unfurnished rooms.

BARBARA HOOD, 28, bookseller, married 3 years. Lives in parents-in-law's house.

JO INGRAM, 26, further education teacher, cohabiting 7 years. Lives in furnished flat.

HILARY JACKSON, 30, catering manager, married 2 years. Lives with her family (mother, older sister) in her mother's house.

DEIRDRE JAMES, 23, jewellery assembler, married 3 years. Lives in unfurnished flat.

PAT JENKINS, 24, shop assistant, married 2 years. Lives in sister-in-law's house.

SUE JOHNSON, 27, photographer, cohabiting 3 years. Lives in unfurnished flat.

TANYA KEMP, 31, medical receptionist, married 5 years. Lives in own house.

ROSALIND KIMBER, 27, social worker, married 3 years. Lives in own house.

ANGELA KING, 26, cashier, married 2 months. Lives in 3 furnished rooms.

JOSEPHINE LLOYD, 23, boutique manager, separated, cohabiting with the baby's father four months. Lives in his mother's council-house.

CHRISTINA LYNCH, 28, traffic warden, married 4 years. Lives in own maisonette.

LOIS MANSON, 29, educational research worker, married 7 years. Lives in own house.

DIANA MEADE, 28, card trimmer, married 3 months. Lives in 1 furnished room.

KIRSTY MILLER, 20, pattern grader, married 5 months. Lives in parents-in-law's council flat.

LILY MITCHELL, 29, civil servant, married 4 years. Lives in own house.

SARAH MOORE, 28, civil servant, married 6 years. Lives in own house.

JULIET MORLEY, 28, rebate officer, married 6 years. Lives in own flat.

SASHA MORRIS, 26, air hostess, married 1 year. Lives in own flat.

ALISON MOUNTJOY, 27, fashion designer, married 2 years. Lives in unfurnished flat in her parents' house.

DAWN O'HARA, 21, packer, married 5 months. Lives in 1 furnished room.

MAUREEN PATERSON, 27, library assistant, married 3 years. Lives in unfurnished flat.

VERONICA PRATT, 27, label puncher, married 4 years. Lives in unfurnished flat.

KATE PRINCE, 27, journalist, married 2 years. Lives in own house.

MARY ROSEN, 25, exhibition organiser, married 4 years. Lives in own house.

MARGARET SAMSON, 30, teacher, married 4 years. Lives in own flat.

CAROLINE SAUNDERS, 28, physiotherapist, married 4 years. Lives in own flat.

RACHEL SHARPE, 27, copywriter, cohabiting 4 years. Lives in furnished flat.

DEBORAH SMYTH, 19, checker, married 3 months. Lives in furnished flat.

JANET STREETER, 25, dance instructor, married 5 years. Lives in own house.

JANE TARRANT, 29, librarian, married 3 years. Lives in own house.

LOUISE THOMPSON, 30, law student, married 10 years. Lives in unfurnished flat.

SHARON WARRINGTON, 21, audiotypist, married 1 year. Lives in 2 unfurnished rooms.

JANETTE WATSON, 19, machinist, married 7 months. Lives in father-in-law's council flat.

ROSE WILLIAMS, 21, insurance agent, married 1 year. Lives in parents-in-law's rented house.

CARY WIMBORNE, 27, sales supervisor, married 3 years. Lives in own house.

SANDY WRIGHT, 28, secretary, married 1 year. Lives in unfurnished flat.